When to Screen in Obstetrics & Gynecology

When to Screen in Obstetrics & Gynecology

edited by

Hajo I. J. Wildschut MD, PhD
Consultant in Obstetrics and Gynecology, Department of Obstetrics and Gynecology, Academisch Ziekenhuis, Rotterdam, The Netherlands

Carl P. Weiner MD
Professor and Chairman, Department of Obstetrics, Gynecology and Reproductive Sciences, University of Maryland School of Medicine, Baltimore, Maryland, USA

and

Tim J. Peters BSc, MSc, PhD
Statistician, Department of Social Medicine, University of Bristol, Bristol, UK

WB SAUNDERS COMPANY LIMITED
London   Philadelphia   Toronto   Sydney   Tokyo

W. B. Saunders Company Ltd 24–28 Oval Road
London NW1 7DX

The Curtis Center
Independence Square West
Philadelphia, PA 19106–3399, USA

Harcourt Brace & Company
55 Horner Avenue
Toronto, Ontario M8Z 4X6, Canada

Harcourt Brace & Company, Australia
30–52 Smidmore Street
Marrickville, NSW 2204, Australia

Harcourt Brace & Company, Japan
Ichibancho Central Building, 22–1 Ichibancho
Chiyoda-ku, Tokyo 102, Japan

A catalogue record for this book is available from the British Library

ISBN 0–7020–1874–0

Typeset by Wyvern Typesetting Ltd, Bristol
Printed in Great Britain by WBC Book Manufacturers, Bridgend,
Mid Glamorgan

Contents

Contributors

Sophie Alexander MD, PhD   Senior Lecturer in Public Health, School of Public Health, Université Libre de Bruxelles, Brussels, Belgium

Cynthia J Berg MD, MPH   Medical Epidemiologist, Division of Reproductive Health, Centers for Disease Control & Prevention, Atlanta, Georgia, USA

Alison Bigrigg FRCS(Ed), MRCOG, DMMFFP   Clinical Director, Family Planning and Sexual Health Directorate, Glasgow, UK

Patrick M M Bossuyt MD, PhD   Senior Lecturer in Clinical Epidemiology, Dept of Clinical Epidemiology & Biostatistics, Academic Medical Centre, Amsterdam, The Netherlands

Heiner C Bucher MD, MPH   Assistant Professor, Department of Clinical Epidemiology & Biostatistics, McMaster University, Hamilton, Ontario, Canada

Delores G Cordle MT(ASCP) SBB   Medical Technician, University of Iowa College of Medicine, Iowa City, Iowa, USA

Harry J de Koning MD, PhD   Lecturer in Public Health, Department of Public Health, Erasmus Universiteit Rotterdam, Rotterdam, The Netherlands

G A Dekker MD, PhD   Senior Lecturer in Obstetrics and Gynecology, Department of Obstetrics & Gynecology, Free University Hospital, Amsterdam, The Netherlands

Richard Depp MD   Professor, Department of Obstetrics & Gynecology, Jefferson Medical College, Philadelphia, Pennsylvania, USA

Paul D DePriest MD   American Cancer Society Clinical Oncology Fellow, Department of Obstetrics & Gynecology, Division of Gynecologic Oncology, University of Kentucky Medical Center, Lexington, Kentucky, USA

Walter Foulon MD   Professor, Division of Maternal Fetal Medicine, Department of Obstetrics & Gynecology, Akademisch Ziekenhuis Vrije Universiteit Brussel, Brussels, Belgium

Holly H Gallion MD   American Cancer Society Clinical Oncology Career Development Awardee, Department of Obstetrics & Gynecology, Divison of Gynecologic Oncology, University of Kentucky Medical Center, Lexington, Kentucky, USA

James E Haddow MD, PhD   Associate, Foundation for Blood Research, Scarborough, Maine, USA

Ian Harvey MRCP, FFPHM   Consultant Senior in Public Health Medicine, Department of Social Medicine, University of Bristol, Bristol, UK

R Phillip Heine MD   Assistant Professor, Obstetrics, Gynecology & Reproductive Science, University of Pittsburgh, Magee-Women's Research Institute, Pittsburgh, Pennsylvania, USA

Stephen K Hunter MD   Fellow Associate, Department of Obstetrics & Gynecology, University of Iowa College of Medicine, Iowa City, Iowa, USA

Susan R Johnson MD, MPH   Professor/Associate Dean, Department of Obstetrics & Gynecology, University of Iowa Hospitals and Clinics, Iowa City, Iowa, USA

Peter Kenemans MD, PhD   Professor, Department of Obstetrics & Gynecology, Academisch Ziekenhuis Vrije Universiteit, Amsterdam, The Netherlands

Christine Kirkpatrick MD, PhD   Senior Lecturer in Obstetrics and Gynecology, Department of Obstetrics & Gynecology, Hôpital Erasme, Université Libre de Bruxelles, Brussels, Belgium

George J. Knight PhD   Director, Prenatal Screening Laboratory, Foundation for Blood Research, Scarborough, Maine, USA

Rudolph W Koster MD, PhD   Senior Lecturer in Cardiology, Department of Cardiology, Academic Medical Centre, Amsterdam, The Netherlands

Ann Laros MD   Clinical Assistant Professor, Department of Obstetrics & Gynecology, University of Iowa Hospitals and Clinics, Iowa City, Iowa, USA

Lambert H Lumey MD, PhD   Division of Epidemiology, American Health Foundation, New York, and Sergievsky Center, Columbia University, New York, USA

George A Macones MD   Assistant Professor of Obstetrics and Gynecology, Center for Clinical Epidemiology and Biostatistics, University of Pennsylvania School of Medicine, Philadelphia, Pennsylvania, USA

Jeanne C McDermott CNM, PhD   Medical Epidemiologist, Centers for Disease Control & Prevention, WHO Collaborating Center in Perinatal Care and Health Services Research in Maternal and Child Health, Atlanta, Georgia, USA

Anne Naessens MD   Department of Microbiology, Akademisch Ziekenhuis, Vrije Universiteit Brussel, Brussels, Belgium

Glenn E Palomaki BS   Director, Biometry, Foundation for Blood Research, Scarborough, Maine, USA

Jeffrey F Peipert MD, MPH   Assistant Professor of Obstetrics & Gynecology, Department of Obstetrics & Gynecology, Brown University School of Medicine, Women and Infants' Hospital, Providence, Rhode Island, USA

Tim J Peters BSc, MSc, PhD   Senior Lecturer in Medical Statistics, Department of Social Medicine, University of Bristol, Bristol, UK

Joanne T Piscitelli MD, FACOG   Associate Clinical Professor, Chief, Division of General Obstetrics-Gynecology, Duke University Medical Center, Durham, North Carolina, USA

Jose A Prieto MD   Fellow, Maternal Fetal Medicine, Magee-Women's Research Institute, University of Pittsburgh, Pittsburgh, Pennsylvania, USA

Dwight J Rouse MD   Assistant Professor, Department of Obstetrics & Gynecology, Division of Maternal–Fetal Medicine, University of Alabama at Birmingham, Birmingham, Alabama, USA

Sicco Scherjon MD, PhD   Senior Registrar in Obstetrics and Gynecology, Department of Obstetrics, Academic Medical Center, Amsterdam, The Netherlands

Johannes G Schmidt MD   Professor, Family Practice and Institute of Clinical Epidemiology, Einsiedeln, Switzerland

Lisan S Schrevel   Junior House Officer, Academic Medical Center, University of Amsterdam, Amsterdam, The Netherlands

Darren Shickle MPH, MFPHM   Senior Lecturer in Public Health Medicine, University of Sheffield, Sheffield, UK

David L Simel MD, MHS   Associate Professor, Co-Director, Women Veterans Healthcare Center, Durham Veterans Affairs Medical Center, Duke University, Durham, North Carolina, USA

Jami Star MD   Assistant Professor of Obstetrics & Gynecology, Department of Obstetrics & Gynecology, Women and Infants' Hospital, Brown University School of Medicine, Providence, Rhode Island, USA

Ronald G Strauss MD   Professor of Pathology and Pediatrics, University of Iowa College of Medicine, Iowa City, Iowa, USA

Paul J van der Maas MD, PhD   Professor, Department of Public Health, Erasmus University Rotterdam, Rotterdam, The Netherlands

John R van Nagell Jr MD   American Cancer Society Professor of Clinical Oncology, Department of Obstetrics & Gynecology, Division of Gynecologic Oncology, University of Kentucky Medical Center, Lexington, Kentucky, USA

Carl P Weiner MD   Professor and Chairman, Department of Obstetrics, Gynecology &

Reproductive Science, University of Maryland School of Medicine, Baltimore, Maryland, USA

Hajo I J Wildschut MD, PhD   Consultant in Obstetrics and Gynecology, Department of Obstetrics & Gynecology, Academisch Ziekenhuis Dijkzigt, Rotterdam, The Netherlands

Clare Wilkinson MB BCh, DRCOG, MRCGP   Senior Lecturer in General Practice, Department of General Practice, University of Wales College of Medicine, Department of General Practice, Llanedeyrn Health Centre, Cardiff, UK

Juriy W Wladimiroff MD, PhD   Professor of Obstetrics & Gynecology, Erasmus Universiteit Rotterdam, Rotterdam, The Netherlands

Kees A Yedema MD, PhD   Consultant in Obstetrics and Gynecology, Department of Obstetrics & Gynecology, Westeinde Ziekenhuis, The Hague, The Netherlands

Introduction

Both the complexity and the cost of modern medicine continue to rise while societal resources to pay for it fall further behind. A growing number of tests are routinely performed in the name of advanced medical care before their advantages and disadvantages have been clearly demonstrated. This is especially true in obstetrics and gynecology, where the risk of litigation is high and physicians fear being held responsible for either an unpreventable or an unpredictable event. However, many screening tests lead to unnecessary interventions that pose a health risk to the patient. Since a screening test is performed on asymptomatic individuals, it must be accurate and safe. Too often, though, the medical practitioner is ill-prepared to evaluate its value. Limited resources require the practitioner to seek the greatest return on investment.

The purpose of this book is to examine objectively many of the screening tests used in obstetrics and gynecology. It was neither pragmatic nor feasible to cover all screening tests. We have focused on more common ones in everyday practice plus a few 'future' screening tests such as that for cystic fibrosis.

Objective evaluation requires that the sensitivity, specificity, and positive and negative predictive values be quantified before even considering the cost of testing and its potential impact. Such an appraisal requires a heavy dose of epidemiology, a subject capable of sedating the most lively individual. As a result, the information often fails to reach those in greatest need of it. Those seeking the typical, in-depth epidemiological approach to screening issues should look elsewhere. We asked our expert contributors to digest the available information and present it in the following standardized format, addressing fundamental questions the practitioner should consider to make an informed decision:

1 **What is the problem that requires screening?**
    a What is the incidence/prevalence of the target condition?
    b What are the sequelae of the condition which are of interest in clinical medicine?
2 **The tests**
    a What is the purpose of the tests?
    b The nature of the tests
    c Implications of testing
        1 What does an abnormal test result mean?
        2 What does a normal test result mean?
    d What is the cost of testing?
3 **Conclusions and recommendations**

Our goal was to produce an easily read text which would help the practitioner to make everyday decisions. The three editors bring a diverse scientific and international background to this effort. Two are obstetricians and gynecologists (one with an interest in public health), while the third is a medical statistician. The authors represent many countries and were asked to take an international approach considering both how the costs of testing and the frequency of the target disorder might vary among locations. Perhaps to the disgruntlement of some contributors, all chapters were heavily edited to give the feel of a 'single author' text. Preparation of the book was truly an educational experience for the editors. Several of the screening tests commonly used in obstetrics and gynecology are unjustified. The usefulness of many remains unclear despite widespread application. In other cases, the tests were adopted before an appropriate evaluation was even attempted. We believe established practitioners, trainees, midwives and nurse practitioners will find the text valuable as they reexamine their current (and plan for their future) practices. In many instances, they will find their practice differs from the recommendations. Considering the need for evidence-based practice, the divergence provides a challenge – confirm the value of a screening test, or cease to use it.

Hajo I.J. Wildschut
Carl P. Weiner
Tim J. Peters

1

Epidemiologic Considerations in Screening

Tim J. Peters, Hajo I. J. Wildschut & Carl P. Weiner

DEFINITIONS AND OBJECTIVES

Screening is defined as a procedure to help identify, in an organized way, a specified disease or condition among asymptomatic individuals. Since most screened individuals will be unaffected, the test must be safe to be acceptable. A **diagnostic test** is defined as the application of a variety of examinations or tests to patients who have actively sought health care services in order to identify the exact cause for their complaints (Sackett and Holland, 1975). The two are not mutually exclusive (e.g. genetic screening). The distinction between the two is whether or not that individual would have sought service for that particular problem. Diagnostic tests are also applied to subjects who seek medical care because of positive or suspicious findings resulting from a screening test. Diagnostic tests should be highly accurate. Screening tests, however, should be relatively simple and quick to perform. For this reason screening tests are allowed to possess higher margins of error and may be less accurate than diagnostic tests (Wilson and Jungner, 1968; Sackett and Holland, 1975).

Population (or mass) screening programs are applied to a general population to detect disease early in order to facilitate effective treatment. Such programs may also be applied for the purpose of separating seemingly healthy individuals into groups with high and low probabilities for a given disorder so that further health care resources can be targeted more efficiently (Sackett and Holland, 1975). The initiative for screening comes from either an investigator or an agency and involves participants with no known or reported symptoms or complaints related to the condition sought (Last, 1988). Subjects with positive or suspicious findings are referred for further investigation, diagnosis and appropriate management.

The objectives of population screening programs are to reduce morbidity and mortality, and improve the quality of life (Morrison, 1985; Last, 1988; Hannigan, 1991). Prerequisites for a successful screening program include a safe and acceptable test; an adequate infrastructure in terms of administrative setting, quality control measures, and systematic data handling; adequate health care services at the referral level which are accessible to those who need it; and clear targets in terms of delineating the problem to be screened. The condition should be amenable to treatment or prevention, with the timing of screening reflecting the opportunities for effective intervention. Finally, the severity or frequency of the target condition should be sufficient to justify the cost of screening.

Targeted screening programs involve the systematic testing of a selected group considered to be at increased risk. Targeted screening programs can be situation-dependent (for example, screening in pregnancy), age-dependent (mammography), inheritance-dependent (for example, screening of family members because the subject has a specified genetic disorder), or ethnic/race-dependent (for example, screening for sickle cell disease in black populations).

What is the problem that requires screening?

A clear, well-defined statement of the target condition being screened for is critical in assessing the value of any screening program. In practice, the true status is often not known for certain and hence effectively the test is evaluated in comparison with some other, more accurate classification – the 'gold standard' (Fletcher *et al.*, 1988; Editorial, 1992).

What is the nature of the screening test result?

Given that the test result is to be used as an indication of the presence or absence of the target condition, the simplest and most common situation is that the test itself classifies individuals into just two groups – those with a positive test result and those with a negative test result. For example, a woman may be either positive or negative for hepatitis B surface antigen. Alternatively, test results may be presented as continuous variables, where the value of a measurement can take any number in a range – for example, the blood glucose level. Given the objective of identifying a subgroup of individuals for further investigation, these measures are usually simplified to a dichotomy according to whether the measurement is above or below a cut-off. In this situation, the selection of the cut-off is critical and often controversial.

The proper evaluation of a screening program should address the following questions (Table 1.1), derived from Wilson and Jungner (1968), Sackett and Holland (1975) and Hannigan (1991).

Is the condition being screened for an important health problem?

Perception of the importance of a health problem needs to be considered from the point of view of the individual, of health care personnel, and of the community. Conceptually, the benefits of screening may signify 'reassurance' to the individual, 'prolonging life' to the physician and 'reduced cost' to policymakers. The following five principles have been suggested (Backett *et al.*, 1984): (1) considerable weight should be accorded to community priorities, preferences and concerns; (2) common problems should have higher priority than ones that occur rarely; (3) serious problems should be given higher priority than minor ones; (4) easily preventable health problems should be given higher priority than ones difficult to prevent; (5) health problems whose frequencies show upward trends should generally be given higher priority than those that are static or decreasing. These principles, however, are to some extent open to interpretation.

As indicated earlier, the importance of a health problem is closely associated with its frequency in the general population. In this context, the terms 'incidence' and 'preva-

Table 1.1   Desirable characteristics for a successful screening program.

1	**Is the condition being screened for an important health problem?**
2	**Is the screening test (and its consequences in terms of further diagnostic testing and subsequent treatment) acceptable to the population?**
3	**Does the target condition have a recognizable latent or early symptomatic phase? Is the natural history of the target condition well understood?**
4	**How valid and reliable is the screening test?**
5	**Are there adequate facilities for confirming the diagnosis and for adequate treatment?**
6	**Is the screening program a continuing process and not just a 'once and for all' project?**
7	**Is 'early' treatment of the target condition effective?**
8	**Do the objectives of the screening program justify the costs?**

Derived from Wilson and Jungner (1968), Sackett and Holland (1975), and Hannigan (1991)

Table 1.2   Characteristics of incidence and prevalence.

	INCIDENCE	**PREVALENCE**
numerator	**new cases occurring during a period of time among a group initially free of disease**	**all cases counted on a single survey or examination of a group**
denominator	**all susceptible persons present at the beginning of the period**	**all persons examined, including affected and non-affected**
time	**duration of period**	**given point or period**
how measured	**cohort study**	**cross-sectional study**

From Fletcher et al. (1988) Clinical Epidemiology: The Essentials, 2nd edn., with permission. Copyright Williams & Wilkins, Baltimore.

lence' are often used. Incidence and prevalence are related but different terms and should not be used interchangeably.

Incidence (Table 1.2) measures the occurrence of newly diagnosed events among previously unaffected persons. Typically, incidence rates are calculated from follow-up studies (cohort studies), where a fixed number of apparently healthy people are observed over a given period of time (usually a year) in order to determine the number of new events which occur during that period (Last, 1988).

Prevalence (Table 1.2) measures the extent to which the condition of interest exists among a specified group of people at a given point (or period) in time. Prevalence is usually given as a proportion – that is, the total number of affected persons per total number of subjects. For example, the annual incidence of pancreatic cancer is likely to be similar to its prevalence since most patients die within a year of diagnosis. In contrast, the prevalence of diabetes in a particular group of individuals will continue to grow even if its incidence remains stable since most patients will live more than a year with disease. Thus, the prevalence depends upon the incidence and duration of the disease. Barker has described incidence as the water flowing into a lake and prevalence as the water in the lake (Barker and Rose, 1990). Incidence and prevalence are frequently confused in obstetrics. For example, the proportion of newborns with trisomy 21 is generally referred to as a birth incidence, whereas in truth it is the birth prevalence.

Are the screening test and its consequences acceptable to the population?

The individual (or community) has a free choice to participate in a screening program. The screening test itself must be safe and acceptable. The individual should be adequately informed prior to testing about the potential benefits and hazards of the program. For instance, therapeutic options may not be acceptable because of ethical concerns, regarding for example termination of pregnancy in the case of Down syndrome, or unwanted side-effects such as unnecessary surgery in ovarian cancer screening programs. Furthermore, with respect to screening programs for certain medical conditions, such as sexually transmitted diseases, it is well known that non-compliance is high, especially among those who would benefit most from the program. If a large proportion of the population do not comply with the medical advice following positive test results, any potentially beneficial effects of the screening program will be undermined.

Does the target condition have a recognizable latent or early symptomatic phase? Is the natural history of the target condition well understood?

Survival rates may appear to improve if earlier diagnosis is achieved as a result of screening, that is, before signs or symptoms of the condition of interest become manifest. This so-called *lead time* is dependent on both the biological rate of disease progression and on the ability of the screening test to detect disease at an early stage. If the lead time is short, screening is unlikely to be of value since treatment of the target condition following detection by screening will be essentially the same as treatment following overt disease (Fletcher *et al.*, 1988).

Overestimation of survival time due to detection of disease in the early – asymptomatic – stage is known as *lead time bias* (Fletcher *et al.*, 1988). It is important not to be misled by lead time bias. For example, if screening could successfully identify women with stage I ovarian cancer but no therapy was instituted, and success was measured by survival time from diagnosis, it might appear that survival was improved by screening although in reality it was unaltered. Where there is no effective treatment, screening only provides an early death sentence. Knowledge of the natural history of the target condition is clearly important for the assessment of the results of early treatment.

How valid and reliable is the screening test?

VALIDITY

Validity is a summary measure of test performance, which is determined by both the underlying quality of the test and the way the test is carried out. Validity refers to the

Table 1.3   Formulae for sensitivity, specificity, prevalence, positive predictive value (PPV) and negative predictive value (NPV).

TEST RESULT	TARGET	CONDITION[1]
	present	absent
positive	a	b
negative	c	d

[1] *True state of the individual, as determined by a relevant 'gold standard'; sensitivity = $a/(a + c)$; specificity = $d/(b + d)$; prevalence = $(a + c)/(a + b + c + d)$; PPV = $a/(a + b)$; NPV = $d/(c + d)$. (For detailed definitions see text.)*

degree to which a test measures what it purports to measure. It therefore requires an independent standard of reference (Fletcher *et al.*, 1988; Editorial, 1992). Both internal and external validity must be considered.

Internal validity is synonymous with accuracy, i.e. the degree to which the test result corresponds with the true state of the phenomenon being measured (Fletcher *et al.*, 1988). The two components of internal validity are sensitivity and specificity (Barker and Rose, 1990).

Sensitivity is defined as the proportion of individuals with the target condition who screened positive (Fletcher *et al.*, 1988; Altman, 1991) (Table 1.3). Sensitivity is a measure of how good the test is at identifying patients with the disease. High sensitivity implies that a large proportion of individuals with the target condition have a positive result on the screening test. Highly sensitive tests are needed when there is an important penalty for missing the disorder (Fletcher *et al.*, 1988). This is particularly true when 'false negative' test results (category *c* in Table 1.3) create harm. Any test that is not 100% sensitive will inevitably result in false reassurance and possibly delay the seeking of medical care once symptoms of the target disorder do appear (Hannigan, 1991). Moreover, the physician or midwife may fear litigation when the target disorder is not detected by the test.

Specificity is defined as the proportion of individuals without the disease who have a negative result on the screening test. Specificity is a measure of how good the test is at identifying unaffected subjects (Fletcher *et al.*, 1988; Altman, 1991) (Table 1.3). It assesses how good it is at excluding the condition of interest. Hence, specificity is related to reassurance about health. High specificity thus reflects a low proportion of individuals falsely labeled as having the disease when they are in fact free of disease (the 'false positives', category *b* in Table 1.3). In contrast, low specificity implies a high proportion of healthy individuals who are labelled as test positive (high false positive rate). In screening programs, false positive test results produce most of the problems since healthy individuals are subjected to often expensive, time-consuming and potentially dangerous diagnostic procedures that would not be experienced without the screening test (Hannigan, 1991). Moreover, false positive test results may create unnecessary anxiety for the patient. For a test involving a continuous measurement, such blood glucose determination, the receiver operating characteristic (ROC) curve is useful when there are many possible cut-off values (Altman, 1991). The ROC curve is a graphical representation, where sensitivity is plotted against the false positive rate (1 − specificity). As is illustrated by such curves, the sensitivity and specificity are inversely related to each other. In a given situation, false positive results are decreased at the cost of increasing false negative results, and vice versa. Sensitivity and specificity, and therefore the ROC curve, do not take into account the prevalence of the condition sought.

Table 1.4   Predictive values of a test with a sensitivity of 90% and a specificity of 99% when the prevalence of the disease is 10%.

TEST RESULT	DISEASE/CONDITION		
	present	absent	total
positive	90	9	99
neagtive	10	891	901
total	100	900	1000

PPV = 90/99 = 90.9%; NPV = 891/901 = 98.9%

In clinical practice, *predictive values* are important since they are the probabilities in a particular setting that someone testing positive really has the condition and someone testing negative does not. In this context, the *positive predictive value* (PPV) is the probability of disease in subjects with a positive test result, whereas *negative predictive value* (NPV) is the probability of absence of the disease in subjects with a negative test result (Table 1.3). Predictive values are affected by test performance, in terms of sensitivity and specificity, *and* by the prevalence of the condition in the target population. As illustrated in Table 1.4, in settings with a relatively high prevalence of disease (for example, 10%), the probability of disease among the test positive subjects is high (the PPV is 91%). On the other hand, in settings with a lower prevalence (e.g. 1%) the probability of disease among test positive subjects is reduced (in Table 1.5, the PPV is 47%). This occurs despite the fact that the sensitivity (90%) and specificity (99%) are identical in each setting. A further general point to be emphasized when considering the above performance statistics is that we are considering the ability of the test to detect *prevalent* cases, whether at a given point in time or over a period of time; hence the relevant measure of frequency in the context of tables such as Tables 1.3 and 1.4 is prevalence not incidence.

Likelihood ratios (LRs) are an alternative way of looking at test performance. They are a reflection of sensitivity and specificity, and are given by the formulae presented in Table 1.6 (Fletcher *et al*., 1988; Altman, 1991). Likelihood ratios can be used to calculate 'post-test probabilities' which are the probabilities of disease after either a positive or a negative test result. For example, LRs allow us to update the pretest probability of intrauterine growth restriction (IUGR) from about 10% of all deliveries to 20% of those with an abnormal uterine artery Doppler ratio and 7% of those with a normal Doppler (see Chapter 10).

Table 1.5   Predictive values of a test with a sensitivity of 90% and a specificity of 99% when the prevalence is 1%.

TEST RESULT	DISEASE/CONDITION		
	present	absent	total
positive	9	10	19
negative	1	980	981
total	10	990	1000

PPV = 9/19 = 47.4%; NPV = 980/981 = 99.9%

Table 1.6 Formulae for the likelihood ratio (LR) associated with a positive (abnormal test result (LR$^{(pos)}$) and LR associated with a negative (normal) test result (LR$^{(neg)}$).

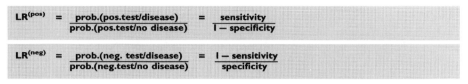

prob. (pos. test/disease) = probability of a positive test result among those with the disease (that is, sensitivity); prob. (neg. test/no disease) = probability of a negative test result among those without the disease (that is, specificity)

First, the value of the pretest odds is computed from the pretest probability (prevalence), using the following formula:

$$\text{pretest odds} = \frac{\text{pretest probability}}{1 - \text{pretest probability}}$$

Note that odds and probability are not the same and should not be used interchangeably. For example, a probability of 1/3 would correspond to odds of 1/2. These pretest odds are then converted to post-test odds by applying the likelihood ratios in the following way:

$$\text{post-test odds}^{(pos)} = \text{pretest odds} \times \text{LR}^{pos}$$

$$\text{post-test odds}^{(neg)} = \text{pretest odds} \times \text{LR}^{(neg)}$$

and the post-test odds values converted to probabilities by:

$$\text{prob. (disease/pos.test)} = \frac{\text{post-test odds}^{(pos)}}{1 + \text{post-test odds}^{(pos)}}$$

$$\text{prob. (disease/neg.test)} = \frac{\text{post-test odds}^{(neg)}}{1 + \text{post-test odds}^{(neg)}}$$

In summary, the prevalence is first expressed as a single odds. In turn, this is converted via the LR$^{(pos)}$ and LR$^{(neg)}$ to *two* post-test odds, which are then reexpressed as post-test probabilities of either a positive or negative test result. This procedure is equivalent to obtaining the positive and negative predictive values from the sensitivity, specificity and prevalence using Bayes' theorem (Altman, 1991). The purpose is to allow the calculation of predictive values in various clinical settings with different prevalence given the under-lying sensitivity and specificity of the test. As illustrated in Table 1.4, even if the sensitivity and the specificity do not change, the predictive values are dependent on the prevalence. Of course, sensitivity and specificity *may* vary in different clinical settings (for example due to varying skills in carrying out the test and varying durations of follow-up – see Chapter 24).

In conclusion, a likelihood ratio different from 1 demonstrates that a test is potentially useful, but does not necessarily imply that the test is a good indicator of disease, especially when the target condition is rare. In this situation, someone testing positive is still more likely to be unaffected than affected (Altman, 1991). Nevertheless, for rare conditions the $LR^{(pos)}$ will be approximately equal to the odds ratio, which in turn approximates to the relative risk (Altman, 1991), and the $LR^{(neg)}$ will be approximately equal to 1.

External validity (generalizability) is the degree to which test results hold true in other settings (Fletcher *et al.*, 1988). Sensitivity estimates are usually derived from carefully controlled research settings and may not apply to everyday situations. Published sensitivity values for a given test or examination tend to be overestimates since the findings are often based on special expertise and novel technologies applied to an atypical clinical population.

Reliability is also a measure of a test's performance. It is synonymous with reproducibility, repeatability, transferability, precision, and consistency. Reliability refers to the degree of stability when a measurement is repeated under the same conditions (Last, 1988). The extent to which a test is reproducible is affected by variation arising from three main sources: the examination (laboratory facilities or equipment), the examiner (skill), and the examined (characteristics) (Sackett and Holland, 1975). Lack of reliability may be the result of measurement errors or instability of the attribute being studied.

Are there adequate facilities for confirming the diagnosis and for treatment?

Several aspects of screening procedures are demanding. These include the recording of the screening result, the proper interpretation of the result, communication between the screening program and the patient/caregiver, and quality control. Results, in particular when abnormal, should be communicated to the individual being screened and to the physician responsible for further evaluation and management. For this purpose, adequate facilities should be accessible to those who need it. Adequate facilities include hospitals and laboratories, which need to be properly staffed and technically equipped to meet the demands of confirmatory testing, diagnosis and subsequent treatment where indicated. For the optimal use of resources, a carefully designed and agreed referral system is imperative for a successful screening program. The total burden on medical, diagnostic and therapeutic resources could be increased by the introduction of a screening program.

Is the testing a continuing process and not a 'once and for all' project?

In some situations, screening is best served by the performance of examinations at regular intervals. An ongoing reminder system should be part of the screening program.

Is 'early' treatment of the target condition effective?

Will 'early' treatment – that is, in the asymptomatic phase – be more effective than 'delayed' treatment – that is, when symptoms appear? The question of whether treatment can work is one of both efficacy and effectiveness (Fletcher *et al.*, 1988; Last, 1988). Efficacy is the performance of an intervention under ideal circumstances, whereas effectiveness is performance under everyday circumstances (Fletcher *et al.*, 1988; Last, 1988). The randomized controlled trial (RCT) is generally accepted as the ideal method to ascertain efficacy (Thacker, 1985). By the use of pragmatic RCTs (Schwartz and Lellouch, 1967), it is possible to bring efficacy as close as possible to effectiveness. Random allocation to intervention groups eliminates the possibility that differences in outcome between the groups are due to differences in underlying risks between the groups.

Of course, the justification for screening requires more than evidence of effective early treatment. In general, the proper evaluation of screening programs should involve an RCT of the screening program compared with an appropriate unscreened group where disease is detected in the usual way. Such RCTs would normally involve randomization of groups rather than individuals. Since such a trial should incorporate all the complexities that would occur in practice – such as variations in attendance, compliance, acceptability, and quality of procedures, among others – a pragmatic approach would invariably be needed. Furthermore, comprehensive evidence about screening is not possible without full attention to cost-effectiveness.

Do the objectives of the screening program justify the costs?

WHAT ARE THE IMPORTANT AND RELEVANT COSTS?

The costs of screening can be both psychological and economic. Psychological costs include the anxiety engendered by participation in the screening program, the wait for test results and subsequent treatment, and knowledge of one's risk status or the future likelihood of overt disease (in particular the unnecessary anxiety produced by a false positive screen). In addition, there may be other psychological stresses caused by indicated follow-up tests and therapy.

Economic costs include direct costs to the health care system (such as organizational and operating costs), direct costs borne by patients and their families (for example, travel expenses) and any indirect costs such as lost work time. In economic evaluations of health care programs, marginal (extra) costs should be used. Marginal cost refers to the extra cost of producing one extra unit of the desired health outcome. For example, the desired outcome might be years of life gained or the number of abnormalities avoided. Hence, when making a comparison of two or more programs, the question is what the extra costs and consequences are of the alternative program over and above the costs of the existing program. In screening, as in many other contexts, marginal costs depend on the size of the program. For example, the introduction of a small-scale screening program targeted at high-risk groups may show a low cost per case detected. If the screening program were to be expanded to groups at lower risk, the number of screening tests required to detect a positive case would rise, resulting in a net increase in the cost per case detected (Cohen, 1994).

WHY IS AN ECONOMIC EVALUATION IMPORTANT?

Choices have to be made concerning deployment of health care programs, services and procedures since resources in terms of personnel, time, facilities, and equipment are limited. Decisions on where to allocate resources should be based on explicit criteria. A systematic economic evaluation is important to identify clearly the costs and consequences of alternative programs (Drummond *et al.*, 1987). Only with systematic evaluation is it possible to estimate and compare the various costs and benefits. In this context, the term 'efficiency' is defined as maximizing the benefit derived from available resources (Cohen, 1994). Hence, costs incurred finding a case, which includes both identification and treatment, should be weighed against the costs of an alternative program (Hakama, 1991).

WHAT STRATEGIES ARE USED FOR A FULL ECONOMIC EVALUATION?

There are two prerequisites for a full economic evaluation. First, two or more alternative programs, services or procedures need to be compared. Second, both costs and health outputs need to be compared. The four types of full economic evaluation considered are cost-minimization analysis, cost-effectiveness analysis, cost-utility analysis, and cost-benefit analysis (Drummond *et al.*, 1987).

Comparative evaluation of health programs solely in terms of costs is called **cost-minimization analysis**. For this approach to be appropriate, some preceding evidence is required to rule out differences in effectiveness of the programs being compared. An example of cost-minimization analysis is the comparison of progesterone versus danazol for the treatment of endometriosis. They are similar in effectiveness, but one is considerably more expensive than the other.

Cost-effectiveness analysis is concerned with determining the least cost to achieve a specified level of effectiveness, or the greatest effectiveness for a given level of expenditure (Last, 1988). Cost-effectiveness analysis is relevant to programs that produce health effects directly, and to those achieving clinical objectives that can be linked to improvements in patient outcome (Drummond *et al.*, 1987). It implicitly assumes that the output in terms of health effects (for example, preventing death, increasing life-years gained or disability days saved) is worth having (Drummond *et al.*, 1987). For instance, the different diagnostic strategies for breast cancer can be compared in terms of the cost per case detected.

In **cost-utility analysis**, utilities are employed as measures of the effects of a program. Utility refers to the perceived value, or worth, of a particular health status. It can be quantified by elucidating individual or societal preferences in relation to specific health outcomes (Drummond *et al.*, 1987). The results of a cost-utility analysis are expressed in terms of the costs per unit of health-related utility, or cost per quality adjusted life year (QALY) gained under one program compared with another (Drummond *et al.*, 1987).

Cost-benefit analysis is the evaluation of health care programs by valuing benefits as well as costs in terms of money. This means that costs and benefits can be compared directly, which in principle allows the assessment of a program's worth in absolute terms rather than just relative to an alternative program (Drummond *et al.*, 1987). In practice, though, cost-benefit analyses almost always involve the comparison of at least two programs, even if one is a 'do-nothing' alternative with more or less minimal intervention (Drummond *et al.*, 1987). In evaluations of screening programs, the 'do-nothing' option includes all the clinical management of patients which will take place even in the absence of screening. For example, in a cost-benefit analysis of screening for neural tube defects, it would be assumed that therapy is given to children with spina bifida under the 'no screening' alternative.

IS AN ECONOMIC EVALUATION ALWAYS NEEDED?

Evaluation is in itself a costly activity; indeed it has been said that even a cost-benefit analysis should itself be subjected to a cost-benefit analysis (Drummond *et al.*, 1987). In addition, economic evaluations are difficult to accomplish, requiring a variety of subjective and qualitative decisions which may greatly affect the final result. When the analysis is mainly descriptive, the term 'partial evaluation' is used. 'Partial evaluation' indicates that the analysis will not determine definitively whether the health program is worth doing (Drummond *et al.*, 1987). A full economic evaluation, however, only seems reasonable in situations where program objectives require clarification, where the competing alternatives are markedly different in nature, or where large resource commitments are under consideration (Drummond *et al.*, 1987). In any case, all economic evaluations should be subjected to a sensitivity analysis, where the assumptions and valuations employed are varied within appropriate bounds of uncertainty in order to ascertain the robustness of the conclusions. One of the objectives of the sensitivity analysis will be to assess the generalizability of the results of the economic evaluation, in particular, how the implications of the evaluation may vary in different local settings.

CONCLUSIONS AND RECOMMENDATIONS

The ultimate objective of screening is to reduce mortality and morbidity (Hannigan, 1991). Conditions screened for should therefore include important causes of mortality or morbidity, in terms of prevalence, severity, or both. Moreover, such conditions should be amenable to either treatment or prevention when detected early. The screening procedure itself should be safe and easy to perform in order to maximize compliance. The ideal screening test should be capable of identifying a large group of subjects with (or susceptible to) disease and should also be capable of excluding the majority of those without disease. Harm should be avoided and adverse psychological effects kept to a minimum. A full description of the screening program should be given: who does what, to whom, where, how often and what are the results (Drummond *et al.*, 1987)? A precise definition of the condition and the target population are essential.

Appropriate action should be taken based on explicit criteria when an abnormal result is obtained. For this reason, adequate health care services should be available for the diagnosis and treatment of confirmed disease. These services should be accessible and affordable. Screening programs are demanding in various respects, including data handling, continuity and communication. Adequate infrastructure and health care facilities at the referral level are essential if a screening program is to be successful.

Finally, individuals should be motivated to comply with medical advice. There is widespread ethical, legal and medical agreement that screening should be preceded – and followed – by counseling, even if a screening test becomes 'routine'. The individual should be adequately informed about the potential benefits and limitations of screening in terms of primary objectives, results and implications. Screening should always be offered as an option, which may be accepted or rejected.

REFERENCES

Altman DG (1991) *Practical Statistics for Medical Research*, pp 409–419. London: Chapman & Hall.
Backett EM, Davies AM & Petros-Barvazian A (1984) The risk approach in health care. With special reference to maternal and child health care planning. World Health Organization Public Health Reports Geneva: WHO.
Barker DJP & Rose G (1990) *Epidemiology in Medical Practice*, 4th edn. Edinburgh: Churchill Livingstone.
Cohen D (1994) Marginal analysis in practice: an alternative to needs assessment for contracting health care. *Br Med J* 309: 781–784.
Drummond MF, Stoddard GL & Torrance GW (1987) *Methods for the Economic Evaluation of Health Care Programmes*. Oxford University Press.
Editorial (1992). Instructions for authors. *JAMA* 268: 43–44.
Fletcher RH, Fletcher SW, & Wagner EH (1988) *Clinical Epidemiology: The Essentials*, 2nd edn. Baltimore: Williams & Wilkins.
Hakama M (1991) Screening. In Holland WW, Detels R & Knox G (eds), *Oxford Textbook of Public*

Health, 2nd edition. *Applications in Public Health* (vol. 3), pp. 91–106. Oxford: Oxford University Press.

Hannigan VL (1991). The periodic health examination. In Diehl AK (ed.). *Prevention and Screening in Office Practice: Contemporary Management in Internal Medicine*, pp. 3–26. New York: Churchill Livingstone.

Last JM (1988) *A Dictionary of Epidemiology*, 2nd edition. Oxford University Press.

Morrison AS (1985) *Screening in Chronic Disease*, 2nd edition. Oxford University Press.

Sackett DL & Holland WW (1975) Controversy in the detection of disease. *Lancet*, ii: 357–359.

Schwartz D & Lellouch J (1967) (Explanatory and pragmatic attitudes in therapeutical trials. *J Chron Dis* 20: 637–648.

Thacker SB (1985) Quality of controlled clinical trials. The case of imaging ultrasound in obstetrics. A review. *Br J Obstet Gynaecol*, 92: 437–444.

Wilson JMG & Jungner G (1968) *Principles and Practice of Screening for Disease*. Public Health Papers 34. Geneva: World Health Organization.

2

Nonvenereal Diseases Acquired During Pregnancy

Walter Foulon & Anne Naessens

WHAT IS THE PROBLEM THAT REQUIRES SCREENING?

NEONATAL GROUP B STREPTOCOCCAL INFECTION.

What is the incidence/prevalence of the target condition?

Early-onset group B streptococcal infection (GBS) of the neonate is defined as a GBS sepsis within 5 days of birth. The incidence of GBS depends on the colonization rate of pregnant women. Group B streptococcus colonizes the lower vagina, vulva or rectum in 15–30% of pregnant women (Christensen *et al.*, 1981; Baker and Barret, 1983).

From 40% to 75% of colonized mothers transmit the bacterium to their fetus either during labor or at birth (Yow *et al.*, 1980; Christensen *et al.*, 1981; Baker and Barret, 1983). Only a small minority (1–2%) of these neonates develop life-threatening sepsis (Table 2.1). The rate of early-onset GBS in the USA is about 1–3 per 1000 live births for all women and 1 per 100 colonized women (Rouse *et al.*, 1994). Risk factors for early-onset GBS are well known and include low birthweight or preterm delivery, prolonged rupture of the membranes (> 12–18 hours), heavy maternal colonization, fever during labor and low serum concentration of the type specific antibody.

Table 2.1 Public health consequences of maternal group B streptococcal (GBS) infection.

NUMBER		PROBABILITY[a]	RANGE[b]
1000	pregnant women		
200	GBS colonized women	0.20	0.15–0.30
100	vertical transmission	0.50	0.40–0.75
2	neonatal GBS infection	0.02	0.01–0.02

[a] *Crude estimates;* [b] *See text*

What are the sequelae of the condition which are of interest in clinical medicine?

Early-onset GBS is one of the most serious newborn infections, causing fulminant septicemia, pneumonia, meningitis, and shock; it is frequently accompanied by respiratory distress. The vast majority (about 90%) occur on day 1 of life, suggesting the infection is acquired in utero. The mortality rate has been reported to be as high as 50% though recent figures are closer to 20%. Surviving infants commonly develop longterm sequelae (e.g. neurologic problems). Preterm infants constitute up to 30% of GBS deaths. Term babies also develop early-onset GBS, and though their individual risk is much lower than that of the preterm infant, they are numerically important because of their large number.

THE TESTS

What is the purpose of the tests?

To identify pregnant women colonized with group B streptococcus.

Early-onset GBS may develop so rapidly that antibiotic therapy begun after birth is too late. Intrapartum antibiotic chemoprophylaxis reduces the neonatal colonization rate from 50% to 10% (Yow et al., 1979). The decrease in colonization appears to be associated with a reduction in early-onset GBS infection (Boyer and Gotoff, 1986).

The nature of the tests

Bacterial culture in selected medium is relatively low in cost and is the 'gold standard'. Since as many as 20% of pregnant women in the second trimester with a negative vaginal culture will have a positive vaginal culture at birth, both the lower part of the vagina and the rectum should be cultured (Pass et al., 1982; Dillon et al., 1987). A major drawback to relying on a culture is that the result will not available for 24–48 hours.

Since a rapid diagnosis of the carrier status is often clinically important, other diagnostic methods have been studied. A Gram stain performed on a vaginal smear, although simple and of low cost, has a too low a sensitivity and specificity to be of value in the detection of the group B streptoccus carrier status (Sandy et al., 1988; Yancy et al., 1992). The rapid antigen detection tests also have poor sensitivity (15–30%), but rather high specificity (> 90%) (Greenspoon et al., 1991; Shall et al., 1991). Many of these tests are not 'user friendly' and most are more expensive than culture.

Implications of testing

Three general approaches to the identification of at-risk pregnancies have been used. Each assumes that at-risk pregnancies will benefit from the administration of intrapartum chemoprophylaxis. The first approach is to assume all women are at high risk and treat them in labor. The second approach is to restrict treatment to pregnancies with *at least one* risk factor (preterm delivery, preterm rupture of membranes, rupture of membranes greater than 12–16 hours, under age 18 years, drug addiction, prostitution, maternal fever during labor, a sibling affected by early-onset GBS). The third approach is to culture all patients for group B streptococcus one or two times during pregnancy (e.g. at 28 and 36 weeks of gestation) and treat either all positive women, or those who are positive and have one or more risk factors. Each approach seems to reduce the incidence of GBS, but not to the same degree (see section on costs). Further, the percentage of pregnant women who would receive antibiotics varies from 15% to 100%. It should be noted that 5–20% of women claim a penicillin allergy. The risk of a maternal death due to anaphylaxis secondary to either penicillin or ampicillin is estimated to be 1 per 57 000 women treated (Rouse *et al.*, 1994).

WHAT DOES AN ABNORMAL TEST RESULT MEAN?

Maternal colonization is a poor predictor of neonatal GBS, which occurs in only in 1% of the infants of group B streptococcus carriers (Easmon *et al.*, 1985). In addition, the rate of colonization can change during pregnancy and the antepartum treatment of carriers with penicillin does not alter their carrier status at delivery (Hall *et al.*, 1976). Group B streptococcus is eradicated from the lower genital tract by penicillin, but remains present in the bowel. The vagina is frequently recolonized from that area after the treatment. While antibiotic treatment does not necessarily eliminate maternal group B streptococcus carriage, it will eliminate it from the vagina during the treatment period. This forms the basis for the only strategy which seems to be effective: intrapartum chemoprophylaxis.

Multiple studies have demonstrated that intrapartum chemoprophylaxis significantly reduces the neonatal colonization rate (Easmon *et al.*, 1983; Boyer and Gotoff, 1986; Matonàs *et al.*, 1991) and several others early-onset disease (Jeffery and McIntosh, 1994; Pylipow *et al.*, 1994). However, there is only one randomized controlled trial demonstrating the efficacy of intrapartum antibiotherapy in preventing early-onset group B streptococci infection (Boyer and Gotoff, 1986). In this study, women carrying group B streptococcus in the third trimester of pregnancy and having risk factors such as premature labor or prolonged rupture of membranes (> 12 hours) were treated with ampicillin 2 g intravenously followed by 1 g every 4 hours until delivery.

There are several problems with basing intrapartum treatment on an antepartum culture result. Group B streptococcus carriage in pregnancy is not a constant and a patient who is positive in the early third trimester may be negative at delivery and vice versa. Secondly, maternal colonization is a very poor predictor of early-onset GBS. If antibiotics are given to all pregnant women harboring group B streptococcus in the vagina or rectum, then the number of pregnant women treated during labor will be large (20–30% of the population).

WHAT DOES A NORMAL TEST RESULT MEAN?

Pregnant women considered at high risk because of demographic factors but with negative vaginal and rectal cultures for GBS need not be treated during labor since the likelihood of early-onset GBS would be low.

What is the cost of testing?

Several investigators have examined the cost-efficacy of the various proposed screening methods (Mohle-Boetani *et al.*, 1993; Rouse *et al.*, 1994; Strickland *et al.*, 1990). Strategies based on the currently available rapid streptococcus identification tests are ineffective at reducing neonatal sepsis and are costly. Thus, antepartum screening relies on some type of culture paradigm. One 'decision tree' analysis concluded that routine culture at 28 weeks with intrapartum treatment of at-risk positives cost US $28 800 per case prevented with a benefit-cost ratio of 1.2. In contrast, intrapartum treatment based on demographic risk factors alone cost $10 200 per case prevented with a benefit-cost ratio of 4.2 (Mohle-Boetani *et al.*, 1993). A similar 'decision tree' analysis of 19 strategies reached a similar conclusion though the estimated cost per case prevented was considerably higher (Rouse *et al.*, 1994). In both analyses, universal culture at 28 weeks and treatment of culture positive, high-risk patients in labor were among the *least* effective methods of reducing early neonatal GBS, and the *most* costly.

CONCLUSIONS AND RECOMMENDATIONS

Asymptomatic vaginal colonization with GBS occurs in 15–30% of pregnant women. Vertical transmission from colonized woman to infant occurs in 40–75%. The incidence of early-onset neonatal GBS infection is about 1% of colonized newborns. Approximately 20% of affected newborns die and 50% of survivors are left with permanent neurologic damage. The goal of group B streptococcal screening during pregnancy is to detect vaginal GBS colonization in order to offer some form of chemoprophylaxis. Antepartal treatment of group B streptococcal colonization is ineffective in reducing the incidence of early-onset GBS. The effectiveness of intrapartum chemoprophylaxis in decreasing the neonatal group B streptococcal colonization rate is established. It is likely but not yet definitively shown that chemoprophylaxis also reduces early-onset GBS.

There is no consensus on the best approach to prevent early-onset GBS. Universal screening for group B streptococcus colonization by culture at 28 weeks' gestation has the lowest benefit-risk ratio and is the most costly of the three general approaches. It cannot be recommended. Treating all women intrapartum seems intuitively undesirable if there is an effective alternative. 'Decision tree' analysis suggests that the intrapartum treatment of women whose babies are at high risk for early-onset GBS based on demographic factors is the best approach.

SUMMARY

1 ## WHAT IS THE PROBLEM THAT REQUIRES SCREENING?

NEONATAL GROUP B STREPTOCOCCAL INFECTIONS.

a What is the incidence/prevalence of the target condition?

The incidence of early-onset GBS is about 1–3 per 1000 life births.

b What are the sequelae of the condition which are of interest in clinical medicine?

Group B streptococcal infection can cause fulminant sepsis, pneumonia, meningitis and shock, and is frequently accompanied by respiratory distress. The mortality is close to 20%. Surviving infants often develop longterm (e.g. neurologic) sequelae.

2 THE TESTS

a What is the purpose of the tests?

To identify pregnant women colonized with group B streptococcus.

b The nature of the tests

The 'gold standard' is culture of the vagina, cervix, and rectum. The rapid antigen test has too low a sensitivity to be clinically useful.

c Implications of testing

Three approaches have been applied to the prevention of early-onset GBS. First, treatment of all pregnant women. Second, selective administration of antibiotic therapy based on the presence of high-risk demographic factors – preterm delivery, preterm rupture of membranes, rupture of membranes greater than 12–16 hours, age under 18 years, drug addiction, prostitution, maternal fever during labor. Third, routine culture of the cervix, vagina, and rectum for group B streptococcus and treatment of culture positive patients.

1 What does an abnormal test result mean?

Maternal colonization is a poor predictor of early-onset GBS which occurs in only 1% of the infants of group B streptococcus carriers. Thus, a positive culture indicates the need for either universal chemoprophylaxis or prophylaxis based on risk factors.

2 What does a normal test result mean?

A negative culture indicates the woman is at low risk for having a child with early-onset group B streptococcal sepsis.

d What is the cost of testing?

Either universal or selective intrapartum maternal chemoprophylaxis based on risk factors has the highest cost-benefit ratio. Universal culture at 28 weeks and treatment of culture positive, high-risk patients in labor is among the least effective approaches to reducing early-onset GBS and is the most costly.

3 CONCLUSIONS AND RECOMMENDATIONS

Intrapartum chemoprophylaxis significantly reduces the neonatal colonization rate and apparently early-onset disease. However, antepartal routine culture is neither the most clinically effective nor cost-effective approach. Rather, intrapartum chemoprophylaxis should be administered, to laboring women with demographic or clinical risk factors which place them at high risk.

REFERENCES

Baker CJ & Barret FF (1983) Transmission of group B streptococci among parturient women and their neonates. *J Pediatr* **83**: 919–925.

Boyer KM & Gotoff SP (1986) Prevention of early-onset neonatal group B streptococcal disease with selective intrapartum chemoprophylaxis. *N Engl J Med* **314**: 1665–1669.

Christensen KK, Dahlander K, Ekstrom A *et al.* (1981) Colonization of newborns with group B streptococci: relation to maternal urogenital carriage. *Scand J Infect Dis* **13:** 23–27.

Dillon HC Jr, Khare S & Gray BM (1987) Group B streptococcal carriage and disease: a 6-year prospective study. *J Pediatr* **110:** 31–36.

Easmon CSF, Hastings MJG, Deeley J *et al.* (1983) The effect of intrapartum chemoprophylaxis on the vertical transmission of group B streptococci. *Br J Obstet Gynaecol* **90:** 633–635.

Easmon CSF, Hastings MJG, Neill J *et al.* (1985) Is group B streptococcal screening during pregnancy justified? *Br J Obstet Gynaecol* **92:** 197–201.

Greenspoon JS, Fishman A, Wilcox JG *et al.* (1991) Comparison of culture for group B streptococcus versus enzyme immunoassay and latex agglutination rapid tests: results in 250 patients during labour. *Obstet Gynecol* **77:** 97–100.

Hall RT, Barnes W, Krishamn I *et al.* (1976) Antibiotic treatment of parturient women colonized with group B streptococci. *Am J Obstet Gynecol* **124:** 630–634.

Jeffery HE & McIntosh ED (1994) Antepartum screening and nonselective intrapartum chemoprophylaxis for Group B streptococcus. *Aust NZ J Obstet Gynaecol* **34:** 14–9.

Matonàs R, Garcia-Perea A, Omeñaca F *et al* (1991) Intrapartum chemoprophylaxis of early-onset group B streptococcal disease. *Eur J Obstet Gynecol Reprod Biol* **40:** 57–62.

Mohle-Boetani JC, Schuchat A, Plikaytis BD, Smith JD & Borrome CJ (1993) Comparison of prevention strategies for neonatal group B streptococcal infection: a population-based economic analysis. *JAMA* **270:** 1442–1448.

Pass MA, Gray BM & Dillon HC Jr (1982) Puerperal and perinatal infections with group B streptococci. *Am J Obstet Gynecol* **143:** 147–152.

Pylipow M, Gaddis M & Kinney JS. (1994) Selective intrapartum prophylaxis for Group B streptococcus colonization: management and outcome of newborns. *Pediatrics* **93:** 631–5.

Rouse DJ, Goldenberg RL, Cliver SP, Cutter GR, Mennemeyer ST & Fargason CA (1994) Strategies for the prevention of early-onset neonatal Group B streptococcal sepsis: a decision analysis. *Obstet Gynecol* **83:** 483–94.

Sandy EA, Blumenfeld ML & Iams JD (1988) Gram stains in the rapid determination of maternal colonization with group B beta-streptococcus. *Obstet Gynecol* **71:** 796–798.

Shall MA, Mercer BM, Baselski V *et al.* (1991) Evaluation of two rapid group B streptococcal antigen tests in labor and delivery patients. *Obstet Gynecol* **77:** 322–326.

Strickland DM, Yeomans ER & Hawkins GDV (1990) Cost-effectiveness of intrapartum screening and treatment for maternal group B streptococci colonization. *Am J Obstet Gynecol* **163:** 4–8.

Yancy MK, Armer T, Clark P & Duff P (1992) Assessment of rapid identification tests for genital carriage of group B streptococci. *Obstet Gynecol* **80:** 1038–1047.

Yow MD, Mason EO, Leeds LJ *et al.* (1979) Ampicillin prevents intrapartum transmission of group B streptococcus. *JAMA* **241:** 1245–1247.

Yow MD, Leeds LJ, Thompson PK, *et al.* (1980) The natural history of group B streptococcal colonization in the pregnant woman and her offspring. I. Colonization studies. *Am J Obstet Gynecol* **137:** 34–38.

WHAT IS THE PROBLEM THAT REQUIRES SCREENING?

CONGENITAL CYTOMEGALOVIRUS INFECTION.

What is the incidence/prevalence of the target condition?

Congenital cytomegalovirus (CMV) infection is a global problem. Serologic surveys indicate that the prevalence of maternal CMV infection varies by geographic location and socioeconomic status – from 30% of women in upper socioeconomic groups of highly industrialized countries, to nearly 100% of lower socioeconomic groups of underdeveloped countries (Stagno *et al.*, 1982a). Approximately 40% of reproductive age women from industrialized countries are seronegative. Approximately 1% of these patients develop a primary CMV infection during pregnancy; fetal infection occurs in 20–50% of cases (Stagno *et al.*, 1982a; Dworsky *et al.*, 1983).

Cytomegalovirus may also be transmitted to the fetus by a seropositive woman after reactivation of latent infection. Though maternal antibodies to CMV do not prevent the transplacental passage of CMV, they reduce the frequency of occurrence and ameliorate the severity of disease when it does occur. The vast majority of congenital CMV infections worldwide are likely to be caused by reactivation and not by primary maternal infection (Stagno et al., 1982b).

In many studies, CMV is the most frequent cause of intrauterine infection. This may be in part due to its ease of culture. The incidence of congenital CMV infection based on either virus isolation or the presence of neonatal immunoglobulin M (IgM) has been estimated to be 2–22 per 1000 of liveborn infants (Stagno et al., 1983).

What are the sequelae of the condition which are of interest in clinical medicine?

It appears that only neonates infected during a primary event during pregnancy are symptomatic at birth (Table 2.2). (Fowler et al., 1992a). Neonatal symptoms at birth include hepatosplenomegaly, thrombocytopenia, purpura, jaundice, hemolytic anemia, hepatitis, microcephaly, chorioretinitis, and cerebral calcifications (1–10 per 10 000 births). Symptomatic disease at birth is more common when the infection occurs during the first half of pregnancy (Stagno et al., 1986). The prognosis for children symptomatic at birth is poor. The mortality rate is as high as 20% and 90% of survivors suffer late sequelae such as hearing loss, mental retardation or both (Stagno and Whitley, 1985). Children asymptomatic at birth are also at risk for sequelae, but their rate is lower (10–15%). After a mean follow-up of nearly 5 years of all congenitally infected infants, one or more sequelae are seen in 25% of the primary infection group and 8% of the secondary infection group (Fowler et al., 1992a). In the latter group, sequelae are usually limited to sensorineural hearing loss which develops over several years.

Table 2.2   Public health consequences of primary cytomegalovirus infection.

NUMBER		PROBABILITY[a]	RANGE[b]
100 000	pregnant women	1.00	
40 000	seronegative women	0.40	0.40 – 0.50
400	maternal infection[c]	0.01	
140	vertical transmission	0.35	0.20 – 0.50
14	symptomatic defects at birth mortality (n = 3) late sequelae (n = 10)	0.10 0.20 0.70	
126 32	asymptomatic at birth; sequelae after mean follow-up of 5 years [c,d] (n=32)	0.90 0.25	 0.09 – 0.30

[a] Crude estimates; [b] See text; [c] Fowler et al., 1992b; [d] Logan et al., 1992

THE TEST

What is the purpose of the test?

To identify pregnant women at risk for primary CMV infection. Implicit in screening is the assumption that the prevention of CMV infection is theoretically possible by good hygiene, since there is no effective antenatal treatment.

The nature of the test

Cytomegalovirus-specific IgM and IgG antibodies are tested for by one of several commercially available assays. Specific IgM antibodies are found in 80% of women with primary CMV infection (Stagno *et al.*, 1985). Those IgM antibodies detected by enzyme-linked immunosorbent assay (ELISA) typically persist for 4 months but may last as long as 7 months. A frequent cause of clinical confusion, CMV-specific IgM antibodies reappear in about 20% of women with a CMV reactivation. Primary infection can be diagnosed with certainty only if either there is a documented seroconversion during pregnancy, or if the IgG is negative and IgM positive when first tested with a subsequent seroconversion in IgG. As a result, a screening program for CMV will require retesting seronegative women (about 40%) later in pregnancy to search for seroconversion.

Implications of testing

WHAT DOES AN ABNORMAL TEST RESULT MEAN?

Women with a primary CMV infection during pregnancy can be offered antenatal diagnosis for the identification of congenitally infected fetuses. Though Donner *et al.* (1993) found that the overall sensitivity for the antenatal detection of a fetal CMV was 81%, they did not routinely culture amniotic fluid which appears to be the most sensitive method. There is only one reported false negative for fetal CMV infection using culture. Though it is likely that the antenatal diagnosis of fetal CMV can be made with high sensitivity and specificity, no test can discriminate – when the ultrasound examination is normal – between the majority of fetuses who will develop normally and the 10% of fetuses who suffer severe sequelae. Furthermore, there is no effective therapy currently available either to protect fetuses exposed to CMV or to treat infected fetuses, as there is for toxoplasmosis. While some practitioners routinely offer pregnancy termination to women with primary CMV infection in the first 20 weeks of pregnancy, the rationale is weak since only 1 in 20 fetuses will develop sequelae. Termination of a wanted pregnancy prior to 20 weeks' gestation should be considered only when antenatal investigation confirms fetal infection (Donner *et al.*, 1993). Counseling the patient with an infected fetus remains problematic in the face of a normal ultrasound scan since most infected fetuses have no sequelae. Postnatally, the diagnosis is confirmed with a culture of the newborn's urine.

WHAT DOES A NORMAL TEST RESULT MEAN?

Seronegative women have not had CMV infection. One aim of screening would be to prevent CMV infection in susceptible pregnant women since it is clearly established that the infection is transmitted through contamination of oropharyngeal or genital secretions. Seronegative women are encouraged to wash their hands thoroughly after contact with either the saliva or urine of young children and other possibly contaminated body fluids. However, there are no studies indicating that such practices reduce the rate of the CMV seroconversion during pregnancy.

What is the cost of testing?

The cost-efficacy of CMV screening has not been examined using any strategy. However, a rough estimate can be made. The typical cost of CMV serology using an ELISA in the USA is US $50–70 for either IgG or IgM. If we assume a patient cost of $120 to measure both IgG and IgM and 40% of the women are seronegative, the cost to screen 100 000 women is $168 million (US, 1995). Based on epidemiologic studies, we would expect there to be 300 infected newborns if 1% of seronegative women contract CMV and 30% of their children are infected. Assuming 100% sensitivity and specificity, the cost of screening all women at their first visit and repeat screening of seronegatives between 16–20 weeks per infected neonate, exclusive of any extra antenatal evaluation, would be $560 000.

CONCLUSIONS AND RECOMMENDATIONS

Although congenital CMV is an important health problem, there are too many unsolved problems before mass screening of pregnant women can be recommended. Indeed, detection of primary infection is difficult and creates needless anxiety in many women who have experienced a reactivation. Counseling the women with either seroconversion or reactivation but a normal ultrasound examination cannot be based on fact. There are no effective therapeutic interventions after a primary CMV infection has been identified. Though recommendations to abstain from close intimate contact with her partner or children may not be acceptable, women at high occupational risk may benefit by paying closer attention to hygiene. The effectiveness of hygienic measures to prevent CMV infection during pregnancy in seronegative women is as yet unproven. Fetal infection can be accurately detected, but in most cases there will be no sequelae from the infection.

If CMV screening during pregnancy is performed, the caregiver will be frequently faced with the evaluation of women with CMV-specific IgM antibodies. Since it is often difficult to distinguish between primary CMV infection and reactivation, screening will probably result in overutilization of both noninvasive and invasive procedures. It can be expected that such a screening program will also lead to abortions of wanted pregnancies, based more on the anxiety of the parents than on the likely sequelae of the fetal infection.

Since there are methodologic problems with the screening tests, there are no sound trials of therapy (for either infected fetuses or uninfected women), and no evidence that the screen negative women will comply with advice that will reduce the chance of their infection, routine screening for CMV during pregnancy is not recommended.

SUMMARY

1 WHAT IS THE PROBLEM THAT REQUIRES SCREENING?

CONGENITAL CYTOMEGALOVIRUS INFECTION.

a What is the incidence/prevalence of the target condition?

The incidence is 2–22 per 1000 deliveries. Maternal seropositivity varies by location and socioeconomic status: approximately 40% of reproductive age women from industrialized countries are seronegative. About 1% of these develop a primary infection during pregnancy causing fetal infection in about 20–50% of cases.

b What are the sequelae of the condition which are of interest in clinical medicine?

Most congenitally infected infants are asymptomatic at birth; 10% experience severe sequelae including thrombocytopenia, hemolytic anemia, hepatitis, microcephaly, and chorioretinitis. Late sequelae such as hearing loss, mental retardation, or both occur in 90% of these survivors. The majority of asymptomatic children remain normal, but 10 to 15% will develop sequelae over several years.

2 THE TESTS

a What is the purpose of the test?

To identify women at risk for primary CMV infection.

b The nature of the test

The measurement of maternal CMV-specific IgG and IgM antibodies.

c Implications of testing

1 What does an abnormal test result mean?

Women with a primary CMV infection during pregnancy can be offered antenatal diagnosis. Amniotic fluid culture appears to be highly sensitive and specific. Much more difficult is the counseling of patients as to the prognosis.

2 What does a normal test result mean?

Women without CMV antibodies have not been previously infected and are thus at risk for a primary episode during pregnancy. These women are encouraged to practice oral-digital hygiene since CMV is transmitted through contamination of oropharyngeal or genital secretions. However, there are no studies indicating such practices reduce the CMV seroconversion rate.

d What is the cost of testing?

Not previously examined. A rough estimate assuming 100% sensitivity and specificity is in excess of US $500 000 per infected newborn.

3 CONCLUSIONS AND RECOMMENDATIONS

Although congenital CMV infection is an important health problem, there are too many unsolved problems to recommend mass screening of pregnant women.

REFERENCES

Donner C, Liesnard C, Content J et al. (1993) Prenatal diagnosis of 52 pregnancies at risk for congenital cytomegalovirus infection. *Obstet Gynecol* **82:** 481–486.

Dworsky ME, Welch K, Cassady G & Stagno S (1983) Occupational risk for primary cytomegalovirus infection among pediatric health care workers. *N Engl J Med* **309:** 950–952.

Fowler KB, Stagno S, Pass RF, Britt WJ, Boll WJ & Alford CA (1992b) The outcome of congenital cytomegalovirus infection in relation to maternal mortality. *N Engl J Med* **326:** 663–667.

Logan S, Tookey P & Ades T (1992) Congenital cytomegalovirus infection and maternal antibody status (letter). *N Engl J Med* **327:** 466.

Stagno S & Whitley RJ (1985) Herpes virus infections of pregnancy. Part I: Cytomegalovirus and Epstein-Barr virus infections. *N Engl J Med* **313:** 1270–1274.

Stagno S, Pass RF, Dworsky ME, Alford CA (1982a) Maternal cytomegalovirus infection and perinatal transmission. *Clin Obstet Gynecol* **25:** 563–576.

Stagno S, Pass RF, Dworsky ME, et al. (1982b) Congenital cytomegalovirus infection. The relative importance of primary and recurrent maternal infection. *N Engl J Med* **306:** 945–949.

Stagno S, Pass RF, Dworsky ME & Alford CA (1983) Congenital and perinatal cytomegalovirus infections. Semin Perinatal **7:** 31–42.

Stagno S, Tinker MK, Ebrod C, et al. (1985) Immunoglobulin M antibodies detected by enzyme-linked immunosorbent assay and radioimmunoassay in the diagnosis of cytomegalovirus infections in pregnant women and newborn infants. *J Clin Microbiol* **21:** 930–935.

Stagno S, Pass RF, Cloud G, et al. (1986) Primary cytomegalovirus infection in pregnancy. Incidence, transmission to the fetus and clinical outcome. *JAMA* **256:** 1904–1908.

WHAT IS THE PROBLEM THAT REQUIRES SCREENING?

CONGENITAL RUBELLA SYNDROME (CRS).

Rubella poses a serious threat to the fetus, and vaccination programs are used to reduce the incidence of CRS.

What is the incidence/prevalence of the target condition?

The incidence of CRS has declined in Western countries since the introduction in 1969 of large-scale rubella vaccination programs. Several approaches to vaccination have been taken. The first is to vaccinate only the population at risk, i.e. teenage girls. This approach reduces the incidence of nonimmune pregnant women from 20% to 5% and decreases the likelihood of a large epidemic (Noah and Fowle, 1988). However, smaller outbreaks still occur because a significant percentage of male children remain susceptible to the rubella virus and provide a reservoir for the wild virus. During these outbreaks, nonimmunized pregnant women (who have either not had the disease or escaped vaccination) are at risk of becoming infected with the virus. This is probably the reason why the UK, where such a vaccination strategy was used, still had 100 cases per year (1 per 6000 live births) recorded in the late 1970s and the early 1980s (Public Health Laboratory Service Communicable Disease Surveillance Centre, 1983).

A second strategy, used in the USA, is to vaccinate all children in an attempt to reduce the circulation of wild rubella virus among the total population. This policy also decreases the likelihood of a rubella epidemic and the incidence of CRS. Data obtained through voluntary notification indicate that 550 children (1 per 5500 live births) were born in the USA with CRS during 1979 (CDC, 1983). Since then, the effort to vaccinate prepubertal children has been intensified and rubella is now incorporated into the childhood vaccination schedule. As a result, the incidence of CRS in the USA has decreased dramatically to an average of 20 cases per year since 1986 (1 per 300 000 live births). Most western European countries and more recently the UK have adopted the American policy of routine immunization of all children at 15 months of age. As a result, the incidence of CRS has dropped to a similar low level.

Nevertheless, CRS remains a problem in developed countries because of either failure to immunize some children or a vaccination failure. In the USA, approximately 10% of reproductive age women are still seronegative, usually because they were not vaccinated as children. Another explanation for the persistence of susceptible pregnant women is that a small proportion of vaccinated women have lost their protective antibody level by the time they become pregnant. Longterm protection (about 15 years) from vaccination is about 98–99% (Chu *et al.*, 1988); thus, about 2% of vaccinees will be negative for rubella antibodies when tested during pregnancy (Forsgren, 1985). Ideally, all vaccinated women would have their serological status determined before becoming pregnant.

What are the sequelae of the condition which are of interest in clinical medicine?

The fetus is infected during the maternal viremia (Table 2.3). Fetal infection is systemic. There is a strong correlation between the timing of the maternal viremia and the likelihood and severity of CRS (Miller *et al.*, 1982). Eighty per cent of fetuses will be infected when the maternal infection occurs in the first trimester, 54% between 13 and 16 weeks, and 40% thereafter. Severe sequelae such as cataracts, deafness, cardiac abnormalities, and neurologic damage are almost universal in fetuses infected prior to 12 weeks' gestation. Between 13 and 16 weeks' gestation, the risk of CRS declines to about 35% and the sequelae are mostly deafness and to a small extent mild neurologic abnormalities

Table 2.3   Public health consequences of maternal rubella infection.

NUMBER		PROBABILITY[a]	RANGE[b]
300 000	pregnant women	1.00	
30 000	seronegative women	0.10	0.02 – 0.12
17	maternal infection[c]	0.0006	?
10	vertical transmission[d]	0.60	0.40 – 0.80
1	congenital rubella syndrome at birth	0.10	0.00 – 0.10

[a] *Crude estimates;* [b] *See text;* [c] *Maternal infection in ongoing pregnancy (no figures are currently available on the number of pregnancy terminations for maternal rubella infection);* [d] *Dependent on the stage of pregnancy at which infection occurs*

(Miller *et al.*, 1982). Though fetal infection occurs after 16–18 weeks' gestation, it does not usually result in either detectable neonatal disease or longterm defects.

THE TESTS

What is the purpose of the tests?

To detect pregnant women who are serologically negative for rubella and thus at risk for infection during pregnancy. All pregnant women should be tested at the time of the first prenatal visit. Susceptible women should be retested between 16 and 20 weeks' gestation to exclude occult infection during the period when CRS could result. Seronegative women should be vaccinated after delivery to protect subsequent pregnancies and to reduce the subject pool available for wild virus.

The nature of the tests

Several types of tests for either the diagnosis or the detection of immunity to rubella are available. The first is the hemagglutination-inhibition (HAI) test. A titer equal to or greater than 1/8 signifies the presence of protective antibodies. The HAI test response to wild virus is longlasting. Other reliable tests for detecting immunity include the IgG-ELISA test, the latex agglutination test and the radial immune hemolysis test. The complement fixation test is not suitable for detecting immunity. Owing to their high sensitivity and specificity and the possibility of automation, the ELISA tests are most often used in clinical practice.

The clinical diagnosis of rubella is based on the appearance of a maculopapular rash over a 3-day period. It is often difficult to be certain of the diagnosis because rubella resembles many other viral exanthemas. Moreover, the clinical signs may be so mild that they go undetected by the patient and physician. Therefore, the diagnosis of a rubella infection should never be based on clinical grounds only. Serologic confirmation is mandatory. Recent rubella infection is diagnosed by the finding of rubella-specific IgM antibodies or by the detection of an IgG seroconversion. Rubella-specific IgM antibodies appear early after the onset of clinical disease, peak at 10 days and remain positive for 4–8 weeks. Rubella-specific IgM antibodies can persist for up to 6 months after a primary infection. Recent rubella infection can also be diagnosed by testing serial samples. The appearance of rubella-specific IgG antibodies in a patient showing no antibodies in the previous serum sample (seroconversion) confirms a recent rubella infection. Seroconversion is detectable by HAI within 10 days of the appearance of a rash.

Implications of testing

WHAT DOES AN ABNORMAL TEST RESULT MEAN?

The presence of rubella-specific IgM indicates a recent infection. If infection occurs during the first 16 weeks of pregnancy, the woman is at risk of delivering a child with CRS and should be offered either antenatal diagnosis or a termination of pregnancy.

Antenatal diagnosis is based on the detection of fetal IgM antibodies after 20 weeks' gestation. Amniotic fluid cultures for rubella are difficult, and the polymerase chain reaction (PCR) for rubella in either amniotic fluid or fetal blood has not yet been tested in clinical settings. Daffos *et al.* (1984) correctly identified 12 of 13 infected fetuses by performing a cordocentesis between 20 weeks and 26 weeks of gestation. However, the experience with the antenatal detection of congenital rubella is limited and false negative diagnosis may occur. Therefore, it remains acceptable in view of the severity of CRS to offer pregnancy termination without antenatal diagnosis after a proven maternal infection during the first 16 weeks of pregnancy.

The pregnant woman without clinical signs who is seropositive for both rubella-specific IgM and IgG antibodies when first tested poses a challenging problem. These patients should be tested with a second and even a third serum sample to evaluate the possibilities for recent rubella infection. The use of a panel of different tests on paired sera will, in most cases, give a definite answer as to whether the infection is recent or not. Women with unclear rubella serology are candidates for a antenatal diagnosis.

WHAT DOES A NORMAL TEST RESULT MEAN?

The presence of rubella-specific IgG without IgM indicates immunity. No further analyses are required.

What is the cost of testing?

The 1994 cost for a single test for both IgM and IgG antibodies in Belgium is estimated at US $7. More relevant is the patient cost, rather than the cost of the test itself. The 1994 patient cost in a large medical center in the USA for rubella-specific IgG is US $32.50. If we assume all women register for care by 10 weeks' gestation (an unlikely event in many geographic areas), 90% of patients are immune, and seronegative patients are rescreened at 16–18 weeks' gestation, the cost per case of CRS identified is approximately $154 000 if the incidence is 1 per 4300 pregnancies, or $10 725 000 if the incidence is 1 per 300 000. This excludes the cost of additional antenatal testing.

Most children with CRS require round-the-clock supervision and help for the rest of their lives. The annual cost per individual was estimated in 1985 to be at least US $31 000 (Appel, 1985). This amount is probably double in 1995 adjusting for inflation. Further, it does not include societal costs such as the loss of income and patient suffering. If we assume an average 50-year lifespan, CRS would add a minimum of US $3 100 000 in excess medical costs.

CONCLUSIONS AND RECOMMENDATIONS

Rubella is a mild disease with potentially devastating consequences for the offspring when infection occurs during the first and early second trimesters. The horizontal transmission rate in the first trimester approximates 80%. Congenital rubella is a totally preventable disease. Vaccination is effective, safe and inexpensive. The global effect of mass vaccination in Western countries is that rubella infections in pregnancy are becoming a rare event, which increases the cost per case identified. While congenital rubella is no longer considered a problem of high priority in developed countries, it is a major problem in less developed countries where vaccination programs are insufficient or nonexistent (Schatzmayer, 1985).

In many Western countries, maternal screening is probably no more longer cost-effective. However, CRS is a very severe and detectable disease and school immunization programs do not ensure all women of childbearing age are immune. Although great progress has been made in the control of congenital rubella, it would be inappropriate to stop pregnancy screening as long as a substantial proportion of women are seronegative, despite the diminution of its cost-efficacy.

Rubella-specific IgG and IgM antibodies should be tested for during the first prenatal visit. Women who are immune can be reassured since there is no documented evidence of reinfection. The addition of IgM antibodies to the screen during the first prenatal visit will detect a small number of women who have rubella in early pregnancy. Screening with only the HAI test or with IgG antibodies only will not detect these recent infections. It seems prudent to screen with the most sensitive and reliable method available – the ELISA. A second sample should be tested in seronegative patients between 16 and 18 weeks of gestation. After this period, repeat testing is unnecessary since the risk to the fetus for CRS is essentially nil. Vaccination should be performed during the postpartum period in all seronegative women.

SUMMARY

1 WHAT IS THE PROBLEM THAT REQUIRES SCREENING?

CONGENITAL RUBELLA SYNDROME (CRS).

a What is the incidence/prevalence of the target condition?
It is 1 per 5500 to 1 per 300 000 depending on the country's vaccination policy.

b What are the sequelae of the condition which are of interest in clinical medicine?
Congenital rubella syndrome includes cataracts, deafness, cardiac abnormalities, and neurologic damage and occurs in about 80% of infected fetuses.

2 THE TESTS

a What is the purpose of the test?
To detect women at risk for rubella during pregnancy.

b The nature of the tests
Measurement of rubella-specific IgG and IgM.

c Implications of testing

1 What does an abnormal test result mean?

Rubella-specific IgM indicates a recent infection. If infection occurs during the first 16 weeks of gestation, the woman is at risk of delivering a child with CRS and should be offered either antenatal diagnosis or a termination of pregnancy.

2 What does a normal test result mean?

The presence of rubella-specific IgG without IgM indicates an infection of at least 1 month earlier.

d What is the cost of testing?

Assuming all women register for care by 10 weeks of gestation, 90% are immune, and seronegative women are rescreened between 16–18 weeks' gestation, the cost per case of CRS identified ranges with the incidence from US $154 000 (1 per 4300 pregnancies) to US $10 million (1 per 300 000 pregnancies) excluding the cost of antenatal testing.

3 ## CONCLUSIONS AND RECOMMENDATIONS

Congenital rubella is a preventable disease. Vaccination is effective, safe and inexpensive. While congenital rubella is no longer considered a problem of high priority in developed countries, it is a major problem in the third world where vaccination programs are insufficient or non-existent. Maternal rubella-specific IgG and IgM antibodies should be screened for during the first prenatal visit.

REFERENCES

Appel MW (1985) The multihandicapped child with congenital rubella: impact on family and community. *Rev Infect Dis* **7**: 17–21.
CDC (1983) Rubella and congenital rubella – United States, 1980–1983. *MMWR* **32**: 505–509.
Chu SY, Bernier RH, Stewart JA *et al.* (1988) Rubella antibody persistence after immunization. *JAMA* **259**: 3133–3136.
Daffos F, Forestier F, Grangeot-Kevos L *et al.* (1984) Prenatal diagnosis of congenital rubella. *Lancet* ii: 1–3.
Forsgren M (1985) Standardization of techniques and reagents. Proceedings of the International Symposium on the Prevention of Congenital Rubella Infection. *Rev Infect Dis* **7**: 129–132.
Miller E, Cradock-Watsen JE & Pollock TM (1982) Consequences of confirmed maternal rubella at successive stages of pregnancy. *Lancet* ii: 781–784.
Noah WD & Fowle SE (1988) Immunity to rubella in women of child-bearing age in the United Kingdom. *Br Med J* **297**: 1301–1304.
Public Health Laboratory Service Communicable Disease Surveillance Centre (1983) Rubella Surveillance. *Br Med J* **287**: 752.
Schatzmayer HG (1985) Aspects of rubella infection in Brazil. *Rev Infect Dis* **7**: 53–55.

WHAT IS THE PROBLEM THAT REQUIRES SCREENING?

MATERNAL-FETAL TRANSMISSION OF HEPATITIS B VIRUS.

What is the incidence/prevalence of the target condition?

Hepatitis B virus (HBV) infection occurs worldwide. Spread usually results from contact with infected body fluids such as blood, semen, vaginal secretions, and saliva. Most people mount an effective immune response and clear the virus after the acute episode. However, a small percentage of infected people become chronic carriers of the virus, as indicated by a positive test for HB surface antigen (HBsAg) and remain infectious. Epidemiological studies reveal wide variation by geographic location in the prevalence

Table 2.4   Public health consequences of hepatitis B chronic carriage during pregnancy.

NUMBER		PROBABILITY[a]	RANGE[b]
100 000	pregnant women		
2 000	HBsAg positive women	0.02	0.02 – 0.15
300	vertical transmission[c]	0.15	0.10 – 0.20
8	acute neonatal hepatitis	0.025	0.02 – 0.03
120	chronic hepatitis	0.40	
75	death due to chronic liver disease	0.25	0.10 – 0.40

[a] Crude estimates; [b] See text; [c] Excluding women positive for HBeAg

of the carrier state. In the USA 0.5–1% of the total population are chronic carriers of HBV. In Australia, the carrier rate is 2–3% (Gilbert, 1984); it rises to 15% in Southeast Asia and the Pacific Islands (Beasley et al., 1981a).

What are the sequelae of the condition which are of interest in clinical medicine?

Neonates are typically infected by their mother – either because the mother experienced an acute HBV infection during the last 3 months of pregnancy, or because she is a chronic carrier who infects the fetus as it swallows infected body fluids during delivery (Table 2.4). Women who have acute hepatitis B in the first or second trimesters rarely transmit the virus to their babies. Transplacental infection accounts for the minority of cases (Wong et al., 1980).

Transmission depends largely on the antigen status of the mother: in HBsAg positive mothers, neonatal infection occurs in 10–20% of the cases. When the mother is also positive for the HB early antigen (HBeAg), transmission is as high as 90% (Okada et al., 1976; Beasley et al., 1977, 1981b).

Neonatal hepatitis often has a mild, even asymptomatic course. Only rarely does it result in fulminant hepatitis with hepatic failure, encephalopathy and death after a few days. The critical public health issue is that nearly 85% of newborns with neonatal HBV become chronic carriers, with serious longterm sequelae. Chronic hepatitis develops in 40%. The children may have mild hepatomegaly, intermittent elevations of liver enzymes and spider angiomas. They are at risk for developing either cirrhosis or hepatocellular carcinoma. As many as 25% of chronic carriers of HBV die from one of these complications. (Beasley et al., 1983).

THE TEST

What is the purpose of the test?

To identify women who are chronic carriers.
The identification of newborns at risk for neonatal HBV relies on the detection of those

pregnant women who are chronic carriers. The best virological marker for infectivity for HBV is the HBs antigen. This test is positive in all acute HBV infections and remains positive in chronic carriers.

Two approaches to screening have been suggested. Screening only those pregnant women with specific risk factors for being a HB carrier (such as women from Southeast Asia, a history of multiple sexual transmitted diseases or injecting drug abuse) will result in 47–67% of the HBsAg positive women being missed (Cruz et al., 1987; Kumar et al., 1987). Universal screening for HBsAg is the best way to control vertical transmission of HBV infection. It is generally recommended that all pregnant women be screened for HBsAg at their first antenatal visit. Retesting late in pregnancy is not necessary except in cases where acute hepatitis during pregnancy occurs or is suspected.

Some institutions still screen for HBsAg in the third trimester. This has the advantage of detecting any asymptomatic HBV during pregnancy. However, this is rare in countries with a rather low incidence of HBV infections like most Western countries. Third-trimester screening has the disadvantage that in cases of preterm delivery, the HBV serology of the mothers will be unknown at the delivery, rendering the prevention of maternal-fetal transmission less effective.

The nature of the test

The detection of the HBs antigen is the cornerstone in the prevention of HBV maternal-fetal transmission.

Implications of testing

WHAT DOES AN ABNORMAL TEST RESULT MEAN?

Should the test be positive for HBs antigen, the subject either has acute hepatitis or is a chronic carrier. Additional testing is warranted to differentiate between acute or chronic HBV infections. These supplementary markers include: the HBe antigen, the HB core antibody (anti-HBc), the anti-HBe and the anti-HBs antibodies.

The HBs antigen is the first serological marker of HB to appear – 10–30 days before clinical symptoms. The HBeAg typically appears shortly thereafter; it indicates a high degree of infectivity. The persistence of HBeAg beyond 10 weeks predicts progression to a chronic carrier state and to probable chronic liver disease. If the HBsAg persists for more than 6 months, the patient is considered to be a chronic carrier. Anti-HBe antibodies are consistent with disease resolution and usually appear 6–8 weeks after the acute HB infection. Patients who clear the virus also develop anti-HBs antibodies. The presence of anti-HBs antibodies is an indicator of clinical recovery and subsequent immunity to HBV infection. They generally appear 1–4 months after the onset of symptoms. The antibody to the HBcAg rises before the appearance of HBs antibody and remains lifelong after a natural HBV infection. In the absence of HBsAg and anti-HBs, its presence indicates a relative recent infection with disappearance of the antigen. Antibody to HBc antigen does not always develop in vaccine-induced immunity.

Infants whose mothers are chronic carriers of HBsAg are exposed to infected maternal reproductive tract secretions during the delivery. Those infants whose mothers carry HBeAg are at high risk of becoming chronic carriers. Neonatal infection can be prevented in 90% of cases (Beasley *et al.*, 1983; Lo *et al.*, 1985; Cruz *et al.*, 1987; Kumar *et al.*, 1987) by a combination of both passive and active immunization immediately after birth. Hepatitis B immunoglobulin (HBIG, 0.5 ml i.m.) should be given within 12 hours after birth. The efficacy of the treatment decreases if delayed longer. The HB vaccine is given in three doses: the first dose must be administered within the first week of life, the second dose after 1 month, and the third after 6 months. It is important to test the child after 1 year since 10% of infants born to seropositive mothers become chronic HBV carriers despite active and passive vaccination.

WHAT DOES A NORMAL TEST RESULT MEAN?

The mother has not been previously exposed to HBV and the newborn is not at risk for congenital HBV.

What is the cost of testing?

The cost-efficacy of HBV screening has been intensively studied. Screening all pregnant women for HBsAg and immunization of the neonates at risk is cost-effective when the prevalence for HBsAg is at least 0.06% (Arevalo and Washington, 1988). Universal screening could save more than US $105 million annually in the USA where the carrier rate of pregnant women is about 1%. Besides the savings, neonatal vaccination will decrease the number of HB carriers, reducing the transmission rate of the virus in the global population.

New prevention strategies are under evaluation to reduce further the transmission of HBV. These include the selective vaccination of at-risk adolescents and adults, and ultimately universal vaccination of older children (age 6 months to 11 years) (Immunization Practices Advisory Committee, 1991; Kraus *et al.*, 1994). Immunization programs to assure that all women of childbearing age are immune to HBV infection are cost-effective (Bloom *et al.*, 1993).

CONCLUSIONS AND RECOMMENDATIONS

Acute maternal hepatitis B virus infection is a rare disease with potentially severe consequences for the neonate when infection occurs in the third trimester. Women who are chronic carriers may infect their child during birth. Combined passive and active immunization of the neonate beginning within 12 hours of birth reduces the risk of neonatal infection by 90%. Thus, all pregnant women should be screened for HBsAg at their first antenatal visit. All infants born to HBsAg positive mothers should receive a 0.5 ml dose of HBIG within 12 hours of birth, followed by the first dose of the three-dose HB vaccine in a separate site. Vaccinated infants should be retested at 1 year to determine the carrier status of the child.

SUMMARY

1

WHAT IS THE PROBLEM THAT REQUIRES SCREENING?

MATERNAL-FETAL TRANSMISSION OF HEPATITIS B VIRUS
INFECTION.

a What is the incidence/prevalence of the target condition?

There is wide variation in the prevalence of the maternal carrier state by geographic location ranging from 0.5% to 15%. Transmission depends on the antigen status of the mother: in HBsAg positive mothers, neonatal infection occurs in 10–20% of the cases.

b What are the sequelae of the condition which are of interest in clinical medicine?

Neonatal hepatitis is usually mild but can cause fulminant hepatitis with hepatic failure and death within a few days. The real health impact of hepatitis B is that nearly 85% of newborns infected with HBV will become chronic carriers, placing them at risk for serious longterm sequelae. Chronic active hepatitis develops in 40%. These individuals are at risk for either cirrhosis or hepatocellular carcinoma. As many as 25% of chronic carriers of HBV will die of complications.

2

THE TEST

a What is the purpose of the test?

The detection of pregnant women who are chronic carriers for hepatitis B virus.

b The nature of the test

The detection of the HBs antigen is the cornerstone in the prevention of HBV maternal-fetal transmission.

c Implications of testing

1 What does an abnormal test result mean?

Infants whose mothers are chronic carriers of hepatitis B virus are exposed to infected secretions at the delivery. Hepatitis B immunoglobulin (0.5 ml i.m.) should be given within 12 hours of birth. The efficacy of the treatment decreases with a longer time interval. B vaccine is administered within the first week of life, then at 1 month and 6 months of age. The immunized infant should be tested after 1 year since 10% become chronic HBV carriers despite treatment.

2 What does a normal test result mean?

The mother has not been previously exposed to HBV and the newborn is not at risk for congenital HBV.

d **What is the cost of testing?**

Universal screening for maternal HBsAg and immunization of the neonates at risk is cost-effective if the prevalence rate for HBsAg is at least 0.06%.

3 CONCLUSIONS AND RECOMMENDATIONS

All pregnant women should be screened for HBsAg at their first antenatal visit. All infants born to HBsAg positive mothers should receive a 0.5 ml dose of HBIG within 12 hours of birth, followed by the first dose of the three-dose HB vaccine in a separate site.

REFERENCES

Arevalo JA & Washington AE (1988) Cost-effectiveness of prenatal screening and immunization for hepatitis B virus. *JAMA* **259**: 365–369.

Beasley RP, Trepo C, Stevens CE & Szmuness W (1977) The e antigen and vertical transmission of hepatitis B surface antigen. *Am J Epidemiol* **105**: 94–98.

Beasley RP, Hwang LY, Lin CC & Chiw CS (1981a) Hepatocellular carcinoma and hepatitis B virus: a prospective study of 22707 men in Taiwan. *Lancet* **ii**: 1129–1133.

Beasley RP, Hwang LJ, Lin CC et al. (1981b) Hepatitis B immune globulin (HBIG) efficacy in the interruption of perinatal transmission of hepatitis B virus carrier state. Initial report of a randomised double-blind placebo-controlled trial. *Lancet* **ii**: 388–393.

Beasley RP, Hwang LY, Lee GC et al. (1983) Prevention of perinatally transmitted hepatitis B virus infections with hepatitis B immunoglobulin and hepatitis B vaccine. *Lancet* **ii**: 1099–1102.

Bloom BS, Hillman AL, Fendrick AM, Schwartz JS. A reappraisal of hepatitis B virus vaccination strategies using cost-effectiveness analysis. *Ann Int Med* 1993; **118**: 298–306.

Cruz AC, Frentzen BH, Beliuke M (1987) Hepatitis B: a case for prenatal screening of all patients. *Am J Obstet Gynecol* **156**: 1180–1183.

Gilbert GL (1984) Prevention of vertical transmission of hepatitis B. The place of routine screening in antenatal care and the case for immunization of infants at risk. *Med J Austr* **141**: 213–216.

Immunization Practices Advisory Committee (1991) Hepatitis B virus: a comprehensive strategy for eliminating transmission in the United States through universal childhood vaccination. Recommendations of the Immunization Practices Advisory Committee. *MMWR*; **40**: 1–25.

Kraus DM, Campbell MM & Marcinak JF (1994) Evaluation of universal hepatitis B immunization practices of Illinois pediatricians. *Arch Ped Adolesc Med* **148**: 936–942.

Kumar ML, Dawson NV, Mc Cullough AJ et al. (1987) Should all pregnant women be screened for hepatitis? *Ann Intern Med* **107**: 273–277.

Lo KJ, Tsai YT, Lee SD et al. (1985) Immunoprophylaxis of infection with hepatitis B virus in infants born to hepatitis B surface antigen positive carrier mothers. *J Infect Dis* **152**: 817–822.

Okada K, Kamiyama I, Inomata M, et al. (1976) e Antigen and anti-e in the serum of asymptomatic carrier mothers as indicators if positive and negative transmission of hepatitis B virus to their infants. *N Engl J Med* **294**: 746–749.

Wong VC, Lee AK & Ip HM (1980) Transmission of hepatitis B antigens from symptom free carrier mothers to the fetus and the infant. *Br J Obstet Gynaecol* **87**: 958–965.

WHAT IS THE PROBLEM THAT REQUIRES SCREENING?

CONGENITAL *TOXOPLASMA* INFECTION.

What is the incidence/prevalence of the target condition?

The incidence of *Toxoplasma* infection during pregnancy ranges widely according to geographic location. The estimated incidence in France is 2–3 per 1000, in Brussels 8 per 1000, in Scotland 2–3 per 1000, and 2 per 1000 in Norway (Stray-Pedersen, 1993). These estimates are based on the average increase in the prevalence of seropositivity in the population per 9 months during childbearing years, or on serological prospective follow-up of gravidas throughout pregnancy to determine the number who become infected (Stray-Pedersen, 1993). Maternal infection occurs only in seronegative women. The frequency of seronegativity ranges from 30% in France, 43% in Belgium, 87% in Norway, to between 70% and 97% in the USA. Fetal infection results from passage of the parasite across the placenta during the parasitemia. After an undefined lag period, transmission to the fetus may occur. Recent data from serological studies indicate that the congenital infection rate varies from 0.2 per 1000 births as observed in Alabama (USA) (Hunter *et al.*, 1983) and Perth (Australia) to 2 per 1000 births as observed in Melbourne (Australia) (Sfameni *et al.*, 1986), and Belgium (Foulon *et al.*, 1984).

What are the sequelae of the condition which are of interest in clinical medicine?

The clinical manifestations of congenital toxoplasmosis vary greatly. Early maternal infection can cause spontaneous abortion or severe sequelae such as hydrocephalus, chorioretinitis, and mental retardation. Other clinical manifestations include intracranial calcifications, icterus, hepatosplenomegaly, and thrombocytopenia. Congenital infections occurring after the 24th week of pregnancy are nearly always subclinical. Nearly all symptomatic newborns have longterm neurologic and/or ophthalmologic sequelae. The problem of subclinical congenital toxoplasmosis should not be underestimated. A significant number of infants who are congenitally infected but asymptomatic at birth suffer delayed complications years later. Based on longterm follow-up studies, it appears that 50% of these infants, if untreated, develop chorioretinitis during adolescence, leading to severe impairment of vision. Moreover, mental subnormality has been recorded in 20% of this group of patients (Stray-Pedersen & Jenum, 1992; Table 2.5).

The time of pregnancy when maternal infection is acquired affects the frequency of transmission and the pattern of congenital infection (Desmonts and Couvreur, 1974).

Table 2.5   Public health consequences of *Toxoplasma gondii* infection.

NUMBER		PROBABILITY[a]	RANGE[b]
10 000	pregnant women	1.00	
5 000	seronegative women	0.50	0.30–0.97
200	maternal infection	0.04	0.02–0.16
100	vertical transmission[c,d]	0.50	0.15–0.80
10	neonatal symptoms at birth	0.10	0.00–0.10
	longterm sequelae in asymptomatic children:		
45	chorioretinitis	0.50	?
18	mental subnormality	0.20	?

[a] Crude estimates; [b] See text; [c] Dependent on the stage of pregnancy at which infection occurs; [d] From: Klapper and Morris (1990)

When infection occurs in the first trimester, the fetus is infected in about 15% of cases. Fetal infection results in 25% of cases when the gravida becomes infected in the second trimester, and in 50% of cases when maternal infection occurs in the third trimester. Though the risk of fetal infection increases with gestational age, the risk of delivering a severely diseased child decreases. As a result of this transmission pattern, congenital toxoplasmosis is subclinical in most cases; only about 10% will have clinical symptoms at birth. Various clinical studies have shown that when the mother is treated during pregnancy, the transmission frequency is lower. Moreover, the administration of pyrimethamine and sulfonamide appear to reduce the severity of the sequelae.

THE TESTS

What is the purpose of the tests?

To identify women who have not in the past had a *Toxoplasma* infection and who are thus at risk of primary *Toxoplasma* infection.

The nature of the tests

Serologic testing for *Toxoplasma* antibodies is the primary method of diagnosis. The methods include the Sabin–Feldman dye test (SF), the immunofluorescent antibody test (IFA), the enzyme immunoassay (EIA), the complement fixation test (CF), and the indirect hemagglutination test. Testing for seroconversion requires repeated sampling of seronegative women.

During acute infection, IgM antibodies first appear in the patient's serum as soon as 5 days after infection. The titers rise to a maximum level and then decrease until the antibodies disappear from the patient's serum. Depending on the serologic test used, IgM levels may be detected for up to several years in some patients. In most instances where the IgM antibodies persist, the levels are low; however, in some patients they may remain high. Immunoglobulin G antibodies appear a few weeks after an acute *Toxoplasma* infection, and, depending on the serological test used, may take 2–6 months to peak. The IgG levels in chronic infection are normally low and remain stable; however, it is not uncommon to find high IgG antibodies in some of these cases (Feldman and Miller, 1956).

Levels of IgG as well as IgM antibodies should be determined for the proper diagnosis of *Toxoplasma* infection by serological techniques. In acute infection, two serum samples obtained 3 or more weeks apart will reveal either a seroconversion in IgM and IgG antibodies (from negative to positive), or high IgM antibody titers with rising IgG antibodies (Remington and Gentry, 1970). In a chronic or latent infection, only a low level of IgG is found.

Good serologic screening for *Toxoplasma* antibodies during pregnancy depends largely on the selection of proper testing methods. The screening test must accurately discriminate between immune and nonimmune patients and requires a sensitive and specific assay for IgM in order to identify women at risk of *Toxoplasma* infection during pregnancy. The most commonly used serological tests for detection of antibodies against *Toxoplasma gondii* are the IFA and the EIA. Both techniques can detect both IgM and IgG antibodies. The interpretation of serological data for toxoplasmosis is not always easy: for example, when sera show high levels of IgG antibodies and/or the presence of IgM antibodies. Supplementary tests (in addition to the determination of IgG and IgM antibodies) should be performed on these sera. The complement fixation test or the Sabin-Feldman dye test, IgG avidity and IgA antibodies are frequently used as additional tests. The difference in the timing of the appearance of these different antibodies in relation to infection can give additional information on the timing of the infection. It is the application of a panel of additional tests, as used in reference laboratories, that permits in most cases the separation between acute or late infection.

Implications of testing

WHAT DOES AN ABNORMAL TEST RESULT MEAN?

When the diagnosis of toxoplasmosis during pregnancy is confirmed (seroconversion) or suspected (high antibody level in a first serum sample), the patient should be placed on an adequate antibiotic regimen aimed at reducing either transplacental passage or the development of sequelae in the already infected fetus. In Europe, spiramycin, a macrolide antibiotic, has been extensively used at a dose of 3 g daily. Spiramycin is concentrated in the placenta and reduces the incidence of congenitally infected infants from 61% to 23% (Desmonts and Couvreur, 1984).

All patients at risk of delivering a congenitally infected child should be offered antenatal diagnosis. In the past, antenatal diagnosis required a multifaceted approach incorporating ultrasonography, amniocentesis and cordocentesis around the 20th week of gestation. The definite diagnosis of fetal infection relies on the isolation of the parasite from the amniotic fluid, the fetal blood, or on the presence of *Toxoplasma*-specific IgM antibodies in fetal blood. Other nonspecific markers of fetal infection include thrombocytopenia, increased total IgM and increased gammaglutamyl transferase levels. The sensitivity of prenatal diagnosis with this methodology is 92% (Daffos *et al.*, 1988; Foulon *et al.*, 1990). More recent work has focused on the application of PCR to the detection of *Toxoplasma* DNA in amniotic fluid. The sensitivity and specificity for PCR reported by Hohlfeld *et al.* (1994) were 97% and 100% respectively. However, since these results have not yet been confirmed by other groups, it seems prudent for the time being to continue to perform both amniocentesis and cordocentesis.

If a fetal infection is diagnosed, therapeutic abortion is an option particularly when there are sonographic abnormalities such as hydrocephalus or brain necrosis. When the ultrasound examination is normal and the patient desires to continue the pregnancy, treatment is initiated with pyrimethamine 25 mg per day combined with sulfadiazine 3 g per day and folinic acid 5 mg two times a week. Most researchers alternate this treatment regimen with spiramycin for the duration of pregnancy; each regimen is given for 3 weeks at a time.

All infected children, symptomatic or asymptomatic, need careful pediatric follow-up and continued antiparasitic treatment. The children considered to be free of disease based on the prenatal diagnosis need also be tested with serial blood samples up to 11 months of age to confirm or exclude congenital toxoplasmosis.

Women without detectable antibodies are susceptible. They should be instructed on preventive measures which include: (1) never eat raw or insufficiently cooked meat; (2) avoid touching the mouth or eyes after handling raw meat and always wash hands thoroughly; (3) avoid contact with cat feces (or possibly contaminated items, e.g. during gardening). These hygienic measures should be fully explained at the first prenatal visit and if possible additional information should be given during the antenatal classes. Health education on how to avoid toxoplasmosis during pregnancy can reduce the seroconversion rate by 63% (Foulon *et al.*, 1994). Seronegative women are followed during pregnancy for the appearance of the *Toxoplasma* antibodies. The best times to retest are between 16 and 20 weeks, around the 30th week and at delivery.

WHAT DOES A NORMAL TEST RESULT MEAN?

Pregnant women with IgG antibodies and absence of IgM antibodies can be considered to be immune. There is no need to retest these women during pregnancy.

What is the cost of testing?

Using a hospital fee of US $40 per specimen, it has been calculated that the initial screening of all pregnant women in the USA would cost US $160 million (Thorpe *et al.*, 1988). If 70% of US women are seronegative, monthly titer assessment would cost $1 billion annually, exclusive of the costs for confirmatory testing, diagnostic evaluation and treatment. This cost estimate is outdated for at least three reasons. First, the laboratory methodology has changed dramatically. The increased sensitivity and specificity of the ELISAs coupled with the ability to automate testing reduces the cost of screening. Second, the monthly titer assessment of seronegative women as advocated originally is unnecessary. More recent approaches screen three times (in the first trimester, at 16–20 weeks, and around 30 weeks). Third, the cost of prenatal diagnosis will decrease further with the application of the PCR methodology. Based on a serological screening program in Norway, retesting the seronegative population once in the second and once in the third trimester, Stray-Pedersen *et al.* (1992) concluded that screening is of economic benefit when the incidence of maternal toxoplasmosis is 1–1.5 per 1000.

CONCLUSIONS AND RECOMMENDATIONS

Congenital toxoplasmosis is a potentially preventable disease. The clinical sequelae of a fetal *Toxoplasma* infection vary markedly. The majority of infected infants develop mild to severe disease, including unilateral or bilateral blindness, hydrocephalus, and/ or psychomotor and mental retardation in early or late childhood. Adequate serological screening is possible and allows detection of seronegative susceptible pregnant women. These women should receive a leaflet at the first prenatal visit instructing them on hygienic measures to reduce the *Toxoplasma* infection rate during pregnancy. With this simple method it is possible to reduce the *Toxoplasma* infection rate during pregnancy by 63%.

Serologic screening can identify women at risk of carrying an infected fetus (Foulon *et al.*, 1990) and prenatal diagnosis allows detection of infected fetuses in most cases. Antenatal medical therapy appears to reduce the risk of a fetal infection and reduces the sequelae in the already infected fetus (Auley *et al.*, 1994). Screening would appear to be cost effective if the incidence of maternal toxoplasmosis is at least 1–1.5 per 1000 (Stray-Pedersen & Jenum, 1992). Serological screening should be encouraged in regions with a high incidence of congenital toxoplasmosis. Affected patients should be referred to centers where toxoplasmosis in pregnancy can be managed in a multidisciplinary fashion.

SUMMARY

1 WHAT IS THE PROBLEM THAT REQUIRES SCREENING?

CONGENITAL *TOXOPLASMA* INFECTION.

a What is the incidence/prevalence of the target condition?

The incidence of toxoplasmosis during pregnancy ranges widely by geographic location – from 8 per 1000 in Brussels to 2 per 1000 in Norway. Recent data from serological studies indicate that the congenital infection rate varies from 0.2 to 2 cases per 1000 births.

b What are the sequelae of the condition which are of interest in clinical medicine?

Only about 10% of infected neonates have symptoms at birth. Early maternal infection may lead to either spontaneous abortion or severe sequelae such as hydrocephalus, chorioretinitis and mental retardation. Other clinical manifestations include icterus, hepatosplenomegaly, and thrombocytopenia. Congenital infections occurring after the 24th week of pregnancy are nearly always subclinical. Nearly all symptomatic newborns will have longterm neurologic and/or ophthalmologic sequelae.

2 THE TESTS

a What is the purpose of the test?

To detect seronegative pregnant women at risk for primary infection during pregnancy.

b The nature of the tests

A variety of serologic tests, none of which is alone definitive.

c Implications of testing

1 What does an abnormal test result mean?

Women without detectable antibodies are susceptible to the infection. They should be instructed on potentially preventive measures and be retested around 16–20 weeks, 30 weeks of gestation and on cord blood in geographic areas of high risk. When toxoplasmosis during pregnancy is confirmed (seroconversion) or suspected (high antibody level in a first serum sample), the patient should receive antibiotic treatment to reduce either the likelihood of transplacental infection or the development of sequelae in an infected fetus.

2 What does a normal test result mean?
Pregnant women with IgG antibodies and absence of IgM antibodies are considered immune.

d What is the cost of testing?

The cost depends on the geographic prevalence and the frequency of retesting.

3   CONCLUSIONS AND RECOMMENDATIONS

Maternal screening for toxoplasmosis using an automated ELISA at first booking with retesting of seronegative women once in the second and once in the third trimester is likely to be cost-effective when the incidence of maternal toxoplasmosis is 1–1.5 per 1000.

REFERENCES

Auley JM, Boyer KM, Dushyant P *et al.* (1994) Early and longitudinal evaluations of treated infants and children and untreated historical patients with congenital toxoplasmosis: the Chicago collaborative treatment trial. *Clin Infec Dis* **18**: 38–72.

Daffos F, Forestier F, Capella-Pavlovsky M *et al.* (1988) Prenatal management of 746 pregnancies at risk for congenital toxoplasmosis. *N Engl J Med* **318**: 271–275.

Desmonts G & Couvreur J (1974) Congenital toxoplasmosis: a prospective study of 378 pregnancies. *N Engl J Med* **1**: 417–422.

Desmonts G & Couvreur J (1984) Toxoplasmose congénitale. Etude prospective de l'issue de la grossesse chez 542 femmes atteintes de toxoplasmose acquise en cours de gestation. *Ann Pédiatr* **31**: 805–809.

Feldman HA & Miller LT (1956) Serological study of toxoplasmosis prevalence. *Am J Hygiene* **64**: 320–335.

Foulon W, Naessens A, Volckaert M *et al.* (1984) Congenital toxoplasmosis: a prospective survey in Brussels. *Br J Obstet Gynaecol* **91**: 419–423.

Foulon W, Naessens A, Mahler T *et al.* (1990). Prenatal diagnosis of congenital toxoplasmosis. *Obstet Gynecol* **76**: 769–772.

Foulon W, Naessens A & Derde MP (1994) Evaluation of the possibilities for preventing congenital toxoplasmosis. *Am J Perinatol* **11**: 57–62.

Hohlfeld P, Daffos F, Coster JH *et al.* (1994) Prenatal diagnosis of congenital toxoplasmosis with a polymerase-chain reaction test on amniotic fluid. *N Engl J Med* **331**: 695–699.

Hunter K, Stagno S, Capps E *et al.* (1983) Prenatal screening of pregnant women for infections caused by cytomegalovirus, Epstein–Barr virus, herpes virus, rubella, and *Toxoplasma gondii. Am J Obstet Gynecol* **145**: 269–273.

Klapper PE & Morris DJ (1990) Screening for viral and protozoal infection in pregnancy. A review. *Br J Obstet Gynaecol* **97**: 974–983.

Remington JS & Gentry LO (1970) Acquired toxoplasmosis: infection versus disease. *Ann N Y Acad Sci* **174**: 1006–1017.

Sfameni SF, Skurrie IJ & Gilbert GL (1986) Antenatal screening for congenital infection with rubella, cytomegalovirus and toxoplasma. *Aust NZ J Gynaecol* **26**: 257–260.

Stray-Pedersen B (1993) Toxoplasmosis in pregnancy. In Gilbert GL (ed.) *Infectious Diseases: Challenges for the 1990s,* pp. 107–137. Baillière's Clinical Obstetrics and Gynaecology, **7**: 1. London: Baillière Tindall.

Stray-Pedersen B & Jenum P (1992) Economic evaluation of preventive programmes against congenital toxoplasmosis. *Scand J Infect Dis* (suppl.) **84**: 86–92.

Thorpe JM, Seeds JW, Herbert WNP, *et al.* (1988) Prenatal management of congenital toxoplasmosis. *N Eng J Med* **319**: 372–373.

3

Sexually Transmitted Diseases: Syphilis, Gonorrhea, HIV & Chlamydia

Jose A. Prieto & R. Phillip Heine

Syphilis

WHAT IS THE PROBLEM THAT REQUIRES SCREENING?

INFECTIOUS AND CONGENITAL SYPHILIS.

What is the incidence/prevalence of the target condition?

The current prevalence of infectious syphilis in the USA is approximately 15 per 100 000 population (Sweet and Gibbs, 1990). Approximately 35 000 cases of primary and secondary syphilis are reported each year and it has been estimated that for every reported case, three cases go unreported (Centers for Disease Control, 1988a; Sweet and Gibbs, 1990). The rate of infectious syphilis in the adult female has increased in recent years (Mascola *et al.*, 1984; Rolfs and Nakashima, 1990). This increase has occurred mainly in heterosexual women of low socioeconomic status who live in the inner city where the disease is more prevalent (Marx *et al.*, 1991). Importantly, the increased rates of infectious syphilis through heterosexual contact have led to an increase in the rate of congenital syphilis in major urban medical centers (Ricci *et al.*, 1989; Rolfs and Nakashima, 1990). Of the 3000 cases reported in 1990, about 80% occurred in Texas, Florida, California, and New York, and 90% of cases occurred among black American and Hispanic women (Sweet and Gibbs, 1990). Over half of these cases occur among women receiving no prenatal care (Sweet and Gibbs, 1990). Reasons for this dramatic increase include the practice of exchanging drugs for sex and a decrease in funding for syphilis control (Centers for Disease Control, 1988a).

Risk factors for contracting syphilis include adolescent age at the time of first sexual intercourse, multiple sex partners and illicit drug use (Centers for Disease Control, 1988a; Sweet and Gibbs, 1990). Epidemiological data suggest that about one-third of the partners having sexual intercourse with an infected person will themselves become infected (Centers for Disease Control, 1988a). The risk of acquiring syphilis from a single sexual exposure is not known. In western Europe almost all of the cases of syphilis are 'imported'.

What are the sequelae of the condition which are of interest in clinical medicine?

The clinical sequelae of infection with the spirochete *Treponema pallidum* (subspecies *pallidum*) are well described. They include primary, secondary, latent, and tertiary stages. After an incubation period of 10–90 days from exposure, a painless chancre develops at the site of inoculum, which is often associated with painless regional lymphadenopathy. This is the primary stage. The chancre disappears spontaneously in 6 weeks to 6 months and is followed by spirochetemia, the second stage. Clinical manifestations of the second stage include a generalized maculopapular rash of the palms and soles, mucous patches, condyloma latum, and generalized lymphadenopathy. These manifestations usually appear about 6 weeks to several months after healing of the chancre. During the second-ary stage, cerebral fluid abnormalities are detected in about 40% of the patients. Within 2–6 weeks, these clinical findings of the second stage clear spontaneously and the latent stage begins. The latency period is characterized by the absence of clinically evident disease and a history of primary or secondary lesions, or the birth of an infant with congenital syphilis. The diagnosis is usually made by the finding of specific treponemal antibodies for syphilis. If treatment of the primary, secondary, or latent stages is not provided, 25–30% of patients develop tertiary syphilis, with systemic involvement of the cardiovascular, central nervous (including tabes dorsalis), and musculoskeletal systems (Musher, 1991).

Syphilis may infect the fetus at any gestational age including the first trimester, and can be transmitted during any stage of maternal disease (Harter and Benirschke, 1976). Untreated primary or secondary syphilis is associated with a 75–95% probability of fetal infection and with approximately 40% perinatal loss (Fiumara *et al.*, 1952). In general, the more advanced the maternal disease, the lower the risk of transmission to the fetus (Fiumara and Lessel, 1970). Manifestations of fetal infection include preterm birth, fetal hydrops, stillbirth, neo-natal death, and clinically apparent congenital syphilis, which often becomes manifest between 2 weeks and 10 weeks after birth. Neonatal manifestations include mucocutaneous lesions, osteochondritis and osteitis, hepatosplenomegaly, anemia, jaundice, thrombocyto-penia, and lymphadenopathy. In most countries, including the USA, Health Department notification of syphilis is required by law.

THE TESTS

What is the purpose of the test?

To identify women with infectious syphilis. Most cases of syphilis are diagnosed by the routine screening of asymptomatic persons, including pregnant women at their first pre-natal visit. Universal screening is especially important for women, in whom most cases of primary syphilis are asymptomatic.

The nature of the tests

Most primary lesions in the female occur on the cervix or posterior fornix and are not seen by the patient. Patients with syphilis usually develop antibodies directed against a poorly defined lipid. Screening for syphilis is based on serologic testing. Initially, the Wassermann test was used for this purpose. The Wassermann test is based on the complement fixation technique to detect the reaction between a lipoid-tissue antigen and an antibody (so-called 'reagin' in syphilitic serum). Presently, related nonspecific antibody tests, i.e. the Venereal Disease Research Laboratory (VDRL) and the rapid plasma reagent (RPR) tests, have replaced the Wassermann test. Cross-reacting lipids, such as cardiolipin extracted from beef heart, currently serve as the basis for the nonspecific tests. These antigens react with IgG and IgM antibodies to cardiolipin which comprises 10% of treponemal lipids. The nonspecific antibody tests may be quantitated and the result expressed as the highest dilution of serum yielding a positive reaction. Unfortunately, these same cardiolipins are also found in mammalian tissues (Musher, 1990). Thus, a reactive VDRL or RPR result must be confirmed by *Treponema pallidum* specific tests which include the *T. pallidum* immobilization (TPI) test, the fluorescent treponemal antibody absorption (FTA-ABS) test and the micro-hemagglutination test for *T. pallidum* (MHA-TP) (Jaffe, 1975). The *T. pallidum* hemagglutination assay (TPHA) is another *T. pallidum* specific test, which is widely used in Canada and Europe, but is not available in the USA. The *T. pallidum* specific tests are usually not quantitated. *Treponema pallidum* cannot be cultured. Visualization of spirochetes by dark field microscopy in a fresh specimen obtained by sampling a suspected lesion is diagnostic of syphilis. However, a single negative examination does not exclude syphilis.

Implications of testing

WHAT DOES AN ABNORMAL TEST RESULT MEAN?

Asymptomatic persons with a highly reactive (positive) nonspecific antibody test (VDRL titers exceeding 1:8) confirmed by reactive (positive) *T. pallidum* specific test (TPI, FTA-ABS, MHA-TP, or TPHA) are likely to have an active treponemal infection, unless they were recently successfully treated for syphilis. (In certain remote parts of the world nonvenereal treponemal infections of childhood, including yaws (syn. framboesia), pinta and bejel, are endemic. These conditions are associated with nonspecific antibody and *T. pallidum* specific reactions similar to syphilis). Crude sensitivity estimates of the VDRL, FTA-ABS and MHA-TP tests are shown in Table 3.1. In fact, the results from both the nonspecific antibody tests (VDRL or RPR) and the *T. pallidum* specific tests (TPI, FTA-ABS, MHA-TP, and TPHA) may be nonreactive (negative) when the syphilitic chancre first appears (Jaffe, 1975).

False positive nonspecific antibody tests (VDRL, RPR) may occur in 10–20% of patients with active lupus erythematosus. False positive nonspecific antibody tests are also seen in patients with other autoimmune diseases, various infectious diseases (such as viral infections, mycoplasma pneumonia, leprosy, and malaria), drug addiction, and preg-

Table 3.1   Crude sensitivity estimates (%) of the various tests used for detecting syphilis.

TEST	PRIMARY SYPHILIS	SECONDARY AND LATENT SYPHILIS	TERTIARY SYPHILIS
VDRL	75	99	70
FTA-ABS	85	100	99
MHA-TP	80	100	98

From: Radolf and Isaacs (1992)

nancy. Generally, these conditions yield borderline or weakly positive results. In patients with false positive nonspecific antibody tests results, syphilis is excluded by a negative *T. pallidum* specific test result.

False positive *T. pallidum* specific tests occur in about 1% of the population (corresponding with a specificity of 99%) and are usually transient, of unknown etiology, but may be associated with systemic, discoid, and drug-induced lupus erythematosus (Shore and Faricelli, 1977). Given the high specificity, the TPI test is conclusive of past or present treponemal infection.

The Centers for Disease Control (CDC) have outlined their current recommendations for the treatment of syphilis (Centers for Disease Control, 1993). Once the diagnosis is suspected, injectable benzanthine penicillin G (2.4 million units, single dose) remains the drug of choice, although it may cause the Jarisch–Herxheimer reaction. Alternatives for nonpregnant patients include tetracycline and erythromycin. Pregnant patients with a history of penicillin allergy should be skin tested with dilute solutions of penicillin (Betts, 1985). If allergic, they should be hospitalized, desensitized in an intensive care setting, and treated with penicillin (Wendel *et al.*, 1985; Ziaya *et al.*, 1986). After successful treatment of primary and secondary syphilis, the VDRL titers progressively decline and often become very low or negative in 3–12 months following treatment. In contrast, the *T. Pallidum* specific tests (FTA-ABS and hemagglutination tests) remain positive in nearly all patients treated for primary and secondary syphilis. Hence, the latter tests are not useful for primary or secondary syphilis. Patients identified with syphilis should be screened for other sexually transmitted diseases including gonorrhea, chlamydia, and human immunodeficiency virus (HIV). Furthermore, sexual contacts should be traced for diagnosis and treatment, where indicated.

Newborns should be evaluated for congenital syphilis if they were born to seropositive women who were treated for syphilis during pregnancy or to women who either have untreated syphilis or do not have a well-documented history of treatment for syphilis (Centers for Disease Control, 1993). In the newborn, positive serological tests for syphilis can represent either active disease or passively transferred antibodies from the mother. In the latter instance, antibody titers will progressively decrease and disappear by 3–4 months of age (Ikeaa and Jenson, 1990). The assessment of IgM-FTA-ABS in cord blood is not recommended because of questionable sensitivity and specificity.

WHAT DOES A NORMAL TEST RESULT MEAN?

Given the low prevalence of treponemal disease in pregnancy and the high specificity of the various serologic tests, syphilis is essentially ruled out in women with negative serologic testing (Table 3.2). However, clinical judgment may dictate repeat testing in

Table 3.2 Test performance of VDRL to identify untreated infectious syphilis; hypothetical example among 100 000 pregnant women, given a test sensitivity of 75%, test specificity of 99% and a prevalence of 15 per 100 000 pregnancies (see Sweet and Gibbs, 1990).

	SYPHILIS PRESENT	SYPHILIS ABSENT	
VDRL test positive	11	1 000	1 000
VDRL test negative	4	98 985	99 000
	15	99 985	100 000

Positive predictive value: 11/1000 × 100 = 1%; Negative predictive value: 98 985/99 000 × 100 = 100%

individuals at risk since it may take 4 weeks from the initial exposure for the serum tests to become positive.

What is the cost of testing?

The typical cost for screening serology (nonspecific antibody tests) in 1995 was approximately US $20. The cost increases to $30–40 if *T. pallidum* specific antibody testing is required. Ernst *et al.* (1992) estimated the cost of screening emergency room patients with another suspected sexually transmitted disease for syphilis was approximately $104 per detected case. This compares well with the costs reported by other screening programs for Veterans Administration employees, psychiatric patients, and the widely used premarital screening program. (Haskell, 1984; Baumgarten and Swigar, 1987; Normand *et al.*, 1988). Active surveillance systems in hospitals are cost-effective in any area with 5 or more cases of syphilis per 100 000 population (Centers for Disease Control, 1988b). The CDC recommends serologic screening for syphilis of all pregnant women. In persons with infectious syphilis all sexual contacts should be traced. Efficient screening prevents the spread of disease, allows for early treatment, and in the pregnant woman, helps prevent the devastating effects of syphilis infection on the fetus.

CONCLUSIONS AND RECOMMENDATIONS

Since primary lesions are usually asymptomatic in women, serologic testing assumes a prominent role in diagnosing syphilis. Authorities now recommend routine serologic testing in all women during the early stages of pregnancy (Centers for Disease Control, 1993). For women at high risk, screening should be repeated in the third trimester (Centers for Disease Control, 1993). Though it is likely that routine screening in low prevalence areas (i.e. less than 5 per 100 000) is not cost-effective, congenital syphilis is a preventable disease with major sequelae to the offspring. Detection and adequate treatment of pregnant women is essential. A disadvantage of serologic screening programs of syphilis is the relatively high proportion of false positive test results (about 1% depending on the population studied). Generally, false positive findings are transient and often of unknown etiology. False positive VDRL titers usually do not exceed 1:8. Patients who were successfully treated for early primary or secondary syphilis in the past will usually remain positive for *T. pallidum* specific antibodies, while the nonspecific antibody tests results are usually negative.

Infected individuals should be educated about syphilis, its sequelae, mode of transmission, and association with other sexually transmitted diseases. Because of the association between ulcerative diseases such as syphilis and concurrent HIV infection, counseling and testing for HIV is essential (Plummer *et al.*, 1991). It is crucial that any recent sexual contacts be concomitantly treated to avoid reinfection.

SUMMARY

1

INFECTIOUS AND CONGENITAL SYPHILIS.

a What is the incidence/prevalence of the target condition?

The current incidence of infectious syphilis in the USA is approximately 15 per 100 000 population. The rate of congenital syphilis has been increasing in major urban centers and over half of these cases occur among women receiving no prenatal care.

b What are the sequelae of the condition which are of interest in clinical medicine?

The clinical sequelae include primary, secondary, latent, and tertiary stages of syphilis. If treatment is not provided, 25–30% of patients develop tertiary syphilis. Syphilis may infect the fetus at any gestational age. Untreated primary or secondary syphilis is associated with a 75–95% probability of fetal infection and with approximately 40% perinatal death.

2

THE TESTS

a What is the purpose of the test?

To identify women with infectious syphilis.

b The nature of the test (s)

Screening for syphilis is based on the identification of two types of antibodies, the nonspecific antibody and *T. pallidum* specific antibody. Identification of spirochetes by dark field microscopy is diagnostic of syphilis. However, negative finding on dark field microscopy does not rule out syphilis.

c Implications of testing

1 What does an abnormal test mean?

Asymptomatic persons with highly reactive nonspecific antibody tests confirmed by positive *T. pallidum* specific antibody test results are considered to have syphilis. In the newborn, positive serological tests represent either active disease or passively transferred antibodies from the mother. In the latter, antibody titers progressively decrease and disappear by 3–4 months of age. A disadvantage of the screening programmes for syphilis is the relatively high proportion (about 1% of the whole population) of false positive test results. Infants born to women with active or suspected syphilis should be serologically evaluated.

2 What does a normal test result mean?

Syphilis is essentially ruled out in women with negative serologic test results.

d What is the cost of testing?

Standard charges for screening serology are approximately $20 (US, 1995) with specific antibody testing being approximately $30–40. The cost for screening for syphilis in emergency room patients with another suspected sexually transmitted disease approximates $104 per detected case. This compares well with costs of other screening programs.

3 CONCLUSIONS AND RECOMMENDATIONS

Congenital syphilis can be largely prevented by identification and treatment of the infected woman during pregnancy. As primary lesions are usually asymptomatic, identification requires serologic screening. Authorities are now recommending serologic testing of all pregnant women. To avoid reinfection, it is crucial that any recent sexual contacts be concomitantly evaluated and treated, when indicated.

REFERENCES

Baumgarten A & Swigar ME (1987) A lack of justification for routine screening assays for syphilis in general hospital psychiatric patients. *Compr Psych* **28**: 127–130.

Betts RF (1985) Skin testing. In Mandell GL, Douglas RG & Bennett JR (eds) *Principles and Practice of Infectious Diseases*, New York: John Wiley and Sons, pp. 149–153.

Centers for Disease Control (1988a) Syphilis and congenital syphilis – United States, (1985–1988). *MMWR* **37**: 486–491.

Centers for Disease Control (1988b) Policy guidelines for the prevention and control of congenital syphylis. *MMWR* p. 46. **37** (suppl. S-1): 1–13.

Centers for Disease Control (1993) Sexually transmitted diseases treatment guidelines. *MMWR* **42** (RR-14): 1–102.

Ernst AA, Samuels JD & Winsemius DK (1992) Emergency department screening for syphilis in patients with other suspected sexually transmitted diseases. *Ann Emerg Med* **20**: 627–630.

Fiumara NJ, Fleming WL, Downing JG & Good FL (1952) The incidence of prenatal syphilis at the Boston City Hospital. *N Engl J Med* **247**: 48–52.

Fiumara NJ & Lessel S (1970) Manifestations of late congenital syphilis. *Arch Dermatol* **102**: 78–82.

Harter CA & Benirschke K (1976) Fetal syphilis in the first trimester. *Am J Obstet Gynecol* **124**: 705–708.

Haskell RJ (1984) A cost-benefit analysis of California's mandatory premarital screening program for syphilis. *West J Med* **141**: 538–541.

Ikeaa MK & Jenson HB (1990) Evaluation and treatment of congenital syphilis. *J Pediatrics* **117**: 843–852.

Jaffe HW (1975) The laboratory diagnosis of syphilis. New concepts. *Ann Intern Med* **83**: 846–851.

Marx R, Aral SO, Rolfs RT, Sterk CE & Kahn JG (1991) Crack, sex and STD. *Sex Transm Dis* **18**: 92–101.

Mascola L, Pelosi R, Blount JH, *et al.* (1984) Congenital syphilis. Why is it still occurring? *JAMA* **252**: 1719–1722.

Musher DM (1990) Biology of Trepomena pallidum. In Holmes KK *et al.* (eds) *Sexually Transmitted Diseases*, pp 206–210. St Louis: McGraw-Hill.

Musher DM (1991) Syphilis, neurosyphilis, penicillin and AIDS. *J Infect Dis* **163**: 1201–1206.

Normand R, Klotz SA & Tudor S (1988) Annual syphilis serology testing in hospital employees: Is it beneficial? *Am J Inf Contr* **16**: 30–33.

Plummer FA, Simonsen JN, Cameron DW, *et al.* (1991) Cofactors in male-female sexual transmission of human immunodeficiency virus type 1. *J Infect Dis* **163**: 233–239.

Radolf JD & Isaacs RD (1992) Syphilis. In Kelly *et al.* (eds) *Textbook of Medicine*, 2nd edition, pp 1440–1445. Philadelphia: Lippincott.

Ricci JM, Fojaco RM & O'Sullivan MJ (1989) Congenital syphilis, The University of Miami/Jackson Memorial Medical Center Experience, 1986–88. *Obstet Gynecol* **74**: 687–692.

Rolfs RT & Nakashima AK (1990) Epidemiology of primary and secondary syphilis in the United States, 1981 through 1989. *JAMA* **264**: 1432–1437.

Shore RN & Faricelli JA (1977) Borderline and reactive FTA-ABS results in lupus erythematosus. *Arch Dermatol* 37–41.

Sweet RL & Gibbs RS (1990) *Infectious Diseases of the Female Genital Tract.* Second edition. pp. 119–126. Baltimore: Williams & Wilkins.

Wendel GD, Stark BJ, Jamison RB *et al.* (1985) Penicillin allergy and desensitization in serous maternal/fetal infections. *N Engl J Med* **312**: 1232.

Ziaya PR, Hankins DV, Gilstrap LC & Halsey AB (1986) Intravenous penicillin desensitization and treatment during pregnancy. *JAMA* **256**: 2651–2652.

Gonorrhea

WHAT IS THE PROBLEM THAT REQUIRES SCREENING?

INFECTIOUS ANOGENITAL GONORRHEA.

What is the incidence/prevalence of the target condition?

Infection by *Neisseria gonorrhoeae*, a Gram-negative diplococcus, continues to be a major public health issue worldwide. This remains true in the USA despite a decline in the number of reported cases since 1975 (Zenilman, 1989). The reported rate is 323 cases per 100 000 population (Zenilman, 1989). The highest rates of disease occur in the 20–24 years age group, in women who are poor, unmarried, promiscuous and exposed to other sexually transmitted diseases. As with syphilis, there may be a link between illicit drug use and the transmission of gonorrhea. The prevalence of positive cultures for *Neisseria gonorrhoeae* varies with the population screened. Twenty-five per cent of women attending sexually transmitted diseases (STD) clinics have positive cultures compared with as few as 1–2% of women seen in private offices (Spence, 1983). During pregnancy, the prevalence of gonorrhea ranges from 0.5% to 7% depending on the population screened (Sarrel and Pruett, 1968).

What are the sequelae of the condition which are of interest in clinical medicine?

Infertility, sepsis, chronic pelvic pain, and perinatal complications including preterm rupture of the membranes and neonatal conjunctivitis.

Gonorrhea is transmitted almost entirely by sexual contact. The incubation period is usually short, 2–6 days following exposure. In the female, the primary site of involvement is the columnar epithelium of the endocervical canal. In 10–20% of infected women, failure to seek treatment or inadequate treatment of the initial gonococcal infection results in ascending infection of the upper reproductive tract (Holmes *et al.*, 1980). Conversely, 10–70% of women with acute salpingitis have *Neisseria gonorrhoeae* isolated from their cervices (Holmes *et al.*, 1980). Of women with gonococcal cervicitis, 50% develop rectal infection with or without a history of penile-anal contact (Dans, 1975). Other clinical manifestations of gonococcal infection include dysuria (often attributed to 'cystitis'), increased vaginal discharge, perihepatitis (Fitz-Hugh–Curtis syndrome, manifested by right upper quadrant abdominal pain and tenderness), bartholinitis and pharyngeal gonococcal infection. Disseminated gonococcal infection develops in 0.5–1% of women with gonococcal cervicitis (Centers for Disease Control, 1987). Disseminated gonococcal infection typically presents during menstruation and late pregnancy, and commonly manifests as a dermatitis-tenosynovitis syndrome and septic arthritis syndrome. Gonococcal endocarditis, meningitis and osteomyelitis are rare manifestations of disseminated gonococcal infection. Several investigators have identified an association between untreated maternal endocervical gonorrhea and perinatal complications, including an increased risk of preterm rupture of the membranes, preterm delivery, chorioamnionitis, neonatal conjunctivitis and sepsis, and maternal postpartum infection (Armstey and Steadman, 1976; Edwards *et al.*, 1978). Gonococcal infection during pregnancy is not associated with an increased risk of fetal structural anomalies.

THE TESTS

What is the purpose of the tests?

To detect patients with *Neisseria gonorrhoeae* infection who are thus potential transmitters of the disease and at risk for the previously noted medical complications. Since many non-pregnant and pregnant women are asymptomatic, obstetric, gynecologic and family planning clinics with high prevalence populations often culture routinely. Women at high risk for infection with *Neisseria gonorrhoeae* include young, unmarried women living in the inner city, drug users, women with prior STDs or multiple sexual partners, and partners of men with gonorrhea or other STDs. Where routine screening is not practiced, high-risk women should be screened. High-risk pregnant women should be screened at their initial visit and again in the third trimester (Centers for Disease Control, 1993). Because co-infection rates are as high as 50%, women positive for *Neisseria gonorrhoeae* should also be screened for other STD organisms including *Chlamydia trachomatis* (Zenilman, 1989).

The nature of the tests

Methods for the diagnosis of *Neisseria gonorrhoeae* include Gram stain, detection of the gonococcal antigen by enzyme immunoassay, nucleic acid hybridization (GEN-PROBE), and culture in Thayer–Martin media. Culture of *Neisseria gonorrhoeae* from potentially infected sites is the 'gold standard' for diagnosis. Specimens for culture should be collected from the endocervix. Additional specimens from the urethra and rectum improve the sensitivity of detection 5–10% and are considered prudent. Thayer–Martin broth consists of a medium base supplemented with bovine erythrocytes and contains vancomycin, colistin, and nystatin. An estimated 90% of infected men are diagnosed by Gram stain. However, in women the sensitivity of this test is only 60% (Sweet and Gibbs, 1990). Although highly specific (97%), detection of gonococcal antigen by enzyme immunoassay has a sensitivity of only 60% (Olsen and Michael, 1986). Nucleic acid hybridization for the detection of *Neisseria gonorrhoeae* reportedly has excellent sensitivity and specificity (Hosein *et al.*, 1992), but it is more costly and no more accurate than culture. Therefore, the laboratory diagnosis of *Neisseria gonorrhoeae* is best accomplished by isolating the organism on a selective medium such as Thayer–Martin broth. Since a small percentage of *Neisseria gonorrhoeae* organisms are sensitive to vancomycin, simultaneous use of a nonselective media such as chocolate blood agar with Thayer–Martin increases the yield. Detection of *Neisseria gonorrhoeae* by amplification techniques such as polymerase chain reaction or ligase chain reaction appears promising, but at this time remains experimental. Amplification techniques have been effective in diagnosing *Neisseria gonorrhoeae* from urine specimens theoretically making noninvasive testing a possibility (Smith *et al.*, 1995).

Implications of testing

WHAT DOES AN ABNORMAL TEST RESULT MEAN?

Women with a positive culture for *Neisseria gonorrhoeae* are infected and should be treated simultaneously with recent sexual contacts. Treatment should consist of a regimen effective against both *Neisseria gonorrhoeae* and *Chlamydia trachomatis*. Combination therapy is more cost-effective than monotherapy when the sequelae of gonococcal infection are considered (Washington *et al.*, 1987). The new β-lactamase-resistant antimicrobial agents are now the preferred treatment with the emergence of resistant strains of *Neisseria gonorrhoeae*. Ceftriaxone, an extended spectrum cephalosporin with a long serum half-life, has proved to be effective for treatment of uncomplicated anogenital gonorrhea (Centers for Disease Control, 1993). Presumptive treatment for chlamydial infection is indicated.

WHAT DOES A NORMAL TEST RESULT MEAN?

A negative culture for *Neisseria gonorrhoeae* excludes the diagnosis. In many countries, including the USA, silver nitrate prophylaxis (1% aqueous solution in a single application instilled in both eyes soon after delivery) is used for the prevention of gonococcal conjunctivitis in the neonate. In industrialized countries *Chlamydia trachomatis* and nonsexually transmitted agents are more common causes of neonatal conjunctivitis. Alternative preparations recommended for prophylaxis of ophthalmia neonatorum include erythromycin (0.5%) ophthalmic ointment or tetracycline (1%) ophthalmic ointment (Centers for Disease Control, 1993).

What is the cost of testing?

Culture is inexpensive to perform with laboratory materials costing less than US $0.25 per test. Personnel time to read the culture and characterize the organism are the most expensive aspects of culture. Patient charges vary depending on location and range from free at health departments to approximately $30 (US, 1995). Charges for antigen detection and nucleic acid detection are consistently higher than for culture. Phillips *et al.* (1989) observed that testing and treating selected women with risk factors for gonorrhea reduces overall medical costs when the prevalence of infection exceeds 1.5%.

CONCLUSIONS AND RECOMMENDATIONS

All high-risk women should be tested for *Neisseria gonorrhoeae* since its identification and treatment reduces medical complications and is cost-effective. Those patients testing positive as well as any recent sexual contacts should be treated for *Neisseria gonorrhoeae* as well as presumptive chlamydial infection. In addition, patients with gonorrhea should have serologic testing for syphilis as well as for HIV infection.

SUMMARY

1 WHAT IS THE PROBLEM THAT REQUIRES SCREENING?

INFECTIOUS ANOGENITAL GONORRHEA.

a What is the incidence/prevalence of the target condition?

The incidence of reported cases is 323 cases per 100 000 population. In pregnancy, the prevalence of gonorrhea ranges from 0.5% to 7% depending on the populations screened.

b What are the sequelae of the condition which are of interest in clinical medicine?

In 10–20% of infected women, failure to seek treatment or inadequate treatment of an initial gonococcal infection will result in ascending infection of the upper reproductive tract. Conversely, 10–70% of women with acute salpingitis will have *Neisseria gonorrhoeae* isolated from their cervices. Several investigators have identified an association between untreated maternal endocervical gonorrhea and poor pregnancy outcome.

2 THE TESTS

a What is the purpose of the test?

To detect patients with *Neisseria gonorrhoeae* infection.

b The nature of the tests?

Methods for the diagnosis of *Neisseria gonorrhoeae* infection include Gram stain, detection of the gonococcal antigen by enzyme immunoassay, nucleic acid hybridization, and endocervical culture in Thayer–Martin media, the last currently being the most efficient screening test for *Neisseria gonorrhoeae* in women.

c Implications of testing

1 What does an abnormal test result mean?

A positive culture for *Neisseria gonorrhoeae* is diagnostic of infection and mandates treatment of the infected individual and her recent sexual contacts.

2 What does a normal test result mean?

A negative culture for *Neisseria gonorrhoeae* excludes the diagnosis.

b What is the cost of testing?

Testing and treating selected women with risk factors for gonorrhea reduces overall medical costs when the prevalence of infection exceeds 1.5%.

3 CONCLUSIONS AND RECOMMENDATIONS

Screening for *Neisseria gonorrhoeae* during pregnancy seems worthwhile because of the potential adverse effects on women and their offspring and since effective treatment is available for women with proven *Neisseria gonorrhoeae* infection. It only appears to be cost-effective, however, if the underlying prevalence of infection exceeds 1.5%.

REFERENCES

Armstey MS & Steadman KT (1976) Symptomatic gonorrhea and pregnancy. *J Am Vener Dis Assoc* **3:** 14–19.
Centers for Disease Control (1987) Disseminated gonorrhea caused by penicillinase-producing *Neisseria gonorrhoeae*–Wisconsin, Pennsylvania. *MMWR* **36:** 161–167.

Centers for Disease Control (1993) 1993 sexually transmitted diseases treatment guidelines. *MMWR* **42** (RR–14): 1–102.

Dans PE (1975) Gonococcal anogenital infection. *Clin Obstet Gynecol* **18**: 103–107.

Edwards LE, Barrada Ml, Hamann AA & Hakanson EY (1978) Gonorrhea in pregnancy. *Am J Obstet Gynecol* **132**: 637–641.

Holmes KK, Eschenbach DA & Knapp JS (1980) Salpingitis: overview of etiology and epidemiology. *Am J Obstet Gynecol* **138**: 893–900.

Hosein lK, Kaunitz AM & Craft SJ (1992) Detection of cervical *Chlamydia trachomatis* and *Neisseria gonorrhoeae* with deoxyribonucleic acid probe assays in obstetric patients. *Am J Obstet Gynecol* **167**: 588–91.

Olsen JV & Michael MF (1986) Experience with the modified solid-phase enzyme immunoassay for detection of gonorrhea in prostitutes. *Sex Trans Dis* **13**: 1–14.

Phillips RS, Safran C, Aronson MD, *et al.* (1989) Should women be tested for gonococcal infection of the cervix during routine gynecologic visits? An economic appraisal. *Am J Med* **86(3)**: 297–302.

Sarrel PM & Pruett KA (1968) Symptomatic gonorrhea during pregnancy. *Obstet Gynecol* **32**: 670–675.

Smith KR, Ching S, Lee H, Ohhashi Y, Hu H–Y, Fisher HC & Hook EW (1995) Evaluation of ligase chain reaction for use with urine for identification of *Neisseria gonorrhoeae* in females attending a sexually transmitted disease clinic. *J Clin Microbiol* **33(2)**: 455–457.

Spence MR (1983) Gonorrhea. *Clinic Obstet Gynecol* **25**: 111–124.

Stamm WE, Guinan ME & Johnson C (1984) Effect of treatment regimens for *Neisseria gonorrhoeae* on simultaneous infections with *Chlamydia trachomatis*. *N Eng J Med* **310**: 545–549.

Sweet RL & Gibb RS (1990) *Infectious Diseases of the Female Genital Tract*, 2nd edn, pp 109–143. Baltimore: Williams & Wilkins.

Washington AE, Browner WS & Korenbrot CC (1987) Cost-effectiveness of combined treatment for endocervical gonorrhea. *JAMA* **257**: 2056–2060.

Zenilman JM (1989) Gonorrhea and the resistance picture. *STD Bull* **9**: 3–10.

HIV Infection

WHAT IS THE PROBLEM THAT REQUIRES SCREENING?

ADULT AND PERINATAL TRANSMISSION OF HUMAN IMMUNODEFICIENCY VIRUS TYPE I (HIV).

What is the incidence/prevalence of the target condition?

Though the overall prevalence of acquired immunodeficiency syndrome (AIDS) is 10 times greater for men than for women (Centers for Disease Control, 1992), trends in HIV infection and AIDS in women are similar to those in men (Centers for Disease Control, 1992). In recent years, the difference has been narrowing and women now account for approximately 13% of all reported cases of AIDS (Centers for Disease Control, 1992). In Africa, where the disease is most prevalent, the male to female ratio of HIV infection is now 1:1 (Centers for Disease Control, 1992a). The male to female ratio in the USA depends on the population screened. The ratio is 5:1 among military recruit applicants in the Midwest, but almost 2:1 in major urban centers (Burte *et al.*, 1987). The prevalence of HIV does not differ appreciably by gender in injecting drug users who constitute the highest risk group that includes women (Centers for Disease Control, 1991a). The male to female ratio of AIDS among heterosexual adults decreases

Table 3.3 Risk factors for HIV.

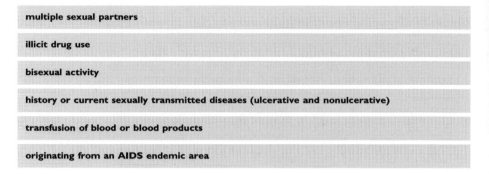

multiple sexual partners
illicit drug use
bisexual activity
history or current sexually transmitted diseases (ulcerative and nonulcerative)
transfusion of blood or blood products
originating from an AIDS endemic area

considerably excluding homosexual and bisexual transmission (Centers for Disease Control, 1992). Risk factors for acquiring HIV infection are listed in Table 3.3.

Acquired immune deficiency syndrome is increasing as a cause of childhood mortality. Gwinn *et al* (1991) estimated that 1.5 per 1 000 women in the USA giving birth in 1989 were infected with HIV. More recent prospective studies show vertical (maternal to fetal) transmission rates of 14–30% (Pizzo and Butler, 1991; European Collaborative Study, 1992; Gabiano *et al.*, 1992). The rate of transmission to infants by infected mothers increases with the clinical severity of maternal disease and is inversely proportional to the maternal CD4$^+$ T-lymphocyte count. Furthermore, disease progression in these infants varies directly with the disease severity in the mother at the time of delivery (Blanche *et al.*, 1994). Factors that may increase the perinatal transmission of HIV include CD4$^+$ cell counts of less than 400 per mm^3 and advanced maternal AIDS-defining illnesses (Blanche *et al.*, 1989).

What are the sequelae of the condition which are of interest in clinical medicine?

Spread of infection to sexual partners and offspring. Infection with HIV leads to a progressive debilitation of the immune system. In cohort studies of adults infected with HIV, clinical symptoms develop in 70–85% of HIV seropositive individuals, and AIDS develops in 55–62% within 12 years after infection (Centers for Disease Control and Prevention, 1993). An HIV infected patient is diagnosed as having AIDS when there is one of several specific opportunistic infections or neoplasia including cervical cancer, pulmonary tuberculosis, recurrent bacterial pneumonias, dementia and encephalopathy, wasting syndrome or CD4$^+$ cell counts of less than 200 mm^3 (Centers for Disease Control, 1991a; Centers for Disease Control and Prevention, 1992).

Patients with early HIV disease typically present without symptoms. As the duration of time infected progresses, laboratory evidence of immune deficiency increases; CD4$^+$ cell count and serum p24 antigen levels may be of prognostic value during this stage (MacDonell *et al.*, 1990). Anemia, neutropenia, or thrombocytopenia may occur. Women with HIV-associated thrombocytopenia can present with epistaxis, petechiae, and menorrhagia. Between 50–90% of individuals with acute primary HIV infection develop a nonspecific syndrome indistinguishable from influenza or infectious mononucleosis (Cooper *et al.*, 1985). Symptoms often include fever, arthralgias, myalgias and fatigue. Physical examination can reveal a diffuse erythematous rash as well as diffuse and symmetric adenopathy (Cooper *et al.*, 1985). As yet there is no specific therapy for patients presenting with this syndrome (Fox *et al.*, 1987; Tindel *et al.*, 1981) It is important for the clinician to initiate counseling and education for the prevention of further HIV transmission as well as facilitating continuing medical care at this time.

Early clinical manifestations of HIV infection in women may center on the genital tract. These manifestations include vulvovaginal candidiasis, pelvic inflammatory disease (PID), and cervical dysplasia (Maiman *et al.*, 1990; Witkin, 1991; Korn *et al.*, 1993). The medical management of vaginal candidiasis is not altered by HIV serostatus, and cure rates are similar to those seen in seronegative women. Pelvic inflammatory disease may pursue a more aggressive course in HIV infected women (Fox *et al.*, 1987). The CDC recommends that HIV infected women who develop PID be hospitalized early and treated aggressively with intravenous antibiotics (Hoegsberg *et al.*, 1990; Centers for Disease Control, 1991b). As with PID, the rate of HPV infection and cervical dysplasia is higher in HIV infected women (Vermund *et al.*, 1992). The Centers for Disease Control and Prevention (1993) recommend Pap smear screening of HIV infected women at their initial evaluation and in 6 months; women with normal Pap smears should thereafter undergo an annual Pap smear.

Patients with late HIV infection have a CD4$^+$ cell count between 50/mm^3 and 200 /mm^3. These patients have AIDS by the revised Centers for Disease Control and Prevention (1992) definition and are at high risk for a wide range of opportunistic infections including *Pneumocystis carinii* pneumonia, toxoplasmosis, lymphoma, and cryptococcal meningitis. Other viral infections such as herpes simplex virus and cytomegalovirus infection seem to be more common in women than men (Fleming *et al.*, 1993).

Patients with advanced HIV disease are defined by a CD4$^+$ cell count of less than 50/mm^3 and are at highest risk of developing a new AIDS-defining illness or dying within a 2 year period (Drew, 1991).

THE TESTS

What is the purpose of the tests?

To detect individuals infected with HIV.

The nature of the tests

There are three screening assays for the identification of HIV infection: enzyme-linked immunosorbent assay (ELISA), the rapid latex agglutination assay, and the dot-blot immunobinding assay (HIV CHEK). The three known confirmatory assays for HIV are Western blot, radioimmunoprecipitation assay (RIPA), and indirect immunofluorescence assay (IFA). The use of the ELISA screening test followed by the Western blot confirmatory test is standard for making the diagnosis of HIV in the USA. In many countries, including the USA, it is legally required that the individual's consent be obtained before HIV testing. In this respect, access to confidential or anonymous testing is advocated (Centers for Disease Control, 1985; Kegeles *et al.*, 1990). The Centers for Disease Control (1985) recommended that all reproductive age women at risk of HIV infection be counseled and tested for HIV.

SCREENING ASSAYS FOR HIV INFECTION

The ELISA detects HIV-specific antibodies in the serum. A similar technique, called capture ELISA, is used to measure the core antigen (p24) of HIV in the plasma of infected individuals. There is evidence that the maternal viral burden, as measured by either PCR or p24 antigenemia, is associated with an increased perinatal transmission risk (St Louis *et al.*, 1993). Furthermore, the risk of developing early and severe disease in the newborn is highest in women with serum p24 antigenemia (Borgard *et al.*, 1992).

The rapid latex agglutination assay and the dot-blot immunobinding assay for HIV infection are rapid tests and because their use does not require expensive laboratory equipment they are frequently used in the field and in less developed countries (Carlson *et al.*, 1987).

CONFIRMATORY ASSAYS FOR HIV INFECTION

A reactive Western blot confirmatory test in individuals with two sequentially positive ELISA screening tests requires the presence of at least two of three major bands: gp160 or gp120, gp41, and p24 (Centers for Disease Control, 1988). The absence of any bands indicates a false positive result, while the presence of a single HIV-1 related band indicates an indeterminate test.

The RIPA technique requires harvested HIV infected cells as well as radioisotopes. Its use is limited to established laboratories experienced in handling radioisotopes (Gaines *et al.*, 1987).

The IFA technique measures the human IgM antibody response and is preferred by some laboratories, having the advantage of being more sensitive than a Western blot (Pyun *et al.*, 1987). It is especially useful for the identification of early infection and active HIV infection in children where it is otherwise difficult to distinguish between the infant's IgM antibodies and passively transferred IgG antibodies of the mother (Lifson *et al.*, 1990).

Polymerase chain reaction is a highly sensitive technique which permits the amplification of the nucleic acid (genome) of HIV (Gaines *et al.*, 1987), and has been used to detect the viral genome in the fetus and neonate. However, contamination is a risk, yielding false positive test results (Lifson *et al.*, 1990).

Culture of HIV from the plasma of infected individuals is expensive, slow, and cumbersome, and therefore not widely used. Finally, the usefulness of serum IgA assay as an early diagnostic test for pediatric HIV infection has been investigated (Quinn *et al.*, 1991).

Implications of testing

WHAT DOES AN ABNORMAL TEST RESULT MEAN?

Data submitted by the manufacturers indicate that the sensitivity and specificity of the immunoassay test currently marketed in the USA are each greater than 99% (Centers for Disease Control, 1988). Repeating each initial reactive test increases the validity of the test by decreasing the likelihood of a laboratory error. A specificity of 99% for the ELISA test has been consistently reported in several laboratories across the USA (Centers for Disease Control, 1988). The use of the ELISA screening assay along with

Table 3.4 Contents of HIV counseling

discussion of the early manifestations of HIV infection
natural history and prognosis of HIV infection
institution of immediate medical care
emphasis on responsible sexual behavior and the notification of sexual partners as well as avoidance of sharing needles
prohibition from donating blood
notification of individual's HIV status in accordance with local statutory requirements

the Western blot confirmatory test for determining infection with HIV has a positive predictive value of 99.5% in both low-risk and high-risk populations (Schwartz *et al.*, 1988). The combined use of these tests for the diagnosis for HIV yields a false positive rate of less than 1 per 1000 individuals tested (Schwartz *et al.*, 1988).

Positive serology means the individual is infected with HIV. An individual with newly diagnosed HIV infection requires specific and extensive counseling at the time the results become known (Table 3.4). Apart from the medical implications, a person who tests positive for HIV may be confronted with the hostile social implications of HIV serostatus, including loss of life and health insurance, employment, friendships and family support. Therefore, HIV reports should be held in strict confidence. For HIV infected pregnant women, information on the risk of perinatal transmission and the possible effects of pregnancy on the progression of the disease is essential. Pregnant HIV infected women with CD4$^+$ cell counts of more than 200/mm^3 should be offered zidovudine (azidothymidine, AZT) treatment after appropriate counseling. Administration of AZT to the mother during pregnancy (100 mg orally five times daily), labor and delivery (2 mg per kg of body weight given intravenously over a 1-hour period, then 1 mg/kg per hour until delivery), and to the newborn (2 mg/kg orally every 6 hours for 6 weeks after delivery) reduces the risk of perinatal transmission of HIV by two-thirds and presents a powerful argument for routine screening (Connor *et al.*, 1994). Although women with HIV infection may transmit the virus through breast milk, the clinical significance of this finding remains to be established (European Collaborative Study, 1992; Gabiano *et al.*, 1992).

Longterm follow-up for women with HIV infection should incorporate the medical, gynecological, psychological, and social implications of HIV infection. These include frequent Pap smears, appropriate vaccination, antiviral therapy and prophylactic antibiotic therapy when needed, and ongoing counseling about HIV infection, as well as referral for psychotherapy or peer support group therapy. Issues concerning physical wellbeing and loss of function, child care and custody arrangements, and death and dying, should be discussed with patients who have advanced HIV disease (Ybarra, 1991). Within the context of a comprehensive AIDS prevention program a discussion of the importance of HIV counseling and testing of sexual partners is also essential (Giesecke *et al.*, 1991; Brandeau *et al.*, 1992).

Repeat testing should be offered to individuals whose test results are inconclusive due to the lack of sufficient criteria for serologic diagnosis (Schwarz *et al.*, 1988). These women will require counseling and reassurance during this additional waiting period.

What does a normal test result mean?

Given the high sensitivity of the currently available immunoassays, HIV infection is virtually ruled out in women with negative test results. Women with HIV infection rarely have negative test results (Table 3.5). The false negative rate is due to the prolonged incubation period of HIV which may last 6–12 weeks (Centers for Disease Control, 1987). Additional testing for HIV type 2 should be conducted in patients with clinical evidence of HIV disease in the absence of a positive test for antibodies to HIV type 1 (Centers for Disease Control and Prevention, 1993). If the individual is engaged in risk behaviors (see Table 3.3) she should be retested within 6 months. Information concerning the probability of a false negative test should be provided to the women at risk (Table 3.5).

Table 3.5 Test performance of screening assays to identify HIV infection. Hypothetical example among 100 000 pregnant women, given a test sensitivity of 99.5%, test specificity of 99.5% and a prevalence of 150 per 100 000 pregnancies (0.15%).

	HIV INFECTION PRESENT	HIV INFECTION ABSENT	
screening test positive	149	499	648
screening test negative	1	99 351	99 352
	150	99 850	100 000

Positive predictive value: 149/648 × 100 = 23%; Negative predictive value: 99 351/99 352 × 100 = 100%; Probability of HIV infection in the individual tested negative: 0.001% (in a population with a HIV prevalence of 0.15%) to 0.005% (in a population with a HIV prevalence of 1%)

What is the cost of testing?

Cost-effectiveness of universal screening for HIV infection depends on the prevalence of the disease. If one considers a screening program in a population with a 1% HIV prevalence, assuming that the cost of screening and counseling is US $40 per woman screened, the cost of identifying 10 HIV positive women is approximately $40 000. If the identification of these 10 women leads to just one less case of HIV infection among their adult contacts, and the discounted future earnings of such an adult equals $500 000, then the $40 000 spent on testing and counseling yields $500 000 in indirect economic savings. Based on similar statistics, sensitivity analyses have revealed that screening women at medium and high risk (i.e. with an underlying HIV prevalence of at least 0.14%) is likely to be cost-beneficial (Brandeau *et al.*, 1992). Screening and institution of AZT during pregnancy and labor and delivery would also be cost-beneficial if one takes into account the enormous cost, both economical and social, of newborn and infant morbidity and mortality from perinatal transmission.

CONCLUSIONS AND RECOMMENDATIONS

The rate of HIV infection and AIDS is increasing in women of reproductive age and their children. For this reason, obstetricians and gynecologists are assuming a central role in the testing and counseling of women at risk for HIV infection. Standard testing in the USA includes an initial ELISA screen which should be repeated if positive. No antibody test result is considered a true positive until a Western blot confirmatory assay has been performed and is reactive.

Counseling of the HIV infected patient should be comprehensive, including medical and psychosocial aspects of coping with the disease. Both asymptomatic and symptomatic patients may transmit HIV to their offspring. Women infected with HIV who are contemplating pregnancy or considering pregnancy termination should be extensively counseled according to their clinical and immunologic status. In HIV infected women with CD4$^+$ cell counts above 200 cells per mm^3, AZT treatment significantly reduces the risk of perinatal transmission (Connor et al., 1994). Women who test negative for HIV but continue to engage in high-risk behaviors should be offered repeat testing for themselves and their sexual partners within 6 months. An emphasis on the need for responsible sexual behavior and the avoidance of sharing needles must be included in their post-test counseling session.

SUMMARY

1 WHAT IS THE PROBLEM THAT REQUIRES SCREENING?

ADULT AND PERINATAL TRANSMISSION OF HUMAN IMMUNODEFICIENCY VIRUS TYPE I (HIV).

a What is the incidence/prevalence of the target condition?

Women account for approximately 13% of all reported cases of AIDS. An estimated 1.5 per 1000 US women giving birth in 1989 were infected with HIV. Several prospective studies show relatively uniform maternal to fetal transmission rates of 14–30%.

b What are the sequelae of the condition which are of interest in clinical medicine?

Infection with HIV causes progressive debilitation of the immune system. An HIV infected patient with one of several specific opportunistic infections or neoplasia, including cervical cancer, tuberculosis, recurrent bacterial pneumonia, dementia, encephalopathy, wasting syndrome, or CD4$^+$ cell counts of less than 200/mm^3, is diagnosed as having AIDS. Early clinical manifestations of HIV infection in women may center on the genital tract. These include vulvovaginal candidiasis, pelvic inflammatory disease (PID), and cervical dysplasia.

2 THE TESTS

a What is the purpose of the tests?

To detect individuals infected with HIV.

b The nature of the tests

The ELISA detects HIV-specific antibodies in the serum of individuals who are tested. An ELISA screening assay coupled to a Western blot test has a positive predictive value of 99.5% in both low-risk and high-risk populations.

c Implications of testing

1 What does an abnormal test result mean?

A possible ELISA screening assay together with a reactive Western blot test indicates that this woman is infected with HIV. The diagnosis requires specific and extensive counseling. Longterm follow-up for women with HIV infection should incorporate the medical, gynecologic, psychological, and social implications of HIV infection. A discussion of the importance of HIV counseling and testing of sexual partners is essential.

2 What does a normal test result mean?

Women with HIV infection rarely have negative test results. The false negative rate is due to the prolonged incubation period of HIV which may last 6–12 weeks. Repeat testing should be offered to women whose tests are inconclusive. Information concerning false negative tests should be provided to women whose results are negative.

d What is the cost of testing?

Screening, sexual contact tracing, and institution of AZT therapy during pregnancy, labor, and delivery is cost-beneficial in women at medium to high risk (i.e. with an underlying HIV prevalence of 0.14%), if one takes into account the enormous cost, both economical and social, of newborn and infant morbidity and mortality from perinatal transmission.

3 CONCLUSIONS AND RECOMMENDATIONS

The rate of HIV infection and AIDS is increasing in reproductive age women and their children. Standard testing in the USA includes an initial ELISA screen which if positive should be repeated. No antibody test result should be considered a true positive unless a Western blot confirmatory assay has been performed and is reactive. The demonstration that AZT dramatically reduces the risk of perinatal transmission strongly favors routine screening for HIV during pregnancy.

REFERENCES

Blanche S, Rouzioux C, Moscato ML *et al.* (1989) A prospective study of infants born to women seropositive for human immunodeficiency virus type 1. HIV infections in newborns French collaborative study group. *N Engl J Med* **320**: 1643–1648.

Blanche S, Mayaux MJ, Rouzioux C *et al.* (1994) Relation of the course of HIV infection in children to the severity of the disease in their mothers at delivery. *N Engl J Med* **330**: 308–312.

Borgard M, Mayaux MJ, Blanche S *et al.* (1992) The use of viral culture and p24 antigen testing to diagnose human immunodeficiency virus infection in neonates. *N Engl J Med* **327**: 1192–1197.

Brandeau ML, Owens DK, Sox CH & Wachter RM (1992) Screening women of childbearing age for human immunodeficiency virus. A cost benefit analysis. *Arch Intern Med* **152**: 2229–2237.

Burke DS, Brundage JF, Herbold JR *et al.* (1987) Human immunodeficiency virus (HIV) infection among civilian applicants for United States military service. October 1985 to March 1986. Demographic factors associated with seropositivity. *N Engl J Med* **317**: 131–136.

Carlson JR, Yee JL, Watson-Williams EJ *et al.* (1987) Rapid, easy, and economical screening tests for antibodies to human immunodeficiency virus. *Lancet* **i**: 361–362.

Centers for Disease Control (1985) Recommendations for assisting in the prevention of perinatal transmission of human T-lymphotropic virus type III/lymphadenopathy associated virus and the acquired immunodeficiency virus syndrome. *MMWR* 34: 721–726, 731–732.

Centers for Disease Control (1987) Public Health Services guidelines for counseling and antibody testing to prevent HIV infection and AIDS. *MMWR* 36: 509–515.

Centers for Disease Control (1988) Update: serologic testing for antibody to human immunodeficiency virus. *MMWR* 36: 833–848.

Centers for Disease Control (1991a) *National HIV Serosurveillance Summary: Results Through 1990.* Atlanta, Ga: Division of HIV/AIDS.

Centers for Disease Control (1991b) Pelvic inflammatory disease: guidelines for prevention and management. *MMWR* 40: 1–24.

Centers for Disease Control (1992a) Update: acquired immunodeficiency syndrome – United States, 1991. *MMWR* 41: 463–468.

Centers for Disease Control and Prevention (1992b) 1993 revised classification system for HIV infection and expanded surveillance case definition for AIDS among adolescents and adults. *MMWR* **41 (RR-17):** 1–19.

Centers for Disease Control and Prevention 1993 sexually transmitted diseases treatment guidelines. *MMWR* **42(RR14):** 1–102.

Connor EM, Sperling RS, Gelber R, *et al.* (1994) Reduction of maternal-infant transmission of human immunodeficiency virus type 1 with zidovudine treatment. *N Engl J Med* 331: 1173–1180.

Cooper DA, Maclean P, Finlayson R, *et al.* (1985) Acute AIDS retrovirus infection. *Lancet* 1: 537–541.

Drew LJ. Cytomegalovirus infection in patients with AIDS (1991) *Clin Infect Dis* 14: 608–615.

European Collaborative Study 1992 Risk factors for mother-to-child transmission *Lancet* 339: 1007–1012.

Fleming PL, Ciesielski C, Byers RH, Castro KG & Berelmen RL (1993) Gender differences in reported AIDS-indicative diagnosis. *J Infect Dis* 168: 61–67.

Fox R, Eldred LJ, Fuchs EJ, *et al.* (1987) Clinical manifestations of acute infection with human immunodeficiency virus in a cohort of gay men. *AIDS* 1: 35–38.

Gabiano C, Tovo P-A, de Martino M *et al.* (1992) Mother-to-child transmission of Human Immunodeficiency Virus type 1: Risk of infection and correlates of transmission. *Pediatrics* 90: 369–374.

Gaines H, von Sydow M, Sonnerberg A, *et al.* (1987) Antibody response in primary human immunodeficiency virus infection. *Lancet* 1: 1249–1253.

Giesecke J, Ramstedt K, Granath F, Ripa T, Rado G & Westrell M (1991) Efficacy of partner notification for HIV infection. *Lancet* 338: 1096–1100.

Gwinn M, Papaioanou M, George JR, *et al.* (1991) Prevalence of HIV infection in childbearing women in the United States. Surveillance using newborn blood samples. *JAMA* 265: 1704–1708.

Hoegsberg B, Abulafia O, Sedlis A, *et al.* (1990) Sexually transmitted diseases and human immunodeficiency virus infection among women with pelvic inflammatory disease. *Am J Obstet Gynecol* 163: 1135–1139.

Kegeles SM, Catania JA, Coates TJ, Pollack LM & Lo B (1990) Many people who seek anonymous HIV-antibody testing would avoid it under other circumstances. *AIDS* 4: 585–588.

Korn AP, Landers DV, Green JR & Sweet RL (1993) Pelvic inflammatory disease in human immunodeficiency virus-infected women. *Obstet Gynecol* 82 765–768.

Lifson AR, Stanley M, Pane J, *et al.* (1990) Detection of human immunodeficiency virus DNA using the polymerase chain reaction in a well-characterized group of homosexual and bisexual men. *J Infect Dis* 161: 436–439.

MacDonell KB, Chmiel JS, Poggensee L, *et al.* (1990) Predicting progression to AIDS: combined usefulness of CD4 + lymphocyte counts and p24 antigenemia. *Am J Med* 322: 166–172.

Maiman J, Fruchter RG, Serur E, Remy JC, Fever G & Boyce JG (1990) Human immunodeficiency virus and cervical neoplasia. *Obstet Gynecol* 38: 377–382.

Pizzo PA & Butler KM (1991) In the vertical transmission of HIV, timing may be everything. *N Engl J Med* 325: 652–653.

Pyun KH, Ochs HD, Dufford MTW, *et al.* (1987) Perinatal infection with human immunodeficiency virus: specific antibody responses by the neonate. *N Engl J Med* 317: 611–614.

Quinn TC, Kline RL, Halsey N, *et al.* (1991) Early diagnosis of perinatal HIV infection by detection of viral specific IgA antibodies. *JAMA* 266 3439–3442.

Schwartz JS, Dars PE & Kinosian BP (1988) Human immunodeficiency virus test evaluation, performance, and use: proposals to make good tests better. *JAMA* 259: 2574–2579.

St. Louis ME, Kamenga M, Brown C, *et al.* (1993) Risk for perinatal HIV–1 transmission according to maternal immunologic, virologic and placental factors. *JAMA* 269: 2853–2859.

Tindall B, Gaines H, Inrie A, *et al.* (1991) Zidovudine in the management of primary HIV–1 infection. *AIDS* 5: 477–484.

Vermund ST, Kelly KF, Klein RS, *et al.* (1992) High risk of human papillomavirus infection and cervical squamous intraepithelial lesions among women with symptomatic human immunodeficiency virus infection. *Am J Obstet Gynecol* 166: 1232–1237.

Witkin SS (1991) Immunologic factors influencing susceptibility to recurrent candida vaginitis. *Clin Obstet Gynecol* **34**: 662–668.
Ybarra S (1991) Women and AIDS: implications for counseling. *J Counsel Dev* **69**: 285–287.

Chlamydial Infection

WHAT IS THE PROBLEM THAT REQUIRES SCREENING?

UROGENITAL TRACT CHLAMYDIAL INFECTION.

What is the incidence/prevalence of the target condition?

Urogenital tract chlamydial infection is the most common sexually transmitted disease in the USA (Cates and Wasserheit, 1991). The prevalence of *Chlamydia trachomatis* infection varies widely from 3% in asymptomatic women to 25% in women attending sexually transmitted disease clinics (Stamm and Holmes, 1990). Approximately 3 million women and 250 000 newborns are infected on a yearly basis (Washington *et al.*, 1986). Exposure to *Chlamydia trachomatis* is more common than to *Neisseria gonorrhoeae*. The prevalence of serum antibodies to *Chlamydia trachomatis* increases up to approximately age 30 years (Stamm and Holmes, 1990). Washington *et al.* (1986) observed that the ratio of *Chlamydia trachomatis* to *Neisseria gonorrhoeae* infection is influenced by age, sex, race, pregnancy status, choice of contraception, proportion of asymptomatic infection, and sexual preference. In Britain 7–12% of women in childbearing years have been found to be infected, but these figures may be biased since they involved clinically based prevalence studies (Taylor-Robinson, 1994). In Sweden, genital chlamydia infection is a notifiable disease. In 1988, the reported rate of 'diagnosed' female genital *Chlamydia trachomatis* infection in Sweden was 603 per 100 000 inhabitants (0.6%) (Ripa, 1990). Since the introduction of a widespread screening programe, involving women below 30 years of age, the prevalence of genital *Chlamydia trachomatis* infection decreased substantially (Ripa, 1990; Taylor-Robinson, 1994).

Chlamydial infection is more common in the young, the poor, unmarried pregnant women, oral contraceptive users, and women with multiple sex partners (Thompson and Washington, 1983; Washington *et al.*, 1985). Young women who use a barrier method of contraception are at reduced risk (Washington *et al.*, 1985). Recently, clinical characteristics predictive of chlamydial infection in women attending sexually transmitted disease clinics have been described (Handsfield *et al.*, 1986). These include women below 24 years of age, those with a new sex partner during the 2 months preceding infection, with a mucopurulent cervical discharge, with bleeding from the cervix on contact with a swab, and sexually active women who either do not use contraception or use a nonbarrier method of contraception.

The epidemiology of *Chlamydia trachomatis* infection has been extensively studied in women attending prenatal clinics (Frommell *et al.*, 1979; Martin *et al.*, 1982). The prevalence of chlamydial infection of the endocervix in pregnant women ranges from 2% to 37% (Cohen *et al.*, 1990). There is an inverse relationship between age and the prevalence of endocervical infection in pregnant women. An association between *Trichomonas vaginalis* infection and concurrent chlamydial endocervical infection has been established (Judson, 1979).

What are the sequelae of the condition which are of interest in clinical medicine?

In women, chlamydial infection is frequently asymptomatic. Numerous clinical conditions have been attributed to *Chlamydia trachomatis* (Schachter and Grossman, 1983). These include acute urethral syndrome, urethritis, mucopurulent endocervicitis, salpingitis, endometritis, and prenatal infection (see below). The endocervix is the most commonly infected organ in the female. In the 1970s, Swedish investigators began the laparoscopic biopsy of the fallopian tubes in women with presumed pelvic inflammatory disease. Their results suggested that *Chlamydia trachomatis* caused up to a third of all PID cases (Mardh *et al.*, 1977). In the USA, rigorous studies employing endometrial biopsy, laparoscopy and fallopian tubes culture in addition to endocervical culture yielded similar results (Wasserheit *et al.*, 1986). Acute PID increases the risk of chronic pelvic pain, infertility and ectopic pregnancy (Westrom, 1980; Svensson *et al.*, 1983). Many experts now believe that *Chlamydia trachomatis* is the most important organism involved in tubal scarring since it appears to cause a mild form of PID associated with delayed diagnosis and treatment.

The natural history of *Chlamydia trachomatis* infection in pregnancy is not well known. Infection may increase the risk of preterm rupture of the membranes, low birthweight and perinatal mortality, but carefully controlled studies are needed to confirm these findings (Ryan *et al.*, 1990). Moreover, there are only limited data regarding the effectiveness of treatment regimens for *Chlamydia trachomatis* infection in pregnancy (Ryan *et al.*, 1990; Centers for Disease Control and Prevention, 1993). Up to 70% of newborns vaginally delivered to infected women acquire chlamydia during birth (Schacter *et al.*, 1986). Conjunctivitis occurs within the first 2 weeks of life in 20–50% of exposed infants; pneumonia occurs within 3–4 months in 10–20% of exposed infants (Schacter *et al.*, 1986).

THE TESTS

What is the purpose of the tests?

To detect urogenital chlamydial infection in asymptomatic and symptomatic women.

The nature of the tests

Methods used for detection of chlamydial infection include tissue culture isolation of the organism, direct fluorescent antibody test (DFA), enzyme immunoassay test (EIA), nucleic acid hybridization assay (Gen-Probe PACE 2 test) and amplification techniques such as polymerase chain reaction (PCR) or ligase chain reaction (LCR). While the currently accepted 'gold standard' diagnostic test is tissue culture isolation, amplification techniques such as PCR and LCR may become the diagnostic test of choice in the future (Wiesenfeld *et al.*, 1994). As most chlamydial infections are asymptomatic, detection requires screening at the time of a pelvic examination. Harrison *et al.* (1985) reported that over 50% of endocervical chlamydial infections are not associated with a clinically detectable inflammatory response. Brunham *et al.* (1984) noted that a yellow discharge on a swab and/or 10 or more white blood cells per oil immersion field on a Gram-stained smear of endocervical secretions is indicative of chlamydial cervical infection. These observations apply to pregnant women, although the predictive value of clinical cervicitis for chlamydial infection during pregnancy appears to be lower than in nonpregnant women (Kiviat *et al.*, 1985).

The currently accepted standard laboratory test for the detection of *Chlamydia trachomatis* is culture in mammalian cell lines. Centrifugation and sensitization of cell monolayers to the polycation diethyl aminoethyl (DEAE) prior to inoculation improves the yield. In addition to proper technique, special precautions must be taken to collect and transport clinical specimens properly. Wooden swabs containing chemicals that are toxic to cell cultures must be avoided; the tips should be constructed of Dacron. Because *Chlamydia trachomatis* is sensitive to temperature and loses viability rapidly at room temperature, specimens should be placed in a refrigerator at 4°C as soon as possible. The specimen should either be transported to the laboratory within 24 hours or frozen at −70°C and shipped on dry ice. These requirements make tissue culture isolation of chlamydia cumbersome and costly.

The nonculture diagnostic tests commonly used for the detection of *Chlamydia trachomatis* include antigen detection tests such as EIA and DFA, nucleic acid hybridization assay that detects chlamydial ribosomal RNA (Gen-Probe PACE 2), and amplification techniques such as PCR or LCR. The DFA test uses fluorescein-labeled monoclonal antibodies directed against major outer membrane proteins of chlamydial elementary bodies. Positive cells are identified under a fluorescent microscope. A positive test has at least 10 complexes. The sensitivity of this test ranges from 68%–100%, while its specificity is greater than 95% (Barnes, 1989; Taylor-Robinson and Thomas, 1991). The DFA test has the advantages of not requiring special storage or transportation, a rapid result, and lower costs compared with culture. Its disadvantages include a higher false positive rate and the need for an experienced microscopist.

Enzyme immunoassays are often used to detect *chlamydia* antigens. The sensitivity of EIA ranges from 64% to 100%, while its specificity ranges from 89% to 100% (Taylor-Robinson and Thomas, 1991). Cross-reactivity with antigenic components in Gram-negative organisms has been reported (Rothburn *et al.*, 1986). Results of EIA tests are available within 4 hours, are objectively interpreted, and require less expertise than DFA or cell culture.

Nucleic acid probes have also been developed for the detection of *Chlamydia*. A study comparing two such probes, the MicroTrak EIA and the Gen-Probe PACE 2, with cell culture revealed that both assays were significantly less sensitive than culture (Clarke *et al.*, 1993). The sensitivity (with culture as the 'gold standard') for the Gen-Probe PACE 2 is 75–80%, while the specificity is greater than 95% (Clarke *et al.*, 1993). In a high-prevalence female population (22.1%) the positive and negative predictive values are 90–94%.

Amplification techniques such as PCR and LCR are perhaps the diagnostic tools of the future. The sensitivity of PCR approaches 100% compared with cell culture (Ostergaard *et al.*, 1990). A study by Roosendaal *et al.* (1994) found that PCR was a suitable method to test for cure, with a specificity approaching 100%. In another study, the positive and negative predictive values of PCR were 100% and 99% (Wiesenfeld *et al.*, 1994). Analysis using PCR is easily performed and gives results within 1 day.

Implications of testing

WHAT DOES AN ABNORMAL TEST RESULT MEAN?

The woman probably is infected with *Chlamydia trachomatis*. The use of commercial assays may be associated with false positive test results. Hence, the patient should be evaluated, counseled and appropriately treated as should any recent sexual partners to prevent reinfection. The recommended treatment for uncomplicated urethral, endocervical or rectal chlamydial infection in the nonpregnant patient is doxycyline (100 mg orally two times daily for 7 days) or azithromycin (1 g orally in a single dose). During pregnancy, either erythromycin base (500 mg orally four times daily for 7 days) or amoxicillin (500 mg orally three times daily for 7–10 days) can be used (Centers for Disease Control and Prevention, 1993). The results of treatment with a single dose of azithromicin during pregnancy are encouraging (Bush and Rosa, 1994).

The patient should also be tested for other sexually transmitted diseases, including syphilis, gonorrhea and HIV. Because resistant organisms have not been reported, a test of cure is currently not recommended by the CDC, unless symptoms persist or reinfection is suspected (Centers for Disease Control and Prevention, 1993). In contrast, repeat testing in pregnancy is recommended preferably by culture, as erythromycin may not be completely effective in eradicating infection. Moreover, the frequent gastrointestinal side effects of erythromycin may have an effect on compliance with treatment.

WHAT DOES A NORMAL TEST RESULT MEAN?

It is unlikely that the woman with a normal test result is infected with *Chlamydia trachomatis*. However, false negative results do occur because of the small numbers of micro-organisms. Furthermore, the sensitivity of the commercially available assays ranges widely. Detection of infection by amplification techniques (PCR or LCR) on urine specimens is noninvasive and may become an attractive screening tool in the future (Lee *et al.*, 1995). The main disadvantage of amplification techniques is their susceptibility to laboratory contamination.

What is the cost of testing?

The total costs (direct and indirect) of female urogenital chlamydial infection in 1986 were estimated to exceed US $2 billion per year (Washington *et al.*, 1987). Women who are culture positive for *chlamydia* frequently have other sexually transmitted diseases. Concomitant testing and treatment for *Neisseria gonorrhoeae* infection is cost effective (Washington *et al.*, 1981).

In low prevalence populations (i.e. with prevalences below 2–7%), several investigators have shown that selective screening based on risk factors is less costly than routine screening and would still detect more than 90% of cases (Phillips *et al.*, 1987; Sellors *et al.*, 1992). These risk factors include cervical friability, a suspicious discharge, urinary frequency, intermenstrual bleeding and a new sexual partner within the past year. Antigen detection techniques such as EIA are of similar sensitivity but cost less than culture (Phillips *et al.*, 1987; Ripa, 1990; Sellors *et al.*, 1992).

Gene amplification techniques such as PCR may become the diagnostic test of choice. The material and labor costs of performing PCR depends on the number of samples. In most centers, the total cost should approximate US $20 per test, somewhat more expensive than the cost of an EIA but much less than cell culture.

CONCLUSIONS AND RECOMMENDATIONS

In women *Chlamydia trachomatis* infection is usually asymptomatic but may cause several common sexually transmitted disease syndromes, including mucopurulent cervicitis, urethritis, and pelvic inflammatory disease. There is strong evidence that *Chlamydia trachomatis* is an important cause of obstructive infertility and ectopic pregnancy and that these complications result from chronic inflammation and secondary scarring elicited by longterm, asymptomatic infection. The effect of chlamydial infection on pregnancy outcome is obscure. In order to prevent postpartum complications and chlamydial infection among newborns, the Centers for Disease Control and Prevention (1993) recommend testing pregnant women below 25 years of age, or those with a new or more than one partner, during the first trimester. The total cost of disease is large. Since treatment with tetracycline, erythromycin or azithromycin is simple, cost-effective and inexpensive, major efforts should be made to identify infected but asymptomatic women. High-risk categories include sexually active young women, older women who are not monogamous, and unmarried pregnant women. Selective screening based on risk factors is effective even in low prevalence settings (i.e. below 2–7%). Male sexual partners of infected women must also be treated, and these women should be screened for other sexually transmitted diseases.

SUMMARY

1 WHAT IS THE PROBLEM THAT REQUIRES SCREENING?

CHLAMYDIAL INFECTION.

a What is the incidence/prevalence of the target condition?

Chlamydial infection is the most common sexually transmitted disease in the USA. Risk factors for chlamydial infection include age, socioeconomic status, number of sexual partners and nonbarrier contraception. Up to 70% of infants delivered vaginally to women with chlamydia acquire the infection.

b What are the sequelae of the condition which are of interest in clinical medicine?

Acute urethral syndrome, urethritis, mucopurulent endocervicitis, salpingitis, endometritis and prenatal infections are attributed to *Chlamydia trachomatis*. However, most chlamydial infections are asymptomatic. The effect of *Chlamydia trachomatis* infection on pregnancy outcome is unclear. Infants born to mothers who have untreated *Chlamydia trachomatis* infection are at increased risk of conjunctivitis and pneumonia.

2 THE TESTS

a What is the purpose of the tests?

To detect urogenital chlamydial infection.

b The nature of the tests

The current 'gold standard' test for the detection of *Chlamydia trachomatis* is culture. The nonculture diagnostic tests commonly used for the detection of *Chlamydia trachomatis* include antigen detection tests such as EIA and DFA, nucleic acid hybridization assay (Gen-Probe

PACE 2) and amplification techniques such as PCR or LCR. Amplification techniques such as PCR and LCR may become the diagnostic tools of choice in the future.

c Implications of testing

1 What does an abnormal test result mean?

The woman probably has an infection with Chlamydia trachomatis and should be treated with antibiotics. Affected patients should be instructed to refer their sexual partners for evaluation and treatment. The nonculture diagnostic tests are associated with false positive results.

2 What does a normal test result mean?

Infection with Chlamydia trachomatis is unlikely, although false negative test results may occur.

d What is the cost of testing?

The total cost of chlamydial infection in women has been projected at over $2 billion (US, 1986) per year.

3 CONCLUSIONS AND RECOMMENDATIONS

Chlamydia trachomatis causes a number of common sexually transmitted disease syndromes, including mucopurulent cervicitis, urethritis, and pelvic inflammatory disease. High-risk categories include sexually active young women, older women who are not monogamous, and unmarried pregnant women. Male sexual partners of infected women should also be treated to prevent reinfection, and infected women should be screened for other sexually transmitted diseases. In low prevalence areas (i.e. with an underlying prevalence of 2% or less) selective screening in nonpregnant women is cost-effective. In pregnant women at increased risk (i.e. those under 25 years of age, and those with a new or more than one partner) testing for Chlamydia trachomatis during the first trimester is recommended.

REFERENCES

Barnes RC (1989) Laboratory diagnosis of human chlamydial infections. *Clin Microbiol Rev* 2: 119–136.
Brunham RC, Paavonen J, Stevens CE *et al.* (1984) Mucopurulent cervicitis: the ignored counterpart in women of urethritis in men. *N Eng J Med* 311: 1–6.
Bush MR & Rosa C (1994) Azithromycin and erythromycin in the treatment of cervical chlamydial infection during pregnancy. *Obstet Gynecol* 84: 61–63.
Cates W Jr & Wasserheit JN (1991) Genital chlamydial infection: epidemiology and reproductive sequelae. *Am J Obstet Gynecol* 164: 1771–1781.
Centers for Disease Control and Prevention (1993) 1993 sexually transmitted diseases treatment guidelines. *MMWR* 42 (RR14): 1–102.
Clarke LM, Sierra MF, Daidone BJ *et al.* (1993) Comparison of the Syva MicroTrak enzyme immunoassay and GEN-PROBE PACE 2 with cell culture for diagnosis of cervical *Chlamydia trachomatis* infection in a high prevalence population. *J Clin Microbiol* 31 (2): 968–971.
Cohen I, Veille JC & Calkins BM (1990) Improved pregnancy outcome following successful treatment of chlamydial infection. *JAMA* 263: 3160–3168.
Frommell OT, Rothenberg R, Wang SP *et al.* (1979) Chlamydial infections of mothers and their infants. *J Pediatr* 95: 28–32.
Handsfield HH, Jasman LL, Roberts PL *et al.* (1986) Criteria for selective screening for *Chlamydia trachomatis* infection in women attending family planning clinics. *JAMA* 255: 1730–1734.
Harrison HR, Costin M, Meder JB *et al.* (1985) Cervical *Chlamydia trachomatis* infection in university

women: relationship to history, contraception, ectopy and cervicitis. *Am J Obstet Gynecol* **153**: 244–251.

Judson FN (1979) The importance of coexisting syphilitic, chlamydial, mycoplasmal, and trichomonal infections in the treatment of gonorrhea. *Sex Transm Dis* **6**(Suppl 2): 112–119.

Kiviat NB, Paavonen JA, Brokway J et al. (1985) Cytologic manifestations of cervical and vaginal infections. I Epithelial and inflammatory cellular changes. *JAMA* **253**: 989–996.

Lee HH, Chernesky MA, Schachter J et al. (1995) Diagnosis of *Chlamydia trachomatis* genitourinary infection in women by ligase chain reaction assay of urine. Lancet **345**: 213–16.

Mardh PA, Ripa T, Svensson L & Westrom L (1977) *Chlamydia trachomatis* infections in patients with acute salpingitis. *N Engl J Med* **296**: 1377–1379.

Martin DH, Koutsky L, Eschenbach DA et al. (1982) Prematurity and perinatal mortality in pregnancies complicated by maternal *Chlamydia trachomatis* infections. *JAMA* **247**: 1585–88.

Ostergaard L, Birkelond S & Christiansen G (1990) Use of PCR for detection of *Chlamydia trachomatis*. *J Clin Microbiol* **28**: 1254–1260.

Phillips RS, Aronson MD, Taylor WC et al. (1987) Should test for *Chlamydia trachomatis* cervical infection be done during routine gynecological visits? *Ann Intern Med* **107**: 188–194.

Ripa T (1990) Epidemiologic control of genital *Chlamydia trachomatis* infection. *Scand J Infect Dis* **69** (suppl): 157–167.

Roosendaal R, Walboomers JMN, Velman OR et al. (1994) Comparison of different sets for detection of *Chlamydia trachomatis* by the polymerase chain reaction. *J Med Microbiol* **38**: 1–8.

Rothburn MM, Mallison H & Multon KJ (1986) False positive ELISA for *Chlamydia trachomatis* recognized by atypical morphology on fluorescent staining. Lancet **1**: 982–983.

Ryan GM Jr, Abdella TN, McNeeley SG, Baselski VS & Brummond DE (1990) *Chlamydia trachomatis* infection in pregnancy and effect of treatment on outcome. *Am J Obstet Gynecol* **162**: 34–39.

Schacter J & Grossman M (1983) Chlamydia. In Remington J & Klein JO (eds) *Infections of the Fetus and Newborn*, 2nd edn, pp 450–463 Philadelphia: WB Saunders.

Schacter J, Grossman M, Sweet RL et al. (1986) Prospective study of perinatal transmission of *Chlamydia trachomatis*. *JAMA* **255**: 3374–3377.

Sellors JW, Pickard L, Gafni A et al. (1992) Effectiveness and efficiency of selective vs universal screening for chlamydial infection in sexually active young women. *Arch Intern Med* **152**: 1837–1844.

Stamm WE & Holmes KK (1990) *Chlamydia trachomatis* infections of the adult. In: Holmes KK, Mardh P-A, Sparling PF, Wiesner PJ, eds. *Sexually Transmitted Diseases*. 2nd ed. New York: McGraw-Hill, 1087–1095.

Svensson L, Westrom L, Ripa KT & Mardh PA (1980) Differences in some clinical and laboratory parameters in acute salpingitis related to culture and serologic findings. *Am J Obstet Gynecol* **138**: 1017–1021.

Svensson L, Mardh PA & Westrom L (1983) Infertility after acute salpingitis with special reference to *Chlamydia trachomatis*. *Fertil Steril* **40**: 322–325.

Taylor-Robinson D (1994) *Chlamydia trachomatis* and sexually transmitted disease. *Br Med J* **308**: 150–151.

Taylor-Robinson D & Thomas BJ (1991) Laboratory techniques for the diagnosis of chlamydial infections. *Genitourin Med* **67**: 256–266.

Thompson SE & Washington AE (1983) Epidemiology of sexually transmitted *Chlamydia trachomatis* infections. *Epidemol Rev* **5**: 96–123.

Washington AE, Browner WS & Korenbrot CC (1981) Cost-effectiveness of combined treatment for endocervical gonorrhea. *JAMA* **257**: 2056–2060.

Washington AE, Gove S, Schacter J & Sweet RL (1985) Oral contraceptives, *Chlamydia trachomatis* infection, and pelvic inflammatory disease: a word of caution about protection. *JAMA* **253**: 2246–2250.

Washington AE, Johnson RE, Sanders LL et al. (1986) Incidence of *Chlamydia trachomatis* infections in the United States: using reported *Neisseria gonorrhea* as a surrogate. In Oriel D, Ridgway G, Schacter J, et al. (eds) *Chlamydial Infections*, p 487 Cambridge University Press.

Washington AE, Johnson RE & Sanders LL (1987) *Chlamydia trachomatis* infection in the United States. What are they costing us? **287**: 2070–2072.

Wasserheit JN, Bell TA, Kiviat NB et al. (1986) Microbial causes of proven pelvic inflammatory disease and efficacy of clindamycin and tobramycin. *Ann Intern Med* **104**: 187–193.

Westrom L (1980) Incidence, prevalence and trends of acute pelvic inflammatory disease and its consequences in industrialied countries. *Am J Obstet Gynecol* **138**: 880–884.

Wiesenfeld HC, Uhrin M, Dixon BW & Sweet RL (1994) Rapid polymerase chain reaction-based test for the detection of female urogenital chlamydial infections. *Inf Dis Obstet Gynecol* **1**: 182–187.

4

Maternal Red Blood Cell Group & Antibody Screen

Delores G. Cordle & Ronald G. Strauss

WHAT IS THE PROBLEM THAT REQUIRES SCREENING?

HEMOLYTIC DISEASE OF THE FETUS AND NEWBORN (HDN), AND POSSIBLE MATERNAL TRANSFUSION AT DELIVERY.

What is the incidence/prevalence of the target condition?

Three to five per cent of pregnant women exhibit red blood cell (RBC) alloimmunization (isoimmunization) (Weinstein, 1982); 1–3% of vaginal deliveries and 3–5% of cesarean deliveries undergo RBC transfusions (Combs *et al.*, 1992).

What are the sequelae of the condition which are of interest in clinical medicine?

Red blood cell alloimmunization is the production of antibodies against foreign antigen loci. It can result in fetal hemolytic anemia leading to stillbirth, preterm delivery, and kernicterus when the fetus is affected. Although the most severe hemolytic disease of the newborn occurs with anti-Rh(D), many other RBC IgG antibodies are able to cause life-threatening disease. The incidence of alloimmunization to Rh(D) can be greatly reduced by the timely administration of anti-D immunoglobulin during pregnancy and postpartum. Red blood cell alloimmunization can greatly delay or even prevent the availability of compatible blood for maternal transfusion.

Because the severity of hemolytic disease of the newborn cannot be predicted precisely, all women should be tested early during pregnancy for the presence and identity of the RBC antibodies (Judd *et al.*, 1990). Only immunoglobulin G (IgG) isotype antibodies, which cross the placenta from mother to fetus and are directed against antigens on fetal/neonatal RBCs cause hemolytic disease of the newborn. Management of sensitized mothers and their fetuses varies with local practices. The decision for an intervention such as amniocentesis, cordocentesis, and intrauterine RBC transfusion is based on antibody specificity, baseline levels and the change in antibody titers, and the severity of hemolytic disease of the newborn in preceding pregnancies (Bowman, 1990).

Less than 3% of women receive an RBC transfusion postpartum. It is unnecessary to perform routine pretransfusion compatibility testing at the time of delivery provided ABO and Rh(D) grouping and RBC antibody screening were normal antenatally, unless a risk factor such as placenta previa or cesarean section is present (Judd *et al.*, 1990). Blood samples for compatibility testing can be obtained at the time transfusions are deemed necessary.

THE TESTS

What is the purpose of the tests?

Antenatal maternal blood grouping identifies women who are Rh(D) negative and thus candidates for Rh immunoglobulin prophylaxis (e.g. completion of pregnancy and those undergoing invasive prenatal diagnosis). The purpose of RBC antibody screening is to detect IgG alloantibodies to RBC antigens which, if present, potentially could cause hemolytic disease of the newborn. In addition, prior knowledge of unexpected antibodies can facilitate the issuance of compatible units of RBCs for transfusion in mothers or their infants during the perinatal period.

The nature of the tests

Blood grouping consists of determining both ABO group and Rh(D) type. These tests should be performed as early as possible in pregnancy, but need not be repeated for subsequent pregnancies, providing the testing facility has records of concordant results on two samples obtained on different occasions (Judd *et al.*, 1990).

The ABO grouping tests distinguish RBCs of four distinct phenotypes: A, B, O, and AB. The ABO group of most adult individuals can be determined by direct agglutination tests (forward grouping) using RBC typing antibodies prepared from either serum of hyperimmunized human subjects (polyclonal antisera) or immunoglobulin-secreting mouse hybridoma cells (monoclonal antisera). All reagents used for both ABO and Rh grouping are required to meet potency and specificity requirements of regulatory agencies, such as the US Federal Food and Drug Administration. The ABO system is the only blood group system in which individuals older than 6 months predictably produce 'natural' antibodies to antigens that they lack. Therefore, serum grouping (reverse grouping) tests are routinely employed to confirm results of RBC antigen grouping procedures. A testing accuracy approaching 100% can be assumed whenever RBC antigen and serum antibody results are complementary. However, discrepancies may occur between the results of antigen and serum grouping, when RBCs either possess unexpected antigens or lack expected ones, and when serum antibodies do not complement the antigens expressed. Certain subgroups of A and B (less than 1%) exhibit reactions weaker than normally seen and, depending on the subgroup, may appear nonreactive (i.e. fail to exhibit presence of the antigen) in normal testing procedures. In addition, antigens may be altered during infection and plasma antibodies may be absent in immunodeficiency states. These discrepancies must be resolved before a final ABO group can be assigned with confidence.

In Rh typing, the terms 'Rh positive' and 'Rh negative' refer to the presence or absence of the Rh(D) RBC antigen. Red blood cells from approximately 85% of whites and 92% of blacks express the Rh(D) antigen. Some Rh positive RBCs fail to directly agglutinate with anti-D typing reagent. To distinguish these D positive cells from those that are truly Rh negative, additional testing for weak D (formerly called D^u) must be performed. Reactions should be read macroscopically, not microscopically, and women testing positively should be considered Rh positive (Judd *et al.*, 1990). Negative reactions obtained at the antiglobulin phase of testing confirm the absence of the weak D antigen, whereas positive reactions suggest the presence of weak D. For technical reasons, RBCs demonstrating a positive direct antiglobulin test cannot be accurately tested for the weak D antigen. Conditions which could result in falsely positive results for D antigen include the presence of strong cold-reactive antibodies or rouleaux-forming factors in the serum.

Red blood cell antibody screening tests are utilized to detect clinically relevant unexpected antibodies (i.e. other than 'expected' anti-A or anti-B). The patient's serum is reacted with RBC screening cells that must bear the following antigens: D, C, E, c, e, M, N, S, s, P$_1$, Le^a, Le^b, K, k, Fy^a, Fy^b, Jk^a and Jk^b. Detected antibodies reactive at 37 °C and/or in the antiglobulin test are more likely to be IgG and clinically significant than those reactive only at room temperature or below. Antibody screening tests do not detect all antibodies of clinical significance. Antibodies to antigens not present on the screening cells (e.g. low-incidence antigens) and those that manifest dosage (react only with RBCs from homozygotes) are likely to be missed.

Implications of testing

WHAT DOES AN ABNORMAL TEST RESULT MEAN?

When screening tests for unexpected RBC antibodies are positive, the antibody must be identified to determine its clinical significance. Antibody titration is an imprecise procedure. When initial titers are high (generally > 8) or the titer is rising, the results are used to determine when either amniocentesis or cordocentesis is initiated. Anti-D is the major antibody for which titration is appropriate, since it is the antibody for which intrauterine intervention or early delivery is most likely to be considered (Judd *et al.*, 1990). Occasionally, other Rh antibodies act similarly (Bowell *et al.*, 1986). In contrast, non-Rh antibodies cause hemolytic disease of the newborn, but early delivery is rarely required. Therefore, routine serial titration of non-Rh antibodies is of questionable value (Judd *et al.*, 1990).

WHAT DOES A NORMAL TEST RESULT MEAN?

A clearly defined RBC type and a negative RBC antibody screening test are the normal result. Although this does not guarantee absence of alloimmunization and/or eliminate the possibility of hemolytic disease of the newborn, clinically significant disease is unlikely. Women who are Rh negative should receive anti-D immunoglobulin (125–375 µg; the practice varies among countries) at 28 weeks' gestation and again at delivery if the newborn is D positive (see Chapter 20). No additional testing is required.

What is the cost of testing?

Institutional charges to the patient can vary markedly, but actual laboratory costs to perform testing should be comparable. As an example, current reagent and supply costs at the authors' center are approximately US $1.50 for each blood type and antibody screen. If the antibody screen is negative, labor is about $3, based on 15 minutes per test at $12 per hour. When the antibody screen is positive, the antibody identification can take 30 minutes to several hours. Thus, laboratory costs can range from $7.50 to $30.

The total patient charges include the sum of the reagent and supply costs, labor costs, and an overhead cost (space, utilities, insurance, etc.), and they often exceed laboratory costs by several times. In our institution, the patient charge for an ABO and Rh type is approximately $50. It is arguably best to rely on laboratory costs rather than patient charges when making economic decisions. Patient charges may vary greatly among hospitals and do not reflect a true picture because of incomplete reimbursement due to capitation and other negotiated pay structures.

It is not necessary to repeat ABO and Rh grouping after the initial prenatal visit, providing the testing facility has records of concordant results on two samples obtained on different occasions (Judd *et al.*, 1990). Patients who are Rh positive should be screened for RBC antibodies once during pregnancy, at the initial visit; Rh negative women should be screened for RBC antibodies at the initial visit and again at 28–30 weeks' gestation prior to administering anti-D immunoglobulin. Repeat antibody screening and identification are recommended during the third trimester whenever unexpected antibodies have been detected (Judd *et al.*, 1990). Titrations need not be repeated after other means of fetal monitoring have been implemented in alloimmunized patients. If one assumes that 95% of pregnant women initially have a negative antibody screen, repeat testing of the 85% who are Rh positive is unnecessary.

CONCLUSIONS AND RECOMMENDATIONS

A maternal blood sample should be obtained early in pregnancy from all pregnant women to determine their red blood cell ABO and Rh(D) groups and to detect unexpected anti-RBC antibodies. Women who are Rh(D) antigen negative and who exhibit no anti-RBC antibodies should be tested for anti-RBC antibodies a second time at 28–30 weeks of gestation, following which anti-D immunoglobulin should be administered to women who have not been immunized to Rh(D). No further testing is needed during a normal pregnancy. Women who are Rh(D) negative and who are immunized to Rh(D) antigen (exhibit anti-D) at the time of initial testing should be referred for additional management according to local practice (antibody titration, ultrasonography, amniocentesis or cordocentesis).

Women who are Rh(D) positive and who on initial testing exhibit no anti-RBC antibodies need no further testing during a normal pregnancy. Women who on initial testing are Rh(D) positive and who exhibit clinically significant anti-RBC antibodies should be retested at least once. Depending on the specificity and titer of the anti-RBC antibody detected on initial testing, the woman should be referred to an appropriate center for management.

SUMMARY

1   WHAT IS THE PROBLEM THAT REQUIRES SCREENING?

HEMOLYTIC DISEASE OF THE FETUS AND NEWBORN (HDN) AND POSSIBLE MATERNAL TRANSFUSION AT DELIVERY.

a What is the incidence/prevalence of the target condition?

Three to five per cent of pregnant women exhibit RBC alloimmunization; 1–3% of vaginal and 3–5% of cesarean deliveries undergo RBC transfusions.

b What are the sequelae of the condition which are of interest in clinical medicine?

Red blood cell alloimmunization can result in fetal hemolytic anemia leading to stillbirth, preterm delivery, and kernicterus when the fetus is affected. Red blood cell alloimmunization can greatly delay or even prevent the availability of compatible blood for maternal transfusion.

2 THE TESTS

a What is the purpose of the tests?

Antenatal maternal blood grouping identifies women who are Rh(D) negative and thus candidates for RhIG prophylaxis. Prior knowledge of unexpected antibodies can facilitate the issuance of compatible units of RBCs for transfusion in mothers or their infants during the perinatal period.

b The nature of the tests

ABO grouping, RBC typing and antibody screening.

c Implications of testing

I   What does an abnormal test result mean?

When screening tests for unexpected RBC antibodies are positive, the antibody must be identified to determine its clinical significance.

2   What does a normal test result mean?

A clearly defined RBC type and a negative RBC antibody screening test are the normal result. No additional testing is required.

3 CONCLUSIONS AND RECOMMENDATIONS

A maternal blood sample should be obtained early in pregnancy from all pregnant women to determine their RBC ABO and Rh(D) groups and to detect unexpected anti-RBC antibodies.

REFERENCES

Bowell PJ, Allen DL & Entwistle CC (1986) Blood group antibody screening tests during pregnancy. *Br J Obstet Gynaecol* **93**: 1038–1043.

Bowman JM (1990) Treatment options for the fetus with alloimmune hemolytic disease. *Transfusion Med Rev* **4**: 191–207.

Combs CA, Murphy EL & Laros RK Jr (1992) Cost-benefit analysis of autologous blood donation in obstetrics. *Obstet Gynecol* **80**: 621–625.

Judd WJ, Luban NLC, Ness PM *et al.* (1990) Prenatal and perinatal immunohematology: recommendations for serologic management of the fetus, newborn infant, and obstetric patient. *Transfusion* **30**: 175–183.

Weinstein L (1982) Irregular antibodies causing hemolytic disease of the newborn: a continuing problem. *Clin Obstet Gynecol* **25**: 321–332.

5

Alpha-fetoprotein Screening for Neural Tube Defects

George J. Knight, Glenn E. Palomaki & James E. Haddow

WHAT IS THE PROBLEM THAT REQUIRES SCREENING?

FETAL NEURAL TUBE DEFECTS.

The phrase 'neural tube defect' describes a family of central nervous system malformations resulting from failure of the neural tube to close anywhere along the neural axis during embryogenesis. Anencephaly occurs when closure is incomplete at the cephalic end of the neural tube. Spina bifida occurs when closure is incomplete more caudally. These two malformations together account for nearly all neural tube defects and occur in approximately equal proportions. Encephalocele, a much less common lesion, is created when neural tube closure fails to occur in the posterior region of the skull.

A neural tube defect is characterized as being closed when it is covered by either skin or a thick membrane. An open neural tube defect is covered by only a thin, permeable membrane or by no membrane at all. Virtually all cases of anencephaly and approximately 80% of spina bifida cases are open. Encephaloceles are nearly always closed. The biochemical tests used to detect neural tube defects for both screening and diagnostic purposes rely on measuring fetal products that transudate across open defects. These tests, therefore, are not capable of detecting closed lesions.

What is the incidence/prevalence of the target condition?

Neural tube defects generally follow a multifactorial inheritance pattern. Both genetic and environmental factors play an etiologic role and the risk of recurrence in future pregnancies rises with each affected pregnancy. For example, a woman who has delivered one child with a neural tube defect is 10 times more likely than a woman in the general population to have a second affected pregnancy. If that same woman delivers a second affected child, her risk with each subsequent pregnancy rises to 20 times that of a woman in the general population (Haddow, 1990).

The birth prevalence of neural tube defects varies according to such conditions as geographic location, racial origin and time. 'Epidemics' have been documented. For example, the birth prevalence approached 8 per 1000 live births in certain areas of the UK in the 1960s (Owens et al., 1991). In the 1970s the birth prevalence of neural tube defects in the northeastern USA was approximately 2 per 1000 and in California was 1 per 1000

(Greenberg *et al.*, 1983). The rate of occurrence of these malformations fell in the USA during the 1970s, prior to the introduction of widespread introduction of prenatal screening and diagnosis (Congenital Malformations Surveillance, 1993). The recent discovery that folic acid supplements are protective helps both to elucidate etiology and to offer the prospect of primary prevention (MRC Vitamin Study Research Group 1991).

What are the sequelae of the condition which are of interest in clinical medicine?

Anencephaly is not compatible with life. Vital functions may continue for hours or days after birth, but viability beyond that time is rare. Nearly all cases of anencephaly are now detected during the second trimester via either biochemical or ultrasound screening. Pregnancy termination is usually chosen.

Spina bifida is variable in severity, but, as a rule, open defects have a worse prognosis than closed ones. With aggressive medical and surgical management, approximately 70% of individuals survive the first 5 years of life. One study reported that at the end of 5 years, survivors had spent an average of more than 6 months in hospital and averaged six major surgical procedures (Althouse and Wald, 1980). The most common problems are hydrocephaly (associated with the Arnold–Chiari malformation), paralysis of the lower limbs (the level of paralysis is defined by the location of the lesion), and problems with bowel and bladder function. Open spina bifida is now regularly detected prenatally during the second trimester. Pregnancy termination is chosen by some; others choose to continue the pregnancy and prepare for managing the medical and surgical problems.

THE TEST

The measurement of alpha-fetoprotein in the maternal serum.

What is the purpose of the test?

The purpose of maternal serum alpha-fetoprotein (AFP) screening is to identify women at increased risk of having a fetus with an open neural tube defect by selecting those with elevated test results.

The nature of the test

The concentration of AFP is measured in a maternal blood sample drawn between 15 weeks and 20 weeks of gestation. The optimum screening window for detecting open spina bifida is 16–18 weeks' gestation. Prior to 15 weeks, the detection rate is reduced. If screening is performed at 21 weeks' gestation or later, the option to terminate after diagnosis is no longer available in many countries (UK Collaborative Study in Relation to Neural Tube Defects, 1977). The woman's AFP value is expressed as a multiple of the laboratory's median AFP value (MoM) at her gestational age. Among other benefits, the conversion of test results to MoM takes into account the normal 15% per week increase. Women with MoM values above specified cut-off levels are considered screen positive and are referred for counseling and diagnostic procedures. Most screening programs use a cut-off of 2.0 or 2.5 MoM, with the latter being more common. At a

2.5 MoM cut-off, approximately 75% of open spina bifida and 90% of anencephalic pregnancies can be detected, with a 2% false positive rate. At a lower cut-off of 2.0 MoM, the detection rates are approximately 85% and 95% respectively, and the false positive rate is approximately 4%.

Several demographic and pregnancy-related factors influence AFP levels and/or prior risk for open neural tube defects. Taking these factors into account enhances screening performance. Questions on the laboratory requisition slip concerning these factors should be carefully answered.

Gestational age: The single most important factor affecting the interpretation of AFP values is the estimation of gestational age. Levels of AFP increase about 15% per week. The estimation of gestational age by physical examination is the least reliable dating method and will decrease screening performance. Use of the first day of the last menstrual period is acceptable for the purpose of prenatal screening. When gestational age is estimated from either first or second-trimester ultrasound measurements, the detection rate of open neural tube defects is increased and false positive rates reduced. Optimal screening performance is achieved when the pregnancy is dated using *only* the biparietal diameter measurement. Because this measurement is smaller than expected in fetuses with open spina bifida (leading to an underestimation of the gestational age), the artifactual increase in the calculated AFP MoM value increases the detection rate (Wald *et al.* 1984).

Maternal weight: On average, heavier women have lower AFP values, and lighter women have higher values. Routine adjustment for maternal weight increases the detection rate for open neural tube defects and reduces the false positive rate (Johnson *et al.*, 1990). There is no known difference in the birth prevalence of open neural tube defects among women of different weight (Haddow and Palomaki, 1995).

Maternal race: The AFP levels of black women are on average 10–15% higher than those of Caucasian women (Baumgarten, 1986). This difference is taken into account either by adjusting individual MoM values from black women (when medians from the Caucasian population are used) or by using race-specific median values. In addition, the birth prevalence of open neural tube defects in black women is approximately half that of Caucasian women (Greenberg *et al.*, 1983). The difference in birth prevalence may be taken into account by raising the screening cut-off for black women (e.g. from 2.5 to 3.0 MoM).

Maternal insulin-dependent diabetes: The AFP levels of women with insulin-dependent diabetes prior to pregnancy are on average 20% lower than those of nondiabetic women (Greene *et al.*, 1988). These differences are taken into account by adjusting the individual MoM values upward. In addition, the birth prevalence of open neural tube defects is three to five times higher than in a comparable nondiabetic population (Adams *et al.*, 1984). This higher prevalence may be taken into account by lowering the screening cut-off level (e.g. from 2.5 to 2.0 MoM).

Multiple fetal pregnancy: Levels of AFP are higher in multiple fetal pregnancy, approximately in proportion to the number of fetuses. For example, levels in twin pregnancies are double those in singleton pregnancies. This difference can be taken into account by raising the screening cut-off (e.g. from 2.5 to 4.0 MoM). However, the screening performance will remain inferior to that achievable with singleton pregnancies (e.g. 58% detection of open spina bifida with an 8% false positive rate) (Cuckle *et al.*, 1990). In addition, the prevalence of neural tube defects is twice as high as in singleton pregnancies (Wald and Cuckle, 1987). The AFP screening performance in triplet or quadruplet pregnancies is poorly defined, and measurements from such pregnancies are usually not interpreted.

Family history of neural tube defects: A woman with a close family member affected by a neural tube defect is at increased risk of having an affected fetus (Haddow, 1990). The risk may be sufficient to warrant a direct offer of diagnostic testing. If AFP screening measurements are performed in such women, it is important to take the increased risk into account by either adjusting the value to reflect the higher individual risk or by lowering the MoM cut-off level (or both).

Implications of testing

WHAT DOES AN ABNORMAL TEST RESULT MEAN?

An elevated AFP level may indicate the presence of an open neural tube defect and suggests the need for additional studies. Until recently, it was common practice to request a second serum specimen when a woman was screen positive. If the second sample tested negative, no further action was recommended. Repeat testing has the effect of reducing the number of women offered diagnostic testing with little loss of detection. Today, the most common practice is to perform a routine ultrasound examination to confirm gestational age, if such testing has not already been performed. When the gestational age estimate by ultrasound is more advanced than that obtained using the last menstrual period (generally defined as being at least 8–14 days), the AFP result is reinterpreted by the laboratory. The routine ultrasound examination can also identify anencephalic pregnancies, along with other conditions associated with elevated AFP levels, such as multiple pregnancy or fetal death.

In the screen positive pregnancies where no explanation can be found (approximately 1% of all pregnancies tested), the women are counseled and offered a high-resolution ultrasound examination by trained personnel and/or amniocentesis. When amniotic fluid is obtained, AFP and acetylcholinesterase are measured (Collaborative Acetylcholinesterase Study, 1989). An elevated amniotic fluid AFP level and a positive acetylcholinesterase test are found in more than 98% of open spina bifida cases with a false positive rate of less than 0.3% (Collaborative Acetylcholinesterase Study, 1989). Though it is common practice to perform chromosomal analysis on these samples, the cost-effectiveness of this practice when associated with a normal high-resolution ultrasound examination is a subject of current debate (Feuchtbaum et al., 1995; Thiagarajah et al., 1995). Women with unexplained serum AFP elevations increasingly opt for high-resolution ultrasound examination in place of amniocentesis (Nadel et al., 1990). This policy has generated some controversy because of the variability in ultrasonographic proficiency between centers (Wald et al., 1991). The optimal policy for any given geographic area and institution requires common sense. When available, high-resolution ultrasound examination by an individual experienced in the diagnosis of fetal malformation can replace the need for most amniocenteses. If such expertise is unavailable, the practitioner will be forced to rely more on amniocentesis.

In addition to its association with open neural tube defects, elevated maternal serum AFP levels are frequently found in cases of open ventral wall defects (omphalocele and gastroschisis) (Palomaki et al., 1988). The maternal serum AFP level tends to be much higher with gastroschisis because omphaloceles are covered by peritoneum and gastroschisis is not. AFP screening, as described above, will detect virtually all cases of gastroschisis and about 70% of cases of omphalocele.

Informed patient counseling is essential to a successful screening program. The patient should understand that this is a screening test. An elevated serum AFP unassociated with structural malformation is associated with a variety of adverse pregnancy outcomes, including spontaneous pregnancy loss and low birthweight (Haddow *et al.*, 1986). Although clinicians should be aware of the increased risk for pregnancy complications and may choose to alter their usual manner of prenatal care, no intervention has yet been shown systematically to be effective in improving pregnancy outcome (Goldenberg *et al.*, 1994).

Prenatal diagnosis of an open neural tube defect will lead to a change in the management of the pregnancy. Some women, after appropriate and nondirective counseling, may choose pregnancy termination. Others choose to continue the pregnancy, but the location of delivery is altered to provide optimal neonatal care.

In contrast to the situation with elevated AFP values, women with unexplained low AFP values are not at increased risk for an adverse outcome once the aforementioned conditions have been ruled out (Haddow *et al.*, 1987). In 1984, reduced AFP levels were found to be associated with fetal Down syndrome (Merkatz *et al.*, 1989), and this association forms the basis of successful prenatal screening programs for Down syndrome. Screening protocols for Down syndrome based on serum AFP measurements are being replaced by more efficient protocols that employ multiple biochemical markers (see Chapter 6).

WHAT DOES A NORMAL TEST RESULT MEAN?

Approximately 20% of cases of fetal open spina bifida are associated with maternal serum AFP levels below the screening cut-off. In addition, cases of spina bifida that are skin-covered are not detectable by AFP screening (closed spina bifida). It is essential, therefore, that both the clinician and the woman understand that a negative screening test reduces, but does not eliminate, the risk of having a fetus with a neural tube defect.

What is the cost of testing?

The American College of Obstetricians and Gynecologists recommends offering AFP testing as part of a screening program (ACOG, 1986). The responsibilities of any screening program include rapid communication of positive test results, availability of expert advice, and access to diagnostic follow-up testing. Though some laboratories provide only an AFP test result (with no support services) at a 'bare bones' charge of US $15–25, it is likely that patient care suffers. When full program services are included, the charge of AFP testing will be in the range of $30 to $50 and includes repeat blood samples where indicated.

A recent survey found that approximately 2 million pregnant women are being offered screening for open neural tube defects in the USA annually (about half the total number of pregnancies) (Palomaki *et al.*, 1993). At an average charge of $40 per serum AFP measurement, screening 2 million women costs $80 million. Using a screening cut-off of 2.5 MoM, 2% of the women (40 000) will be screen positive. An estimated 50% of these women would receive a routine dating ultrasound examination (at $100 per woman), totaling $2 million. At the completion of screening, 1% of the women (20 000) would remain screen positive, and these would be counseled and offered amniocentesis/karyotyping ($1000) or high-resolution ultrasonography ($500). Assuming complete uptake of diagnostic testing, the charges if 10 000 women opt for amniocentesis and the remaining 10 000 women opt for high-resolution ultrasound examination would be $10 million and $5 million, respectively. Overall, the screening and diagnostic charges would be $97 million. At an open neural tube defect birth prevalence of 1 per 1000 and an overall detection rate of 80% (75% for open spina bifida and 90% for anencephaly), 1600 of 2000 cases would be detected. Thus, the charge per case detected would be $61 000. In countries with either a higher birth prevalence and/or lower charges (such as in Britain), the charge per case detected would be lower.

A recent study using actual costs incurred by the State of California in 1988 estimated that the average excess cost of medical care, developmental services, and special education over the entire lifespan of an individual with spina bifida was $258 000 at a 5% discount rate (Waitzman *et al.*, 1994). Societal cost-effectiveness evaluations assume a percentage of women choose pregnancy termination after being informed and appropriately counseled by trained personnel.

CONCLUSIONS AND RECOMMENDATIONS

Spina bifida is variable in severity, but clearly has a long term impact upon family members and society. More than 95% of neural tube defect cases occur to women with no prior history of these abnormalities. Thus, a patient history is not a useful screening tool. Screening using AFP levels is sensitive and specific when part of an organized screening program. Available data suggest that if at least 25% of women opt for pregnancy termination, the net cost to society will be reduced. Consequently, nearly all pregnant women seen for prenatal care prior to 20 weeks' gestation should be offered AFP evaluation. Women with a prior history of neural tube defects, with a suspicious ultrasonographic finding, or with insulin-dependent diabetes mellitus prior to pregnancy, should be considered candidates for diagnostic testing.

SUMMARY

1 ### WHAT IS THE PROBLEM THAT REQUIRES SCREENING?

FETAL NEURAL TUBE DEFECTS.

a What is the incidence/prevalence of the target condition?

The birth prevalence of neural tube defects varies according to such conditions as geographic location, racial origin and time. A commonly reported level is 1–2 per 1000.

b What are the sequelae of the condition which are of interest in clinical medicine?

Anencephaly is not compatible with life. Spina bifida is variable in severity, but, as a rule, open defects have a worse prognosis than closed: 30% die within the first 5 years despite medical care.

2   THE TEST

a **What is the purpose of the test?**

To identify pregnancies at high risk for a fetus with an open neural tube defect.

b **The nature of the test**

Measurement of the maternal serum alpha-fetoprotein level between 15 weeks and 20 weeks of gestation.

c **Implications of testing**

1   What does an abnormal test result mean?

An elevated AFP level may indicate the presence of an open neural tube defect and suggests the need for additional studies. In the screen positive pregnancies where no explanation can be found (1–2% of pregnancies tested), the women are counseled and offered a high-resolution ultrasound examination by trained personnel, and/or amniocentesis.

2 What does a normal test result mean?

A negative screening test reduces but does not eliminate the risk of having a fetus with a neural tube defect.

d **What is the cost of testing?**

The charge per case detected approximates US $61 000. The average excess cost of medical care, developmental services, and special education over the entire lifespan of an individual with spina bifida was $258 000 US at a 5% discount rate in California in 1988.

3   CONCLUSIONS AND RECOMMENDATIONS

Spina bifida has a longterm impact upon family members and society. More than 95% of neural tube defect cases occur to women with no prior history of these abnormalities. Screening using AFP is sensitive and specific when part of an organized screening program.

REFERENCES

ACOG (1986) *Prenatal Detection of Neural Tube Defects*. Technical Bulletin 99. Washington DC: American College of Obstetricians and Gynecologists.

Adams MJ, Windham GC & James LM (1984) Clinical interpretation of maternal serum α-fetoprotein concentrations. *Am J Obstet Gynecol* 148: 241–254.

Althouse R & Wald N (1980) Survival and handicap of infants with spina bifida. *Arch Dis Child* 55: 845–850.

Baumgarten A (1986) Racial differences and biological significance of maternal serum alpha-fetoprotein. *Lancet* ii: 573.

Congenital Malformations Surveillance (1993) Data for birth defects prevention from: MACP 1968–1991; *BDMP* (1970–1991). Centers for Disease Control and Prevention. Atlanta: Georgia.

Collaborative Acetylcholinesterase Study (1989) Second report. *Prenat Diagn* 9: 813–829.

Cuckle H, Wald NJ, Stevenson JD *et al.* (1990) Maternal serum alpha-fetoprotein screening for open neural tube defects in twin pregnancies. *Prenat Diagn* 10: 71–77.

Feuchtbaum LB, Cunningham G, Waller DK, Lustig LA, Tompkinson DG & Hook EB (1995) Fetal karyotyping for chromosome abnormalities after an unexplained elevated maternal serum alpha-fetoprotein screening. *Obstet Gynecol* **86:** 248–254.

Goldenberg RL, Cliver SP & Bronstein J *et al* (1994) Bed rest in pregnancy. *Obstet Gynecol* **84:** 131–136.

Greenberg F, James LM & Oakley GP (1983) Estimates of birth prevalence rates of spina bifida in the United States from computer-generated maps. *Am J Obstet Gynecol* **145:** 570–573.

Greene MF, Haddow JE, Palomaki GE & Knight GJ (1988) Maternal serum alpha-fetoprotein levels in diabetic pregnancies. *Lancet* **ii:** 345.

Haddow JE (1990) Fetal disorders associated with elevated MSAFP values. In Haddow JE (ed.) *Prenatal Screening for Major Fetal Defects*, vol. 1, section 1:12–4. Scarborough: Foundation for Blood Research.

Haddow JE & Palomaki GE (1995) Is maternal obesity a risk factor for open neural tube defects? *Am J Obstet Gynecol* **172:** 245–247.

Haddow JE, Knight GJ, Kloza EM & Palomaki GE (1986) Alpha-fetoprotein, vaginal bleeding, and pregnancy risk. *Br J Obstet Gynaecol* **93:** 589–593.

Haddow JE, Hill LE, Palomaki GE & Knight GJ (1987) Very low versus undetectable maternal serum alpha-fetoprotein values and fetal death. *Prenat Diagn* **7:** 401–406.

Johnson AM, Palomaki GE & Haddow JE (1990) The effect of adjusting maternal serum alpha-fetoprotein levels for maternal weight in pregnancies with fetal open spina bifida: a United States collaborative study. *Am J Obstet Gynecol* **163:** 9–11.

Merkatz IR, Nitowsky HM, Macri JN & Johnson WE (1984) An association between low maternal serum alpha-fetoprotein and fetal chromosome abnormalities. *Am J Obstet Gynecol* **148:** 886–894.

MRC Vitamin Study Research Group (1991) Prevention of neural tube defects: results of the Medical Research Council Vitamin Study. *Lancet* **338:** 131–137.

Nadel AS, Green JK, Holmes LB, Frigoletto FD Jr & Benacerraf BR (1990) Absence of need for amniocentesis in patients with elevated levels of maternal serum alpha-fetoprotein and normal ultrasonographic examinations. *N Engl J Med* **323:** 557–561.

Owens JR, Harris F, McAllister E & West L (1991) 19-year incidence of neural tube defects in area under constant surveillance. *Lancet* **ii:** 1032–1035.

Palomaki GE, Hill LE, Knight GJ, Haddow JE & Carpenter M (1988) Second trimester maternal serum alpha-fetoprotein levels in pregnancies associated with gastroschisis and omphalocele. *Obstet Gynecol* **71:** 906–909.

Palomaki GE, Knight GJ, McCarthy J, Haddow JE & Eckfeldt JH (1993) Maternal serum screening for fetal Down syndrome in the United States: a 1992 survey. *Am J Obstet Gynecol* **169:** 1558–1562.

UK Collaborative Study in Relation to Neural Tube Defects (1977) Maternal serum alpha-fetoprotein measurements in antenatal screening for anencephaly and spina bifida in early pregnancy. *Lancet* **i:** 323–332.

Thiagarajah S, Stroud CB, Vavelidis F, Schnorr JA, Schnatterly PA, Ferguson JE (1995) Elevated maternal serum α-fetoprotein levels: what is the risk of fetal aneuploidy? *Am J Obstet Gynecol* **173:** 388–392.

Waitzman NJ, Romana PS, Scheffler RM (1994) Estimates of the economic costs of birth defects. *Inquiry* **31:** 188–205.

Wald NJ & Cuckle HS (1987) Recent advances in screening for neural tube defects and Down's syndrome. *Baillière's Clinical Obstetrics and Gynecology* **1:** 649–676.

Wald NJ, Cuckle HS & Boreham J (1984) Alpha-fetoprotein screening for open spina bifida: Effect of routine biparietal diameter measurement to estimate gestational age. *Revue d'Epidemiol Sante Publ (Paris)* **32:** 62–69.

Wald NJ, Cuckle HS, Haddow JE *et al.* (1991) The ultrasonographic diagnosis of fetal open spina bifida. *N Engl J Med* **324:** 770–771.

6

Triple Marker Screening for Fetal Down Syndrome

George J. Knight, Glenn E. Palomaki & James E. Haddow

WHAT IS THE PROBLEM THAT REQUIRES SCREENING?

FETAL DOWN SYNDROME.

Down syndrome most often arises from nondisjunction of chromosome 21 during meiotic cell division. As a result, the cells of the fetus contain three instead of two copies of the number 21 chromosome (trisomy 21). Occasionally, Down syndrome results from an unbalanced translocation where a parent's chromosome pattern includes a piece of chromatin from the number 21 chromosome attached to another chromosome. This rearrangement causes no clinical problem in the parent as long as the total complement of chromatin material from the number 21 chromosome is unaltered (balanced translocation). However, the amount of this material can become unbalanced during the formation of ova or sperm. One possible result of such an unbalanced translocation is the transmission of extra chromatin material from chromosome 21, with Down syndrome resulting.

What is the incidence/prevalence of the target condition?

Overall, Down syndrome occurs in approximately 1 in 850 births. Maternal age is the most important factor influencing the birth prevalence, which ranges from 1 in 1500 in a 20-year-old woman to 1 in 28 in a 45-year-old woman (Cuckle *et al.*, 1987). The overall rate will therefore vary according to the average age of the pregnant population. For example, there has been a consistent trend in the last decade for women to become pregnant at more advanced ages (National Center for Health Statistics, 1986, 1993). The prevalence of Down syndrome would thus be expected to increase proportionally. However, studies from various geographic regions and in various racial and ethnic groups have documented uniformity in prevalence rates and a consistent relationship with maternal age (Hook, 1981). One other major consideration in Down syndrome prevalence which relates to prenatal screening is that approximately 23% of Down syndrome fetuses are spontaneously lost between the second trimester and term (Cuckle and Wald, 1990). Thus, the second-trimester prevalence is considerably higher than the prevalence at term.

What are the sequelae of the condition which are of interest in clinical medicine?

All individuals with Down syndrome are affected with some degree of mental retardation. About 40% of individuals with Down syndrome have clinically significant malformations of the heart; 40% of Down syndrome individuals with heart lesions and 20% of those without heart lesions die by age 5 years (Baird and Sadovnick, 1987). Major malformations of the gastrointestinal tract occur in about 10% of affected individuals; hypothyroidism occurs approximately 30 times more often than in the general population, leukemia about 20 times more often (Fort *et al.*, 1984; McGrother and Marshall, 1990). More recently, it has been recognized that Alzheimer's disease affects the majority of Down syndrome individuals by 40–50 years of age (Franceschi *et al.*, 1990). A number of other less serious medical conditions are associated with Down syndrome. These can be detected and managed by ongoing monitoring.

THE TESTS

What is the purpose of the tests?

The purpose of measuring biochemical markers in maternal serum is to identify women at sufficient risk of having a fetus with Down syndrome to warrant offering antenatal testing of fetal chromosomes (most frequently by amniocentesis).

The nature of the tests

Alpha-fetoprotein (AFP) and unconjugated estriol (uE$_3$) values average lower, and beta-human chorionic gonadotropin (β-hCG) values average higher, when fetuses are affected with Down syndrome. Since each of the markers provides relatively independent information, the Down syndrome risk for each individual woman can be calculated by combining the three measurements with her age-related risk for Down syndrome. This patient-specific risk, rather than the individual analyte measurements, forms the basis of interpreting test results and for defining screening cut-offs (Wald *et al.*, 1988).

A maternal blood sample is drawn at 15–20 weeks' gestation, and the concentrations of AFP, uE$_3$, and β-hCG determined. All three measurements are converted to their respective multiple of the median analyte levels (MoM) for unaffected pregnancies of the same gestational age. The AFP measurement is used alone as a screening test for open neural tube defects (see Chapter 5). Down syndrome risk is calculated using the woman's age at her estimated date of delivery in combination with the AFP, uE$_3$, and β-hCG MoM values. Risks may be expressed as the probability of giving birth to a baby with Down syndrome (term risk) or the probability of carrying an affected fetus at the time of amniocentesis (second-trimester risk). For example, the risk for a 31-year-old woman is 1 in 650 at term, but is 1 in 500 in the second trimester. One or the other of these two conventions will be used by a given screening program. The cut-off most frequently used by screening programs is equivalent to the risk of a 35-year-old woman – 1 in 270 in the second trimester, 1 in 365 at term. This cut-off was chosen to be consistent with the current practice of offering amniocentesis to all women aged 35 years and older. In an unselected population of pregnant women, approximately 70% of cases of fetal Down syndrome and 8% of all pregnant women will have risks greater than this cut-off. An alternative cut-off, used less commonly, is a 1 in 250 term risk (1 in 190 second-trimester risk). This cut-off is associated with a lower false positive rate (5%) along with a lower detection rate (60%), resulting in a more favorable ratio of amniocenteses performed per case detected (Haddow *et al.*, 1992).

Several demographic or pregnancy-related factors influence the biochemical levels. Taking these factors into account will enhance screening performance. Questions on the laboratory requisition slip concerning these factors should be carefully answered.

Gestational age: Because levels of all three of the markers are strongly associated with gestational age in the second trimester, this variable is the most important of the factors affecting the interpretation. Estimating gestational age by physical examination is the least reliable dating method and will reduce screening performance. Use of the first day of the last menstrual period is acceptable for the purpose of prenatal screening. However, the detection of fetal Down syndrome is higher and the false positive rates are lower when gestational age is based on a first- or second-trimester ultrasound measurement (Wald *et al.*, 1992a, 1993b). Optimal screening performance is achieved when the pregnancy is dated using the biparietal diameter measurement. This is because other second-trimester ultrasound measurements (such as humerus or femur length) are known to be systematically smaller in fetuses with Down syndrome. The resulting underestimation of the gestational age decreases detection (Biagotti *et al.*, 1994). If the false positive rate is kept constant at 5%, Down syndrome detection is 60% when dating is by last menstrual period and 69% when dating is by biparietal diameter (Wald *et al.*, 1993b).

Maternal weight: On average, heavier women have lower values and lighter women have higher values of AFP, uE_3, and β-hCG. Routine adjustment for maternal weight will have only a small impact on overall screening performance, but will be an important consideration for women at extremes of weight (Palomaki *et al.*, 1990). Increasingly, screening laboratories adjust AFP and β-hCG values for maternal weight, and sometimes uE_3 values as well. There is no known effect of maternal weight on the birth prevalence of Down syndrome (Wald and Cuckle, 1987).

Maternal race: AFP levels in black women average 10–15% higher than in Caucasian women (Baumgarten, 1986). A similar difference may exist for β-hCG measurements, but the extent of the difference is unclear (Burton and Nieb, 1991). Currently, most laboratories adjust AFP values for maternal race, but few programs make adjustments for uE_3 or β-hCG. The birth prevalence of Down syndrome appears not to differ by maternal race (Hook, 1981).

Maternal insulin-dependent diabetes: AFP levels average 20% lower in women with insulin-dependent diabetes mellitus prior to pregnancy (Greene *et al.*, 1988). Laboratories routinely adjust values for this difference. Values of β-hCG and uE_3 in women with insulin-dependent diabetes appear not to be affected to the same extent (Wald *et al.*, 1992b), and few laboratories adjust measurement of these analytes.

Multiple fetal pregnancy: Levels of all three analytes are higher in multiple pregnancy, approximately in proportion to the number of fetuses. In twin pregnancies, the levels of AFP, uE_3, and β-hCG are approximately 2, 1.7 and 2 times the levels in singleton pregnancies, respectively (Wald *et al.*, 1991). It is possible to screen twin pregnancies for Down syndrome by dividing the MoM levels by these factors and interpreting the pregnancy as if it were singleton. Screening performance for Down syndrome in triplet or quadruplet pregnancies is poorly defined, and measurements from such women are usually not interpreted.

Family history of Down syndrome: Younger women who have had a previous pregnancy affected with Down syndrome have a risk for recurrence at the time of amniocentesis of 0.8% (Warburton *et al.*, 1987). If such women are screened, it is necessary to take this increased risk into account in the interpretation. In the small percentage of cases with an inherited chromosomal translocation, the recurrence risk is 50%.

Implications of testing

WHAT DOES AN ABNORMAL TEST RESULT MEAN?

The woman is at increased risk of having a fetus with Down syndrome. It is not recommended that a serum sample be redrawn if a woman is classified as high risk. Repeat testing provides no appreciable improvement in screening performance. Repeat tests cannot be interpreted as though they were initial samples (Cuckle *et al.*, 1994). If a woman is classified as being at increased risk for fetal Down syndrome and her pregnancy is dated by ultrasound, the next step is to offer genetic counseling and fetal chromosomal analysis. If her gestational dating is not ultrasonographic, the next step is to determine gestational age by ultrasound examination, preferably based on the biparietal diameter since it has been shown to be an unbiased estimate of gestational age in both affected and unaffected pregnancies (Wald *et al.*, 1993b). (Dating by biparietal diameter also has an advantage in screening for open neural tube defects, see Chapter 5.) If the gestational age is significantly earlier than that calculated using menstrual dates (generally by at least 8–14 days), the revised gestational age is transmitted to the screening program and a new risk calculated. A common reason for an initially positive test result is overestimated gestational age. When gestational age is overestimated, spuriously lower AFP and uE_3 and spuriously higher βhCG MoM values occur, and all are associated with increased Down syndrome risk (a difference of 2 weeks in gestational age can result in up to a ten-fold change in the calculated risk). Screen positive test results based on last menstrual period dating should be regarded as provisional until an ultrasound examination is performed. Upon reassessment of gestational age, between 25% and 50% of the positive results will be reclassified as screen negative (the revised risk is lower than the risk cut-off) or the results are uninterpretable (the sample was obtained prior to 15 weeks' gestation) (Haddow *et al.* 1992). When the blood sample has been obtained prior to 15 weeks' gestation, a new sample needs to be drawn at 15–20 weeks' gestation. Although ultrasound reclassification will markedly reduce the false positive rate, the process will occasionally reclassify a fetus with Down syndrome as well. This loss in detection can only be avoided if no reclassification is attempted. One way to reduce the number of women being reclassified is to ensure that the original Down syndrome risk is based on an ultrasound-derived gestational age. Another benefit of routine ultrasound dating is that the false positive rate will be reduced by up to 40%, because discrepant menstrual dates will be identified before test interpretation. If a woman remains screen positive after ultrasound determination of gestational age, she is counseled and offered amniocentesis.

WHAT DOES A NORMAL TEST RESULT MEAN?

Women who have a Down syndrome risk below the screening program's risk cut-off are offered no further testing. It is essential, however, that both the clinician and the woman understand that a negative screening test does not eliminate the risk of having a fetus with Down syndrome. Approximately 30–40% of cases of fetal Down syndrome are associated with risks falling below the screening cut-off and will not be detected.

What is the cost of testing?

The same specimen is used for both open neural tube defects and Down syndrome screening. Therefore, the fixed charges for drawing and transporting the specimen, logging-in the sample and reporting the screening test results are shared. Consequently, the incremental charges for adding two biochemical tests is considerably less than the charge if each were tested in separate specimens. For the purposes of these calculations, an incremental charge of US $40 (range $30–50) is reasonable. The total cost for prenatal screening for both open neural tube defects and Down syndrome is about US $80 (range $60–100).

A survey by Palomaki et al. (1993) found that approximately 2 million pregnant women are offered prenatal serum screening for Down syndrome in the USA annually (about half the total number of pregnancies). At an average incremental charge of $40 per triple test, screening 2 million women costs $80 million. Using a screening cut-off equivalent to the risk of a 35-year-old woman, 8% of the women (160 000) will be screen positive. An estimated 50% of these women would receive a routine dating ultrasound examination (at $100 per woman), totaling $8 million. At the completion of screening, 5% of the women would remain screen positive (100 000) and these would be counseled and offered amniocentesis or chorionic villus sampling (CVS) for fetal karyotyping. These procedures are associated with a low risk of fetal loss – 0.2% to 1.0%, depending upon the gestation. Assuming complete uptake of diagnostic testing, the charges for the 100 000 women opting for amniocentesis would be $100 million. Overall, the screening and diagnostic charges would be $188 million. Using a second-trimester Down syndrome prevalence of 1 in 650 and an overall detection rate of 70%, the screening would detect 2154 of 3076 cases. Thus, the charge per case detected in the second trimester would be about $87 000. Since only 77% of these detected cases would be expected to be liveborn, the charge per viable Down syndrome case would be $113 000. If a second-trimester risk of 1 in 190 (or 1 in 250) is used, the charge per case detected is lower. The charges would be lower in countries where the costs for both the initial serum screen and genetic amniocentesis are less. Two recent studies in Britain estimated the cost per viable Down syndrome case to be £29 000 (US $44 000), less than half that estimated in the USA (Sheldon and Simpson, 1991; Shackley et al., 1993).

The costs of maternal analyte screening for Down syndrome can be put into context by comparing the charge per case detected with traditional maternal age criteria to select women for amniocentesis, i.e. offering amniocentesis to women aged 35 years or more. In the USA, this would allow the detection of 25–30% of fetal Down syndrome cases and would require that amniocentesis be performed on 8–10% of all pregnant women. The charge per viable Down syndrome case detected using this protocol can be calculated to be $195 000 (Haddow et al., 1994).

A recent study using actual costs incurred by the State of California in 1988 estimated that the average *excess* cost of medical care, developmental services, and special education over the entire lifespan of an individual with Down syndrome was $410 000 US at a 5% discount rate (Waitzman et al., 1994). These costs substantially exceed the cost of detection if 25–50% of couples with an affected fetus chose pregnancy termination.

CONCLUSIONS AND RECOMMENDATIONS

Multiple serum marker screening for Down syndrome is superior to maternal age alone for Down syndrome screening. Societal cost-effectiveness evaluations assume a percentage of women choose pregnancy termination when informed of the abnormality and appropriately counseled by trained personnel. Serum screening for chromosomally abnormal fetuses is highly effective and cost-effective.

SUMMARY

WHAT IS THE PROBLEM THAT REQUIRES SCREENING?

FETAL DOWN SYNDROME.

a What is the incidence/prevalence of the target condition?

One in 850 births (birth prevalence ranges from 1 in 1500 at maternal age 20 years to 1 in 28 at age 45 years).

b What are the sequelae of the condition which are of interest in clinical medicine?

Mental retardation, major structural malformations.

THE TESTS

a What is the purpose of the tests?

To identify pregnancies at high risk for a fetus with Down syndrome.

b The nature of the tests

Measurement of maternal serum AFP, uE_3 and β-hCG levels between 15 and 20 weeks of gestation.

c Implications of testing

1 What does an abnormal test result mean?

The AFP, uE_3 and β-hCG measurements, combined with maternal age, identifying a group of women at risk for fetal Down syndrome. After gestational age is confirmed by ultrasound (if this is not already the case) these women are counseled and offered amniocentesis and fetal karyotyping.

2 What does a normal test result mean?

Women who have a Down syndrome risk below the screening program's risk cut-off are offered no further testing. It is essential, however, that both the clinician and the woman understand that a negative screening test does not eliminate the risk of having a fetus with Down syndrome.

d What is the cost of testing?

Assuming an incremental cost of US $40 for triple screening and $100 for ultrasonography, the cost per viable Down syndrome case identified would be $113 000. This compares favorably to the additional lifetime cost of $410 000 for each individual with Down syndrome.

CONCLUSIONS AND RECOMMENDATIONS

Down syndrome has a longterm impact on family members and society. More than 70% of cases occur to women below the age of 35. Screening using AFP, uE_3 and β-hCG, combined with maternal age, is a sensitive and specific test when part of an organized screening program.

REFERENCES

Baird PA & Sadovnick AD (1987) Life expectancy in Down syndrome. *J Pediatr* 110: 849–854.

Baumgarten A (1986) Racial differences and biological significance of maternal serum alpha-fetoprotein. *Lancet* ii: 573.

Biagotti R, Periti E & Cariati E (1994) Humerus and femur length in fetuses with Down syndrome. *Prenat Diagn* 14: 429–434.

Burton BK & Nieb B (1991) Effect of maternal race and weight (wt) on hCG and uE3 levels in the mid-trimester. *Am J Hum Genet* 49 (suppl.): a1144.

Cuckle HS & Wald NJ (1990) Screening for Down's syndrome. In Lilford RJ (ed.) *Prenatal Diagnosis and Prognosis*, pp 67–92. London: Butterworth.

Cuckle HS, Densem J & Wald NJ (1994) Repeat maternal serum testing in multiple marker Down's syndrome screening programs. *Prenat Diagn* 14: 603–607.

Cuckle HS, Wald NJ & Thompson SG (1987) Estimating a woman's risk of having a pregnancy associated with Down's syndrome using her age and serum alpha-fetoprotein level. *Br J Obstet Gynaecol* 94: 387–402.

Fort P, Lifshitz F & Bellisario R (1984) Abnormalities of thyroid function in infants with Down syndrome. *J Pediatr* 104: 545–549.

Franceschi M, Comola M, Piattoni F, Fualandri W & Canal N (1990) Prevalence of dementia in adult patients with trisomy 21. *Am J Med Genet* 7: 306–308.

Greene MF, Haddow JE, Palomaki GE & Knight GJ (1988) Maternal serum alpha-fetoprotein levels in diabetic pregnancies. *Lancet* ii: 345.

Haddow JE, Palomaki GE, Knight GJ et al. (1992) Prenatal screening for Down's syndrome with use of maternal serum markers. *N Engl J Med* 327: 588–593.

Haddow JE, Palomaki GE, Knight GJ et al. (1994) Reducing the need for amniocentesis in women 35 years of age or older with serum markers for screening. *New Engl J Med* 330: 1114–1118.

Hook EB (1981) Down syndrome: frequency in human populations and factors pertinent to variation in rates. In de la Cruz F & Gerald PS (eds) *Down Syndrome: Research Perspectives*, pp 3–18. Baltimore: University Park Press.

McGrother CW & Marshall B (1990) Recent trends in incidence, morbidity and survival in Down's syndrome. *J Ment Def Res* 34: 49–57.

National Center for Health Statistics (1986) *Vital Statistics of the United States, 1982*, vol. 1, *Natality*. DHHS Publication (PHS) 87–1100. Washington, DC: Government Printing Office.

National Center for Health Statistics (1993) *Vital Statistics of the United States, 1989*, vol. 1, *Natality*. DHHS Publication (PHS) 93–1100. Washington, DC: Government Printing Office.

Palomaki GE, Panizza DS & Canick JA (1990) Screening for Down syndrome using AFP, uE3, and hCG: effect of maternal weight. *Am J Hum Genet* 47: a282.

Palomaki GE, Knight GJ, McCarthy J, Haddow JE & Eckfeldt JH (1993) Maternal serum screening for fetal Down syndrome in the United States: a 1992 survey. *Am J Obstet Gynecol* 169: 1558–1562.

RCOG (1993) *Report of the RCOG Working Party on Biochemical Markers and the Detection of Down's Syndrome*. London: Royal College of Obstetricians and Gynaecologists.

Shackley P, McGuire A, Boyd PA et al. (1993) An economic appraisal of alternative screening programmes for Down's syndrome. *J Publ Health Med* 15: 175–184.

Sheldon TA & Simpson J (1991) Appraisal of a new scheme for prenatal screening for Down's syndrome. *Br Med J* 302: 1133–1136.

Waitzman NJ, Romana PS & Scheffler RM (1994) Estimates of the economic costs of birth defects. *Inquiry* 31: 188–205.

Wald NJ & Cuckle HS (1987) Recent advances in screening for neural tube defects and Down's syndrome. *Baillière's Clinical Obstetrics and Gynaecology* 1: 649–676.

Wald NJ, Cuckle HS, Densem JW et al. (1988) Maternal serum screening for Down's syndrome in early pregnancy. *Br Med J* 425: 883–887.

Wald N, Cuckle H, Wu T & George L (1991) Maternal serum unconjugated estriol and human chorionic gonadotrophin levels in twin pregnancies: Implications for screening for Down's syndrome. *Br J Obstet Gynecol* 98: 905–908.

Wald NJ, Cuckle HS, Densem JW, Kennard A & Smith D (1992a) Maternal serum screening for Down's syndrome: the effect of routine ultrasound scan determination of gestational age and adjustment for maternal weight. *Br J Obstet Gynaecol* 99: 144–149.

Wald NJ, Cuckle HS, Densem JW et al. (1992b) Maternal serum unconjugated estriol, human chorionic gonadotrophin and alpha-fetoprotein levels in pregnancies with insulin-dependent diabetes: implications for Down's syndrome screening. *Br J Obstet Gynaecol* 99: 51–53.

Wald N, Densem J & Stone R (1993a) The use of free β-hCG in antenatal screening for Down's syndrome. *Br J Obstetr Gynaecol* 100: 550–557.

Wald NJ, Smith D, Kennard A et al. (1993b) Biparietal diameter and crown-rump length in fetuses with Down's syndrome: implications for antenatal serum screening for Down's syndrome. *Br J Obstet Gynaecol* 100: 430–435.

Warburton D, Kline J, Stein Z et al. (1987) Does the karyotype of a spontaneous abortion predict the karyotype of a subsequent abortion? Evidence from 273 women with two karyotyped spontaneous abortions. *Am J Hum Genet* 41: 465–463.

7

Screening for Cystic Fibrosis Carrier Status

Darren Shickle & Ian Harvey

WHAT IS THE PROBLEM THAT REQUIRES SCREENING?

CYSTIC FIBROSIS.

What is the incidence/prevalence of the target condition?

Cystic fibrosis (CF) is the most common autosomal recessive disorder among Caucasians, occurring in 1 in 2500 live births in the UK (Dodge, 1988). About 1 in 25 Caucasians is a carrier of a CF mutation. The disease is much rarer among nonwhites – 1 in 14 000 live births among American blacks, 1 in 25 500 among Asians and 1 in 11 500 Hispanics (FitzSimmons, 1993). Six thousand individuals were estimated in 1992 to have cystic fibrosis in the UK (Dodge *et al.*, 1993).

What are the sequelae of the condition which are of interest in clinical medicine?

The mutant gene responsible for CF is located on the long arm of chromosome 7 (Rommens *et al.*, 1989). More than 400 mutations are known, the frequency of which varies among populations. The gene product is a 1480 amino acid membrane protein (cystic fibrosis transmembrane regulator, CFTR) which acts as a cAMP regulated chloride channel (Bye *et al.*, 1994). Patients with cystic fibrosis have defects of exocrine secretion characterized by a low water content and thus a high concentration of electrolytes (e.g. diagnostically high sodium and chloride levels in sweat) and protein, which leads to increased secretion viscosity and blockage of ducts. There is also an increased electrical potential difference across epithelial surfaces. Multiple organs are affected by this single mutation.

Lungs: Bronchial and bronchiolar obstruction by viscid secretions leads to recurrent distal infection and ultimately to right-sided heart failure (cor pulmonale). Respiratory symptoms are the dominant symptoms at the time of diagnosis in 45% of patients (FitzSimmons, 1993).

Pancreas: Inspissated pancreatic secretions lead to destruction of secretory tissue in 85–90%; pancreatic insufficiency with diabetes mellitus, gastrointestinal malabsorption and slow weight gain occurs in 10–12% of cases. Ketoacidosis is rare.

Gut: Meconium ileus leads to intestinal obstruction in 10–20% of affected neonates. Rectal prolapse occurs in 20% of affected children.

Liver: Bile duct blockage can cause prolonged obstructive neonatal jaundice. Symptomatic biliary cirrhosis occurs relatively rarely in up to 5% of cases.

Testes: Spermatogenesis is normal but blockage of the vas deferens and epididymis leads to azospermia. Fertility is also reduced in females.

These pathophysiological alterations allow the early diagnosis of affected individuals. The 'sweat test' involves the analysis of sweat produced by pilocarpine iontophoresis. An abnormal sweat sodium or chloride value (usually in the range of 50–70 mmol/l) indicates CF. The sweat test is the diagnostic tool nearest to a 'gold standard' for the detection of homozygotes in the absence of a complete library of gene probes (Bye *et al.*, 1994; Webb and David, 1994). However, sweat tests are difficult to perform in the newborn since 100 mg of sweat is needed. Affected newborns also have raised blood levels of pancreatic trypsin owing to leakage from the obstructed pancreas. Immunoreactive trypsinogen (IRT) can be measured in the dried blood spot obtained from neonates for phenylketonuria/hypothyroidism/galactosemia testing in many countries. If the value is above the 99th centile for the normal population, the positive predictive value of this test is 3% (Ranieri *et al.*, 1994). These children should undergo a sweat test at a later date.

Mortality rates from CF are highest during the first year of life. The median survival from birth is 24 years for females and 25 years for males, excluding recipients of lung, heart, and pancreas transplants (Dodge *et al.*, 1993). Birth cohort analysis reveals that survival continues to improve – probably owing to a combination of earlier detection and improved treatment. The median survival of a child born with CF today may be as high as 40 years (Elborn *et al.*, 1991). Gene therapy to correct the fundamental genetic defect using a helper virus to insert the gene is on the horizon (Zabner *et al.*, 1993). A recent study of UK cystic fibrosis sufferers over 16 years old showed that 54% were in paid employment, indicating a reasonable functional capacity (Walters *et al.*, 1993).

THE TEST

What is the purpose of the test?

The purpose of CF carrier screening is to identify couples at high risk of having a child with CF. Couples are considered to be at high risk if both are carriers of a detectable *CFTR* gene mutation.

The nature of the test

Genetic testing for the CF gene mutations.

The *CFTR* gene was first cloned in 1989 (Kerem *et al.*, 1989; Riordan *et al.*, 1989; Rommens *et al.*, 1989). Over 400 different mutant CFTR alleles have been described (Mennie *et al.*, 1992; Cystic Fibrosis Genetic Analysis Consortium, 1994). The ΔF508 mutation accounts for 70–80% of all CFTR mutations among white UK residents (Cystic Fibrosis Genetic Analysis Consortium, 1990), but only 50% among British residents of Asian origin, 37% among African-Americans in Baltimore and 27% among Turks in Germany. The subject's DNA is extracted from either cells collected from mouthwashes or EDTA blood samples, and analyzed by polymerase chain reaction (PCR) assays. Only a limited number of the common mutations are tested for during screening. Testing centers must select the mutations tested for based on their target population. It is generally feasible to test for at least 85% of the known mutations, thus permitting detection of at least 70% (0.85 × 0.85) of carrier couples.

There are two principal models for genetic carrier testing: 'inwards-out' (also known as cascade screening) and 'outwards-in' (Shickle and Harvey, 1993). The first approach involves identification of an index case either homozygous or compound heterozygous for the *CFTR* mutation and then offering testing to immediate relatives and their family members if carriers. The alternative 'outwards-in' model involves screening individuals in an at-risk population as part of a population genetics screening program (sometimes called community genetics or primary care genetics). Holloway and Brock (1994) estimated that inwards-out screening would identify a high ratio of carriers to people tested (1 in 3 compared with 1 in 25 for general population screening). Unfortunately, fewer than 20% of pregnancies at risk for an important single gene disorder are identifiable from the family history. Thus, inwards-out screening would identify only 4–13% of carriers in the population, or 8–24% of all carrier couples. In contrast to the inwards-out model, outwards-in CF screening programs (Mennie *et al.*, 1992; Wald *et al.*, 1993; Livingston *et al.*, 1994) detect at least 50% of carrier couples and can be applied any time during life. Neonatal screening has been done (Lyon *et al.*, 1983; Boland and Thompson, 1990; Rock *et al.*, 1990) but usually by IRT testing to detect homozygotes (rather than carriers) for the purpose of early treatment. Pilot programs of preconceptual carrier screening within primary care have been conducted (Watson *et al.*, 1991a; Bekker *et al.*, 1993). However, many primary health care professionals have inadequate knowledge to provide the counseling support necessary for any genetic screening. While preconceptual screening maximizes reproductive autonomy, it will not be desirable until these training and support issues have been addressed. The advantages and disadvantages of the main strategies are outlined in Table 7.1.

Antenatal CF carrier screening seeks to identify during pregnancy couples who both have a *CFTR* mutation. Antenatal diagnosis is based on fetal DNA obtained either by amniocentesis or chorionic villus sampling (CVS) and allows the couple the opportunity to make an informed choice on the outcome of the pregnancy.

Livingstone *et al.* (1994) asked pregnant women and their mates the preferred time for CF screening. The majority (54%) of those agreeing to carrier screening preferred to be screened during pregnancy; 45% preferred to be screened before pregnancy simultaneously with their partner and only 1% said they would have liked to be tested before they had met their partner. Among the women who declined antenatal testing, 40% stated that the antenatal period was the best time, about half preferred preconceptual screening as a couple, and 11% preferred testing before they met their partner. Botkin and Alemango (1992) surveyed the attitudes of 306 pregnant women towards CF carrier screening: 98% of the 214 respondents said that screening should be provided before pregnancy and 69% said that they would have wanted to be screened.

A survey in northwest London indicated a high level of support for cystic fibrosis carrier screening (Watson *et al.*, 1991). All relatives of patients with cystic fibrosis believed that carrier screening was a good idea and 89% stated that they would want to be tested. A

Table 7.1 Comparison of screening strategies at different times in the life-cycle.

	ADVANTAGES	DISADVANTAGES
neonatal screening	mechanisms already exist for collection of blood samples community midwife/health visitors provide counseling early treatment possible	autonomy increased in subsequent pregnancies only parents give consent on behalf of the child knowledge that child not 'perfect' can affect parent/baby relationship knowledge of carrier status only of importance for the next generation information may be lost/ misunderstood before child reaches reproductive age problem of detection of nonpaternity or sex chromosome abnormalities
antenatal screening	easy to organize most pregnant women attend antenatal clinic performed along with other antenatal tests only offered to people of reproductive age more receptive to issues affecting their children	consent may not be fully informed. availability of partner may be a problem limited period to perform counseling, etc. anxiety about pregnancy may make counseling more difficult termination may not be an acceptable option
childhood (teenager) screening	aware of being a carrier before longterm relationship formed could choose to avoid having children with another known carrier	consent a problem adolescence already a time of sexual confusion stigmatization
young adults of reproductive age	maximizes autonomy and reproductive choice informed choice easiest to obtain	primary care staff may not have skills or time to devote to counseling many young adults do not visit their primary caregiver many pregnancies not planned may be a middle-class bias if individuals have to request screening

high percentage of family planning clinic attendees and school pupils supported screening (90% and 82%, respectively) and most would want to be screened (75% and 77%, respectively). Approximately three-quarters of general practitioners and family planning clinic staff supported the introduction of CF screening. In a survey of 14–16-year-olds (Cobb et al., 1991), 86% thought that carrier testing should be offered routinely and 88% felt that antenatal diagnosis should be offered if both parents were found to be carriers.

Implications of testing

WHAT DOES AN ABNORMAL TEST RESULT MEAN?

A positive test indicates the tested individual is a carrier for one of the *CFTR* mutations. There are two general approaches to screening: two-step and couple (Figure 7.1). The woman is tested first in the two-step approach. The partners of carrier women are subsequently tested after appropriate genetic counseling. In contrast, both the man and

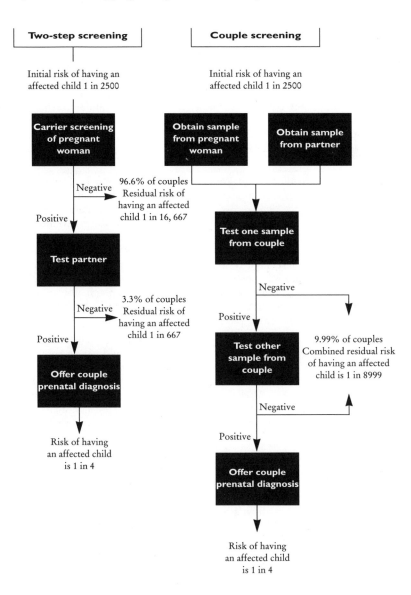

Figure 7.1 Two-step and couple screening for cystic fibrosis carrier status.

woman are sampled simultaneously in couple screening. One specimen is tested first, and the second tested only if the first is positive. The couple is usually told to assume they are at low risk unless they are contacted (Livingstone *et al.*, 1994). They are not told their individual results unless specifically requested.

A major disadvantage of antenatal screening is the limited time available to provide counseling and testing before a decision on pregnancy termination is required. It would be desirable either for women to book earlier or for the screening itself to be conducted within primary care. Primary care-based antenatal screening has been successfully piloted (Harris *et al.*, 1993), although the knowledge base of primary care staff remains an issue.

There are generally more ethical concerns about couple screening because the couple are given a combined risk result, rather than their individual gene status. The residual risk may be as high as 1 in 667 for couples where one member is a confirmed carrier, a risk higher than background (1 in 2500). In addition, carriers whose partners do not have a *CFTR* gene mutation may be falsely reassured that they cannot have an affected child even if they change partners. Therefore, counseling should include the residual risk and the need for retesting if the couple form new relationships. Couple screening does not eliminate the need for counseling; it only changes the timing – pretest counseling is particularly important. The main advantage of couple screening is that women found to be carriers do not experience anxiety while they wait for their partner to be tested (Figure 7.1).

One randomized controlled trial compared two-step and couple screening (Miedzybrodzka *et al.*, 1995). A similar percentage of couples accepted two-step and couple screening (91% and 89% respectively). Subject anxiety during screening was assessed by the short form of the Spielberger State-Trait Anxiety Inventory. Women identified as carriers as part of two-step screening had very high levels of anxiety which returned to normal when they learned of their partner's noncarrier status. Women offered couple screening were slightly more anxious at recruitment than those offered two-step screening ($P = 0.02$). Women who underwent couple screening tended to remain more anxious after receiving negative results than women individually screened. Thus, couple screening allows some carriers to avoid transient high levels of anxiety, but is associated with a higher level of overall anxiety.

Many screen negative women did not fully appreciate they could either still be carriers (21% two-step and 13% couple screening, respectively) or could have a baby with cystic fibrosis (19% and 17%, respectively). Twenty-one per cent of women in the couple screening group had forgotten that repeat testing was indicated should there be a future pregnancy with a new partner. Miedzybrodzka *et al.* (1995) concluded that two-step screening was better than couple screening because it generates less anxiety, less false reassurance, and provides important information to the carriers and their families for future pregnancies.

Mennie *et al.* (1992) offered two-step CF carrier screening to 4348 pregnant women, using cells from a mouthwash sample. Fourteen per cent declined screening and 13% were not tested, typically because of late booking. One in 29 women was found to be a carrier; four of these had carrier partners. All four high-risk couples chose prenatal diagnosis and one pregnancy with an affected fetus was terminated. Psychological status was assessed by the General Health Questionnaire (GHQ). Anxiety was significantly higher among those screened compared with unscreened controls at the time the test result was given. However, their anxiety levels dropped to control levels when their partners' results became known (most of whom were negative). This same group also conducted a couple screening program (Livingstone *et al.*, 1994). Eight per cent of couples approached were considered ineligible because of either late booking or the absence of their partner. A quarter of the remainder declined to participate. The overall

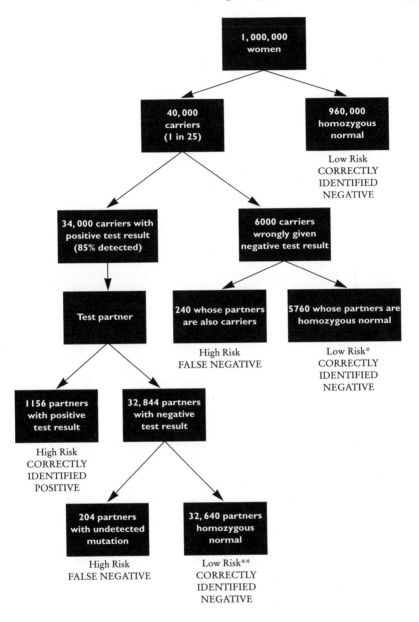

Figure 7.2 Flowchart of screening outcomes in a notational population of 1 million women and their partners. Single asterisk identifies couples correctly described as 'low risk', even though the mutation was missed, because the partners were homozygous normal. Double asterisk: couples correctly described as 'low risk'. Carrier females screened by the two-step approach may experience anxiety until their partner is shown to be normal. This problem does not arise with couple screening because the couple are not given the diagnosis.

Table 7.2   Validity of individual test results.

INDIVIDUAL'S TEST RESULT	CF GENE STATUS		
	CF carrier	Normal	
positive	34 000	0	34 000
negative	6 000	960 000	966 000
	40 000	960 000	1 000 000

Sensitivity = 34 000/40 000 = 85%; Specificity = 960 000/960 000 = 100%

Table 7.3   Validity of couple test results.

COUPLE'S TEST RESULT	CF GENE STATUS		
	BOTH PARTNERS CARRIERS	ZERO OR ONE PARTNER CARRIER	
positive	1 156	0	1 156
negative	444	998 400	998 844
	1 600	998 400	1 000 000

Sensitivity = 1156/1600 = 72.3%; Specificity 998 400/998 400 = 100%

uptake of screening (67%) was slightly lower than for two-step screening (73%). Four couples were found to be high risk; each elected to undergo antenatal diagnosis. Three pregnancies with affected fetuses were terminated. 1.5% of screened couples requested information on individual carrier status despite not being encouraged to do so. No excess anxiety was detected among the first 300 couples screened, and 99% of participants surveyed were satisfied with the concept of couple screening.

Figure 7.2 illustrates the various outcomes of screening a notional population of 1 million couples (Tables 7.2 and 7.3). Ninety-six per cent will be homozygous normal with a negative test result (true negatives). However, 15% of carriers with one of the less common mutations will also have a negative result (false negative). Of the 3.4% of carriers correctly identified, 4% will have a partner who is also a carrier (although 15% of these mutations will also be missed). Thus, 0.12% of couples (1156/1 000 000) will be diagnosed as 'high risk' (correctly identified positives) while 0.04% (444/1 000 000) will be incorrectly described as 'low risk' (false negatives). Those couples with a negative result have only a 0.04% chance of actually being positive (444/998 844). There is a 1 in 4 chance of an 'at risk' couple having an affected child in any given pregnancy. At best, 289 of 400 CF fetuses (1 in 2500 births) will be detected. In practice, the number detected will be lower because the uptake of screening is less than 100%.

WHAT DOES A NORMAL TEST RESULT MEAN?

Couples who test negative for a known *CFTR* mutation are at low risk of having a child with CF. Some risk remains since not all mutations are yet detectable and it is not feasible to screen for all known mutations.

What is the cost of testing?

Lieu *et al.* (1994) examined the cost-effectiveness of antenatal CF carrier screening among women with no family history of CF and under the age of 35 years (it was assumed older women would be offered amniocentesis because of risk of Down syndrome, see Chapter 6). Other assumptions included an uptake rate of 78%, sensitivity of 85%, and an uptake of CVS or amniocentesis among high-risk couples of 80%. As a result, just over a half of the affected fetuses in the cohort would be detected. They estimated that the cost for each test was about US $100 based on a 1992 survey of four diagnostic laboratories. For a cohort of 1 million pregnant women, the total cost of the screening program including follow-up was estimated at $82.7 million (Table 7.4).

Among the hypothetical cohort of 1 million women without screening, 400 children with cystic fibrosis would be born each year. Lieu *et al.* (1994) calculated that the lifetime cost of medical care for a patient with cystic fibrosis (assuming a 5% discount rate) was $243 650 (US 1993). They further assumed, perhaps somewhat conservatively, that 30% of couples would choose to abort an affected fetus. As a result, screening would lead to a 16% reduction in the number of CF births, saving $15.6 million in medical costs. The net (incremental) cost of the screening program relative to no screening would be $67 million per 1 million pregnant Caucasian women, $82 000 per high-risk pregnancy identified or $1.4 million per unwanted cystic fibrosis birth averted. Based on their calculations, they concluded that an antenatal CF carrier screening program 'would not save the healthcare payer money under most assumptions'. However, two pilot carrier screening programs conducted in the UK found that virtually all couples chose to terminate an affected pregnancy (Cystic Fibrosis Genetic Analysis Consortium, 1990; Brock, 1994). Hence, it is likely that a large-scale screening program would be substantially more cost-effective than calculated by Lieu *et al.* (1994) and analogous to the costs of other genetic screening programs.

Table 7.4   Projected costs of CF carrier screening program.

ITEM	COST ($, 1994)	% OF TOTAL PROGRAM COSTS
pretest education	3 000 000	3.6
CF carrier screening tests	74 402 000	90.0
telephone follow-up	304 000	0.4
genetic counseling	750 000	0.9
chorionic villus sampling or amniocentesis	4 222 000	5.1
procedure-associated spontaneous abortions	22 000	0
therapeutic abortions	21 000	0
Total	82 720 000	100

From: Lieu et al. (1994)

The above conclusion is supported by a cost-benefit analysis by Ginsberg et al. (1994) using rather different assumptions. They concluded that the benefit-to-cost ratio exceeds 1. The main differences between Ginsberg's and Lieu's studies are that the former's unit cost of testing was substantially lower ($72), the proportion of those offered screening who accepted was lower (50%), and the proportion of those with an affected fetus accepting termination was higher (92%). They extended the analysis to other countries by altering costs and benefits in proportion to changes in gross national product. For developed countries with Caucasian populations, they suggest that as long as the test is able to detect 73% of mutations in that population, the direct benefits exceed the direct costs.

Are women willing to bear the cost of screening? The cost of the Amplification Refractory Mutation System (ARMS) kit (Newton et al., 1989) produced by Johnson & Johnson is approximately UK £30 (US $47, 1995) per person. Though this excludes the significant costs of labor to collect and perform the test, it compares with a stated willingness of women undergoing antenatal CF carrier screening to pay up to £22 for the test (Miedzybrodzka et al., 1994). However, patients asked such hypothetical questions about a disease with which they are not familiar in a publicly funded health care system may not give valid responses.

CONCLUSIONS AND RECOMMENDATIONS

Despite popular support for CF screening, some caution is necessary. Neither the cost of the anxiety, albeit transient, induced by two-step screening nor the possible stigma attached to positive couples has been taken into account by either of the economic evaluations discussed. A full evaluation of a CF screening program should attempt to consider all the costs and benefits of being classified correctly or a false positive or negative (Shickle and Chadwick, 1994). The conclusions drawn from an economic evaluation are critically dependent on the assumptions used for the calculations – for example the cost of the test, uptake of screening and the proportion of affected fetuses terminated. The differing conclusions of the evaluations considered here underline this point.

The low sensitivity of screening (85% for individual screening and 72% for two-step or couple screening) will mean that careful counseling is essential. The sensitivity of screening will increase as more mutations are included within the routine testing kits, although this may increase the cost. Explaining the meaning of 'low risk' to couples where one partner is a carrier is particularly difficult. The shortage of specialist counseling skills means that general practitioners, midwives and obstetricians would be likely to have a lead involvement in antenatal CF carrier screening if it were to be routinely introduced. However, experience with antenatal maternal serum screening for Down syndrome has shown that midwives do not feel confident about genetic counseling (Khalid et al., 1994) and that additional training in explaining risk information is required (Marteau et al., 1992).

There is at present no agreement as to whether antenatal testing is preferable to pre-conceptual screening. The authors therefore consider that it is premature to introduce antenatal CF carrier screening until the sensitivity of testing improves and the counseling offered to couples is adequate to minimize induced anxiety.

SUMMARY

1 WHAT IS THE PROBLEM THAT REQUIRES SCREENING?

CYSTIC FIBROSIS

a What is the incidence/prevalence of the target condition?

Cystic fibrosis (CF) is the most common autosomal recessive disorder affecting Caucasians, with a frequency of 1 in 2500 live births. About 1 in 25 Caucasians is a carrier of a CF mutation.

b What are the sequelae of the condition which are of interest in clinical medicine?

Patients with cystic fibrosis have defects of exocrine secretions characterized by low water content and thus high concentrations of electrolytes (notably the diagnostically high sodium and chloride levels in sweat) and protein (leading to increased secretion viscosity and blockage of ducts). Multiple organs are affected by this single mutation.

2 THE TEST

a What is the purpose of the test?

To identify couples at high risk of having a child with CF.

b The nature of the test

Genetic testing (usually by PCR) for the CF gene mutations.

c Implications of testing

1 What does an abnormal test result mean?

There are two general approaches to screening: two-step and couple (see Figure 7.1). In a two-step approach, the woman is tested first and her partner tested subsequently only if she is shown to be a carrier. Both the man and woman are sampled simultaneously in couple screening. One specimen is tested, the other examined only if the first is positive. The couple are usually told to assume they are at low risk unless they are contacted. The couple are not told their individual results unless specifically requested. A major disadvantage of antenatal screening is the limited time available to provide counseling and testing before a decision on pregnancy termination is required. It would be desirable either for women to book earlier or for the screening itself to be conducted within primary care. Primary care-based antenatal screening has been successfully piloted, although the knowledge base of primary care staff remains an issue.

2 What does a normal test result mean?

Couples who test negative for a known CF mutation are at low risk of having a child with CF. Some risk remains for low-risk pregnancies screened by either method since not all mutations are yet detectable, and it is not feasible to screen for all known mutations.

d What is the cost of testing?

Estimates range from $250 000 to $1.2 million per birth of a child with CF averted depending upon the assumptions made regarding screen acceptance, sensitivity, and abortion rates.

3 CONCLUSIONS AND RECOMMENDATIONS

It is premature to introduce antenatal CF carrier screening until the sensitivity of testing improves and the counseling offered to couples is adequate to minimize induced anxiety.

REFERENCES

Bekker H, Modell M, Denniss G et al. (1993) Uptake of cystic fibrosis testing in primary care: supply push or demand pull? Br Med J 306: 1584–1586.

Boland C & Thompson NL (1990) Effects of newborn screening of cystic fibrosis on reported maternal behaviour. Arch Dis Child 65: 1240–1244.

Botkin JR & Alemango S (1992) Carrier screening for cystic fibrosis: A pilot study of the attitudes of pregnant women. Am J Publ Health 82: 723–725.

Brock DJH (1994) Heterozygote screening for cystic fibrosis. J Med Screen 1: 130–134.

Bye MR, Ewig JM & Quittell LM (1994) Cystic fibrosis. Lung 172: 251–270.

Cobb E, Holloway S, Elton R & Raeburn JA (1991) What do young people think about screening for cystic fibrosis? J Med Genet 28: 322–324.

Cystic Fibrosis Genetic Analysis Consortium (1990) Worldwide Survey of the △F508 Mutation – Report from the Cystic Fibrosis Genetic Analysis Consortium. Am J Hum Genet 47: 354–359.

Cystic Fibrosis Genetic Analysis Consortium (1994) Population variation of common cystic fibrosis mutations. Hum Mutat 4: 167–77.

Dodge JA (1988) Cystic fibrosis in the United Kingdom 1977–85: an improving picture. Br Med J 297: 1599–1602.

Dodge JA, Morison S, Lewis PA, Coles EC, Geddes D, Russell G, Jackson AD & Bentley B (1993) Cystic fibrosis in the United Kingdom, 1968–1988: incidence, population and survival. Paed Perinat Epidemiol 7: 157–166.

Elborn JS, Shale DJ & Britton JR (1991) Cystic fibrosis: current survival and population estimates to the year 2000. Thorax 46: 881–885.

FitzSimmons, SC (1993) The changing epidemiology of cystic fibrosis. J. Pediatr. 122: 1–9.

Ginsberg G, Blau H, Kerem E et al. (1994) Cost-benefit analysis of a national screening programme for cystic fibrosis in an Israeli population. Health Econ 3: 5–23

Harris H, Scotcher D, Hartley N, Wallace A, Craufurd D & Harris R (1993) Cystic fibrosis carrier testing in early pregnancy by general practitioners. Br Med J 306: 1580–1583.

Holloway S & Brock DJH (1994) Cascade testing for the identification of carriers of cystic fibrosis. J Med Screen 1: 159–164.

Kerem B, Rommens JM, Buchanan JA et al. (1989) Identification of the cystic fibrosis gene: genetic analysis. Science 345: 1073–80.

Khalid L, Price SM & Barrow M (1994) The attitudes of midwives to maternal serum screening for Down's syndrome. Publ Health 108: 131–136.

Lieu TA, Watson SE & Washington AE (1994) The cost-effectiveness of prenatal carrier screening for cystic fibrosis. Obstet Gynecol 6: 903–912.

Livingstone J, Axton RA, Gilfillan A et al. (1994) Antenatal screening for cystic fibrosis: a trial of the couple model. Br Med J 308: 1459–62.

Lyon ICT, Crossley JR & Smith PA (1983) Screening for cystic fibrosis. N Z Med J 96: 673–675.

Marteau TM, Slack J, Kidd J & Shaw RW (1992) Presenting a routine screening test in antenatal care: practice observed. Publ Health 106: 131–141.

Mennie ME, Gilfillan A, Compton M et al. (1992) Prenatal screening for cystic fibrosis. Lancet 340: 214–6.

Miedzybrodzka Z, Shackley P, Donaldson C & Abdalla M (1994) Counting the benefits of screening: a pilot study of willingness to pay for cystic fibrosis carrier screening. J Med Screen 1: 82–83.

Miedzybrodzka Z, Hall MH, Mollison J et al. (1995) Antenatal screening for carriers of cystic fibrosis: randomisation trial of stepwise v couple screening. Br Med J 310: 353–7.

Newton CR, Heptinstall LE, Summers C, et al. (1989) Amplification refractory mutation system for prenatal diagnosis and carrier assessment in cystic fibrosis. Lancet ii: 1481–83.

Ranieri E, Lewis BD, Gerace RL et al. (1994) Neonatal screening for cystic fibrosis using immunoreactive trypsinogen and direct gene analysis: four years' experience. Br Med J 308: 1469–72

Riordan JR, Rommens JM, Kerem B, *et al.* (1989) Identification of the cystic fibrosis gene: cloning and characterization of complementary DNA. *Science* 1066–1073.

Rock MJ, Mischler EH, Farrell PM, *et al.* (1990) Newborn screening for cystic fibrosis is complicated by age-related decline in immunoreactive trypsinogen levels. *Pediatrics* 85: 1001–1007.

Rommens JM, Iannuzzi MC, Kerem B, *et al.* (1989) Identification of the cystic fibrosis gene: chromosome walking and jumping. *Science* 1059–1065.

Shickle D & Chadwick R (1994) Is 'screeningitis' an incurable disease. *J Med Ethics* 20: 1–7.

Shickle D & Harvey I (1993) 'Inside-out', back-to-front: a model for clinical population genetic screening. *J Med Genet* 30: 580–582.

Wald NJ, George LM & Wald NM (1993) Couple screening for cystic fibrosis. *Lancet* 342: 1307–8.

Walters S, Britton J & Hodson ME (1993) Demographic and social characteristics of adults with cystic fibrosis in the United Kingdom. *Br Med J* 306: 549–52

Watson EK, Mayall E, Chapple J, *et al.* (1991a) Screening for carriers of cystic fibrosis through the primary care services. *Br Med J* 303: 504–507.

Watson EK, Williamson R & Chapple J (1991b) Attitudes to carrier screening for cystic fibrosis: a survey of health professional, relatives of sufferers and other members of the public. *Br J Gen Pract* 41: 237–240.

Webb AK & David TJ (1994) Clinical management of children and adults with cystic fibrosis. *Br Med J* 308: 459–62.

Zabner J, Couture LA, Gregory RJ, Graham SM, Smith AE & Welsh MJ (1993) Adenovirus mediated gene transfer transiently corrects the chloride transport defect in nasal epithelia of patients with cystic fibrosis. *Cell* 75: 207–16.

8

Routine Ultrasonography for Dating

Heiner C. Bucher & Johannes G. Schmidt

WHAT IS THE PROBLEM THAT REQUIRES SCREENING?

POOR PERINATAL OUTCOME SECONDARY TO POSTMATURITY, UNRECOGNIZED MULTIPLE GESTATION, OR GROWTH RESTRICTION.

This chapter focuses on the effectiveness of routine second-trimester ultrasonography for dating – that is, the detection and management of post-term pregnancy and its relation to maternal and neonatal outcome. It should be recognized, however, that ultrasonography for accurate dating of gestation is not separable from ultrasonography to diagnose multiple gestation, malformations (Chapter 9), and growth restriction. In addition, the effective detection and diagnosis of adverse pregnancy conditions through ultrasonography will affect the outcome of pregnancy only if effective therapies to alter the course of these conditions are available. A critical appraisal of routine ultrasound examination in pregnancy must consider the entire spectrum of potential benefits and risks and be based on the understanding that it is the 'net' outcome of pregnancy which matters in the end.

What is the incidence/prevalence of the target condition?

A post-term pregnancy is arbitrarily defined as one of 42 completed weeks of gestation (294 days) or more (World Health Organization, 1977; FIGO, 1986). This definition is a statistical surrogate for the clinically known problem of 'prolonged' pregnancies and their well-known obstetric complications. However, the best data available indicate that complications during spontaneous delivery increase progressively from 37 weeks' gestation and not particularly after 42 weeks (Saunders and Paterson, 1991). This observation, together with the notion that the length of pregnancy may be subject to natural biologic variation, makes it difficult to see how meaningful the current definition of 'post-term' really is in clinical terms. In many instances, a gestation of more than 42 weeks may constitute nothing but a normal variant without any pathological bearing.

The occurrence of post-term delivery varies widely from 4% to 14% (Bakketeig and Bergsjø, 1989), possibly due in part to differences among the examined populations and in part to differences in the measurements used. Labor induction policies also affect the rate. In Great Britain, the incidence of post-term pregnancy fell from 11.5% in 1958 to 4.4% in 1970, while the incidence of labor induction increased from 13% to 26% during the same period (Chamberlain et al., 1978).

Many population-based studies have relied on the first day of the last menstrual period to date the gestation. Such dates are often unreliable. In a study representative of all births in Sweden, the overall incidence of post-term pregnancy was 12.2% (Bakketeig and Bergsjø, 1989). In pregnancies with known dates, the incidence was 10.2%, whereas for pregnancies with an uncertain estimated date of confinement, the incidence went up to 22.3%. There is only one series examining the incidence of post-term pregnancy in women whose dates were based on basal body temperatures. The incidence was 1%. Thus, the vast majority of women deliver prior to 294 days of gestation.

What are the sequelae of the condition which are of interest in clinical medicine?

Maternal complications are found to be more common after 42 weeks of gestation compared to deliveries before 42 weeks in a study of over 90 000 births in Sweden (Bakketeig and Bergsjø, 1989). An analysis of 75 000 consecutive deliveries in the UK found 'longterm' pregnancies in primiparae to be associated with a progressively higher rate of labor complications, such as forceps use, cesarean section, hemorrhage, meconium staining, and neonatal intubation from 37 weeks' gestation onward (Saunders and Paterson, 1991). The effect of gestational age on the rate of operative delivery in this study was independent of birthweight.

Perinatal mortality and morbidity are also more common with an increasing length of gestation. Higher rates of fetal distress, shoulder dystocia, and meconium aspiration have been observed in babies delivered after 42 weeks' gestation compared with babies delivered before 42 weeks (Mead and Markus, 1964; Eden et al., 1987; Boyd et al., 1988). Perinatal mortality has been reported to be almost double in pregnancies lasting more than 42 weeks compared with term pregnancies (Bakketeig and Bergsjø, 1989). However, two other studies which make an explicit distinction between pregnancies with certain and uncertain dates found only a slight increase in the perinatal mortality rate in pregnancies lasting more than 42 weeks with precise dating (Bierman et al., 1965; Bakketeig and Bergsjø, 1989). In the Norwegian study, based on almost 31 000 deliveries with a certain expected date of confinement, the perinatal mortality rate (stillbirths plus first week deaths) of pregnancies in the 42nd week was 3.0 per 1000 pregnancies, only slightly higher than the 2.3 and 2.4 per 1000 pregnancies in term births of 40 and 41 weeks' gestation. It is possible, therefore, that the association between late deliveries after 42 weeks' gestation and perinatal mortality may be confounded by characteristics found in pregnancies with uncertain dates. This hypothesis is supported by data from the Cardiff Births Survey in which pregnancies with uncertain dates were found to have a higher perinatal mortality than those with certain dates at all gestational ages (Chalmers, 1975).

These associations between maternal and perinatal complications and the length of gestation, if critically appraised, must not be misunderstood as a necessary causal relationship. Lethal congenital malformations, for example, are more frequently found in long-term pregnancies (Evans et al., 1963; Zwerdling, 1967). Approximately 25% of perinatal deaths in deliveries after 42 weeks' gestation are due to malformations (Naeye, 1978), a finding that may confound the apparent association between prolonged pregnancy and adverse outcome. To control for such bias, obstetric policies confronting the problem of statistically or clinically defined post-term deliveries, and the role of ultrasound for dating in particular, need to be studied in randomized controlled trials.

The frequency of induction in 'term' and 'post-term' pregnancies varies greatly according to local obstetric policy. For example, in a population-based Norwegian study Bakketeig noted over a 10-year period an increase in induction rates from 11.1% to 14.9%. This increased use of induction applied to both 'post-term' pregnancies and to pregnancies of shorter duration (Bakketeig and Bersgjø, 1989). This variation in policy, together with the already mentioned confounding bias, makes the rate of induction an invalid surrogate for perinatal outcome. What matters in the end is the question of whether routine ultrasonography for dating – in connection with a well-defined and finely balanced induction policy (Crowley, 1989) – will improve the outcome in terms of whether perinatal and maternal complications can be effectively prevented and the number of live and healthy babies can be increased.

THE TEST

What is the purpose of the test?

Ultrasound can be used for accurate dating of gestation (Campell et al., 1985) to possibly reduce the incidence of post-term pregnancies (Waldenström et al., 1988), and for the diagnosis of multiple gestation (Grennert et al., 1978), malformations (Chapter 9) (Chitty et al., 1991), and growth restriction (Mintz and Landon, 1988). While anatomical measurements can be reliably performed with ultrasound, such measurements cannot compensate for the lack of clarity of how to define 'post-term' pregnancy (or growth restriction) and their uncertain therapeutic implications. Accurate gestational age assessment, however, facilitates the application of serological screening for markers of Down syndrome and neural tube defect, as the interpretation of these markers requires a precise estimate of gestational age (see Chapters 5 and 6).

The nature of the test

A reference standard for the assessment of gestational age is available from pregnancies with exact dating by induced ovulation (MacGregor et al., 1987). Compared with this standard, estimates derived by using second-trimester ultrasonography have proved to be within ± 3.7 days of the known duration of gestation.

Several sonographically derived fetal parameters are used to date the pregnancy. These include fetal crown-rump length, biparietal diameter, head circumference, femur length, and abdominal circumference. The variability in the mean of all these estimates for dating is smaller prior to the 20th week of gestation. A scan performed prior to 20 weeks' gestation is more accurate than one performed after that time. In the third trimester, biparietal diameter in comparison to menstrual history is a superior predictor in women with suspect menstrual history.

About 75–85% of pregnant women deliver within 2 weeks of their clinically estimated date of confinement (Grennert et al., 1978; Kloosterman, 1979). In a study of over 4000 pregnancies from a socioeconomically mixed population, the accuracy of the clinical predicted date of confinement in women with known menstrual history did not differ from that predicted by ultrasound examination up to the 20th week of gestation (Campell et al., 1985). According to menstrual history 84.7% and according to ultrasound 84.6% of the women delivered within 2 weeks of their estimated date of confinement. Among women with a suspect menstrual history, 69.7% with clinically assessed and 81.2% with sonographically assessed date of confinement delivered within 2 weeks of the anticipated date. Thus, when the dates are in doubt, ultrasonography improves the accuracy of gestational age dating.

Implications of testing

Ultrasonography for dating is confronted with the problem inherent in any screening procedure of false positive or false negative results – for example, pregnant women may be labeled 'post-term' in cases when this may constitute a normal variant and not a pathological condition. However, this problem is rather a matter of possible fallacies in the current obstetrical reasoning (of the 'hard data creed' of 42 weeks) than a problem of ultrasound per se. Ultrasound allows some improvement of dating, especially if menstrual history and the recall of women is unclear. Whether ultrasound dating of gestational age and possible changes in the rate of induction improve perinatal and maternal outcome, however, is another question. Ultrasound, clearly, is a diagnostic tool (Romero, 1993) and its routine application can improve outcome only if there are effective therapies for the conditions it can detect. There is little benefit to diagnosis if there is no effective therapy available.

The impact of routine ultrasound scanning on the induction rate and the overall pregnancy outcome has been assessed in a meta-analysis of four randomized controlled trials comparing routine with selective ultrasound examinations (Bucher and Schmidt, 1993a), and in the RADIUS trial, a large, randomized controlled trial of a *low-risk* population which was published after the meta-analysis (Ewigman *et al.*, 1993). In the meta-analysis, the number of induced labors was not consistently and statistically significantly reduced by screening – odds ratio 0.9, 95% confidence interval (CI) 0.82 to 1.01 – although single trials resulted in a significant reduction of the rate of induced labor (Waldenström *et al.*, 1988) – 64 versus 79 induced labors per 1000 randomized pregnancies (odds ratio 0.64, 95% CI 0.51 to 0.81). The live birth rates in both the screening and the control group were identical (odds ratio 0.99, 95% CI 0.88 to 1.12) – that is, screening did not significantly prevent fetal fatalities during pregnancy and birth. Especially in the Helsinki trial (Saari-Kemppainen *et al.*, 1990), routine ultrasound examination was also used for the early identification and the consequent termination of pregnancies with a malformed fetus (Chapter 9). As these fetuses were not counted as perinatal deaths this resulted in an overall significant reduction of perinatal mortality in the ultrasound group (odds ratio 0.64, 95% CI 0.43 to 0.97), but without a change in the live birth rate as already mentioned. Ultrasound was not associated with a reduction in perinatal morbidity as measured by the frequency of a 1-minute Apgar score below 7 (odds ratio 1.05, 95% CI 0.93 to 1.19) or by the rate of admission to a neonatal care unit (odds ratio 0.92, 95% CI 0.80 to 1.06) (Bucher and Schmidt, 1993b).

In the RADIUS trial of low-risk pregnancies, the numbers of induced labors in the screening and control groups were 251 and 247 per 1000 pregnancies, respectively, a nonsignificant difference (LeFevre *et al.*, 1993). Both of these proportions are considerably higher than in the European studies. In the ultrasound screening group 3.2% of all pregnancies were judged as at least 42 weeks' gestation whereas in the control group 4.6% of all pregnancies according to the last period were judged to be 'post-term', a difference of 1.39% (95% CI 0.77% to 2.01%). Using routine sonography to estimate gestational age at delivery resulted in a 1.4% reduction in pregnancies reaching 42 weeks' gestation. Thus, the reduction in inductions due to overterm pregnancies in this trial had a very modest impact on the overall induction rate. In addition, the trial showed no difference in neonatal outcome or in the rate of any maternal complications such as induced labor and cesarean section in the screening group. The rate of adverse perinatal outcome, defined as fetal or neonatal death up to 28 days of age or severe neonatal morbidity according to a 19 item list, was 5.0% in the screening group and 4.9% in the control group (relative risk 1.0, 95% CI 0.9 to 1.2). Nor were there any significant differences in perinatal outcome in the subgroup of women with post-term pregnancies.

The result of no change in the perinatal mortality rate in this trial has to be seen together with the comparatively low detection rate of fetal malformation and a low rate of pregnancy termination once the diagnosis of a congenital malformation was made.

What is the cost of testing?

Routine ultrasound screening in a low-risk population as examined in the RADIUS trial added on average 1.6 scans per pregnancy. Screening more than 4 million pregnant women a year in the USA (National Center for Health Statistics, 1990, 1991) at $200 per scan would increase costs by US $1.28 billion if there were no other indications for scanning. If only the 72% women who were eligible for this study are considered, total costs for routine sonographic screening would still add up to $921 million without any demonstrable benefit in perinatal and maternal outcome. These estimates may further vary according to the number of selective scans effected in usual care – that is, in the control group in the trials. In the RADIUS trial 44.8% of the control group had at least one ultrasound examination, whereas in other trials the use of selective ultrasound in the control groups ranged from 10.2% to 77.0% (Bucher and Schmidt, 1993a). More important than the direct financial costs is a cost-utility analysis to determine the value pregnant women give the early diagnosis of malformations and reassurance of normal pregnancy in comparison with the risk of false positive diagnosis of malformations or of possibly spurious labeling of growth retardation or other conditions in which diagnosis does not lead to an effective therapy and improved outcome. The incidence and intangible costs of labeling and of false positive diagnosis in routine care outside centers of excellence is a crucial factor in proper economic evaluation.

CONCLUSIONS AND RECOMMENDATIONS

Routine ultrasonography can improve the dating of gestational age, especially in the case of suspect menstrual history. As a consequence, it appears to decrease the incidence of 'post-term' pregnancies. This decrease, however, is a decrease in labeling of post-term pregnancy and must not be mistaken for a true change. Furthermore, since induction of labor in 'post-term' pregnancies defined as 41 or more weeks' duration reduces both the rate of cesarean section and perinatal mortality (Hannah *et al.*, 1992; Crowley, 1991), it is postulated that ultrasound for dating is useful (Romero, 1993). On the other hand, how can improved diagnosis change perinatal and maternal outcome in the absence of unequivocal understanding and definition of 'post-term' as a true pathological condition, particularly if a confounding bias through an increase in lethal malformations with increasing length of gestation cannot be ruled out? In practice, therefore, the theoretical advantage of routine ultrasonography for dating in the management of post-term gestation remains a matter to be evaluated in controlled trials.

Five randomized trials, showing no improvement in the outcome of pregnancy, cast considerable doubt on this theoretical advantage. However, these studies may not always have used routine induction of labor as the standard care in 'post-term' pregnancies, which makes it possible that routine ultrasonography could do more if combined with a clear and effective obstetric policy on management following improved diagnosis through ultrasound examination. Further studies would be needed to provide evidence that this is the case.

There is growing awareness that preventive and therapeutic efforts in low-risk populations may often do as much (if not more) harm as good; also that only preventive efforts targeted at populations with high risks of complications are worthwhile (Davey-Smith and Egger, 1994). Research efforts should therefore be directed to determine the benefit of serial pregnancy ultrasound scans in pregnancies with well-defined risk factors where ultrasonography is likely to improve outcome. Before such studies are done, however, it remains uncertain whether a more selective sonographic screening can truly improve the outcome of pregnancy. Routine obstetric ultrasonography may reduce perinatal mortality if severe congenital anomalies are appropriately identified and if the pregnant mothers choose early termination (Saari-Kemppainen *et al.*, 1990). If the goal is not dating of gestational age but the detection of congenital malformations, the available evidence demonstrates that routine scanning by *experienced* obstetric sonographers can accomplish this objective (Chapter 9). A woman's choice of whether or not to have an ultrasound examination should be based on the best available information as to possible benefits and hazards. This information should include advice that the effectiveness of routine ultrasound scanning is limited to the screening for malformations and its use for this purpose has several implications such as the risk of a false positive diagnosis and ethical issues.

Routine obstetric ultrasound scanning may perhaps be useful as a screening tool for malformations. No other clear benefits have been demonstrated. Its use for this purpose must be made explicit, and pregnant women must be asked to consent.

ACKNOWLEDGEMENT

This work was supported by a grant from the Swiss National Research Foundation (No. 32–38793.93).

SUMMARY

1 WHAT IS THE PROBLEM THAT REQUIRES SCREENING?

POOR PERINATAL OUTCOME SECONDARY TO EITHER POSTMATURITY, UNRECOGNIZED MULTIPLE GESTATION, FETAL ANOMALIES, OR GROWTH RESTRICTION. THE FOCUS HERE IS ON THE POST-TERM PREGNANCY.

a What is the incidence/prevalence of the target condition?

The incidence of post-term pregnancy varies widely, from 4% to 14%, possibly due in part to differences among the examined populations and in part to differences in the measurements used.

b What are the sequelae of the condition which are of interest in clinical medicine?

Post-term pregnancies are associated with adverse outcomes such as a higher rate of induced labor and maternal complications, and increased perinatal mortality and morbidity.

2 THE TEST

a ▶ What is the purpose of the test?

Routine, second-trimester ultrasonography reduces the incidence of post-term pregnancy by accurately dating the gestation. However, routine ultrasound screening is not separable into ultrasound for accurate dating to reduce the incidence of post-term pregnancies, and ultrasound to diagnose multiple gestation, malformations and growth restriction.

b ▶ The nature of the test

Fetal ultrasonography at 14–20 weeks' gestation.

c ▶ Implications of testing

I What does an abnormal test result mean?

An important difference between the age assigned based on the last menstrual period and that based on the sonographic biometric parameters indicates that the estimated date of confinement should be changed to reflect that estimated ultrasonographically.

d ▶ What is the cost of testing?

A cost-utility analysis is required to determine the value to the health care system of routine obstetrical ultrasound scanning.

3 CONCLUSIONS AND RECOMMENDATIONS

Routine ultrasonography for dating reduces the incidence of post-term pregnancy. Information on correct dating may be helpful for the management of 'true' post-term pregnancies because inducing labour in post-term pregnancies (41 or more weeks' duration) reduces cesarean section and perinatal mortality rates. Based on the available studies, routine one-stage ultrasound screening up to 20 weeks' gestation does not improve perinatal outcome assessed by the live birth rate or by a composite index of adverse perinatal outcomes. Routine ultrasound scans may, however, be effective for the detection of fetal malformations. Thus, a definitive answer regarding the advisability of routine second-trimester ultrasound screening is not yet possible.

REFERENCES

Bakketeig L & Bergsjø P (1989) Post-term pregnancy: magnitude of the problem. In Chalmers I, Enkin M & Keirse MJNC (eds) *Effective Care in Pregnancy and Childbirth*, pp 765–774. Oxford: Oxford University Press.
Berkowitz RL (1993) Should every pregnant woman undergo ultrasonography? (editorial). *N Engl J Med* **329:** 874–875.
Bierman J, Siegel E, French FE & Simonian K (1965) Analysis of the outcome of all pregnancies in a community Kauai pregnancy study. *Am J Obstet Gynecol* **91:** 37–45.
Boyd ME, Usher RH, McLean FH & Kramer MS (1988) Obstetric consequences of postmaturity. *Am J Obstet Gynecol* **158:** 334–338.
Bucher HC & Schmidt JG (1993a) Does routine ultrasound scanning improve outcome in pregnancy? A meta-analysis of various outcome measures. *Br Med J* **307:** 13–17.
Bucher HC & Schmidt JG (1993b) Routine ultrasound scanning in pregnancy. *Br Med J* **307:** 559–560.
Campell S, Warsof SL, Little D *et al.* (1985) Routine ultrasound screening for the prediction of gestational age. *Obstet Gynecol* **65:** 613–629.

Chalmers I (1975) *Description and Evaluation of Different Approaches to the Management of Pregnancy and Labour 1965–1973*. MSc Thesis, University of London.

Chamberlain G, Philip E, Howlett B *et al*. (1978) *British Births 1970*. Vol. 2: *Obstetric Care*, p. 292. London: Heinemann.

Chitty LS, Hunt GH, Moore J & Lobb MO (1991) Effectiveness of routine ultrasonography in detecting fetal structural abnormalities in a low risk population. *Br Med J* 303: 1165–1169.

Crowley P (1989) Post-term pregnancy: induction or surveillance? In: Chalmers I, Enkin M, Keirse MJNC (eds) *Effective Care in Pregnancy and Childbirth*, pp 776–791. Oxford University Press.

Crowley P (1991) Elective induction of labour at 41 + weeks gestation. In Chalmers I (ed.) *Oxford Database of Perinatal Trials*. Version 1.2, disk issue 5; record 4144. Oxford University Press.

Davey-Smith G & Egger M (1994) Who benefits from medical interventions? *Br Med J* 308: 72–74.

Eden RD, Seifert LS, Wineger A *et al*. (1987) Perinatal characteristics of uncomplicated postdated pregnancies. *Obstet Gynecol* 69: 296–9.

Evans TN, Koeff ST & Morley GW (1963) Fetal effects of prolonged pregnancy. *Am J Obstet Gynecol* 85: 701–12.

Ewigman BG, Crane JP, Frigoletto FD *et al*. (1993) Effect of prenatal ultrasound screening on perinatal outcome. *N Engl J Med* 329: 821–8.

FIGO (International Federation of Gynecology and Obstetrics) (1986) Report of the FIGO subcommittee on perinatal epidemiology and health statistics following a workshop in Cairo, November 11–18, 1984, on the methodology of measurement and recording of infant growth in the perinatal period. London: International Federation of Gynecology and Obstetrics, p. 54.

Grennert L, Persson PH & Gennser G (1978) Benefits of ultrasonic screening of a pregnant population. *Acta Obstet Gynaecol Scand* (suppl.) 78: 5–14.

Hadlock FP, Harrist RB & Hohler CW (1985) Determination of fetal age. In Athey PA, Hadlock FP (eds) *Ultrasound in Obstetrics and Gynecology*, pp. 22–37. St Louis: CV Mosby.

Hannah ME, Hannah WJ, Hellmann J *et al*. (1992) Induction of labour as compared with serial antenatal monitoring in post-term pregnancy. *N Engl J Med* 326: 1587–92.

LeFevre ML, Bain RP, Ewigman BG *et al*. (1993) A randomized trial of prenatal ultrasonographic screening: impact on maternal management and outcome. *Am J Obstet Gynecol* 169: 483–9.

Kloosterman GJ (1979) Epidemiology of postmaturity. In Keirsre MJNC, Anderson ABM & Bennebroek Gravenhorst J (eds) *Human Parturition*, pp. 247–61. The Hague: Leiden University Press.

MacGregor SN, Tamura RK, Sabbagha RE *et al*. (1987) Underestimation of gestational age by conventional crown-rump length dating curves. *Obstet Gynecol* 70: 344–8.

Mead PB & Marcus SL (1964) Prolonged pregnancy. *Am J Obstet Gynecol* 89: 495–502.

Mintz MC & Landon MB (1988) Sonographic diagnosis of fetal growth disorders. *Clin Obstet Gynecol* 31: 44–52.

Naeye R (1978) Causes of perinatal mortality excess in prolonged gestations. *Am J Epidemiol* 108: 429–33.

National Centre for Health Statistics (1990) *Vital Statistics of the United States, 1988*. Vol. 1, *Natality*. DHHS Publication PAS 90–1100. Washington, DC: Government Printing Office.

National Centre for Health Statistics (1991) *Vital Statistics of the United States, 1988*. Vol. 2, *Mortality*, Part A. DHHS Publication PAS 91–1101. Washington, DC: Government Printing Office.

Romero R (1993) Routine obstetric ultrasound. *Ultrasound Obstet Gynecol* 3: 303–307.

Saari-Kemppainen A, Karjalainen O, Ylostalo P *et al*. (1990) Ultrasound screening and perinatal mortality: controlled trial of systematic one-stage screening in pregnancy. *Lancet* 336: 387–91.

Sabbagha RE & Hughey M (1978) Standardization of sonar cephalometry and gestational age. *Obstet Gynecol* 53: 402–6.

Saunders N & Paterson C (1991) Effect of gestational age on obstetric performance: when is 'term' over? *Lancet* 338: 1190–2.

Waldenström U, Axelsson O, Nilson S *et al*. (1988) Effects of routine one-stage ultrasound screening in pregnancy: a randomised controlled trial. *Lancet* ii: 385–388.

World Health Organization (1977) *Manual of the International Statistical Classification of Diseases, Injuries, and Causes of Death*, 9th ed. Geneva: WHO.

Zwerdling M (1967) Factors pertaining to prolonged pregnancy and its outcome. *Pediatrics* 40: 202–9.

9

Routine Ultrasonography for the Detection of Fetal Structural Anomalies

Juriy W. Wladimiroff

FETAL STRUCTURAL ANOMALIES.

Perinatal mortality is now in the range of 10 per 1000 births in the industrialized countries. The improvement reflects predominantly enhanced intrapartum and neonatal care. Intrauterine growth restriction (IUGR), preterm delivery and congenital disease are still major determinants of perinatal mortality and morbidity. Thus, the prevention and early detection of congenital anomalies has become an important part of maternal health care.

What is the incidence/prevalence of the target condition?

About 2–3% of newborns have detectable congenital structural anomalies, 20–30% of which result in perinatal death (Morrison, 1985).

What are the sequelae of the condition which are of interest in clinical medicine?

Major fetal structural anomalies are potentially associated with preterm delivery, perinatal mortality and morbidity, unwarranted obstetric surgery, prolonged postnatal hospitalization, all of which exact emotional, social and financial hardship upon the involved families and upon society. Prenatal detection of a malformed fetus allows the woman a range of options varying from pregnancy termination to possible intrauterine treatment and adjustment of obstetric management. The latter concerns the immediate availability of sophisticated neonatal care of the structurally abnormal infant. The potential advantage of prenatal diagnosis of a major but nonlethal fetal malformations is modification of the timing, mode, and geographic location of the delivery. Forewarned, the parents can avert the delivery of a child in a hospital ill-prepared to care for the problem.

THE TEST

Routine ultrasound examination.

What is the purpose of the test?

To diagnose major fetal structural anomalies prior to 24 weeks and thus preserve the full range of options to the woman. Other potential benefits of routine ultrasound examination are covered in chapter 8. When evaluating the role of ultrasound scanning for the early detection of fetal structural anomalies it is important to distinguish between standard – level 1 – ultrasound investigations aimed at women attending a general antenatal clinic (screening-based investigations) and 'detailed' – high-resolution, real-time – ultrasound investigations targeted at women who are at increased risk of fetal structural anomalies (indication-based investigations), the latter being usually conducted in secondary or tertiary referral centres with a high level of expertise in ultrasonography.

The nature of the test

SCREENING-BASED ULTRASOUND EXAMINATION

The vast majority of malformed fetuses result from pregnancies not known to have clinical risk factors. Screening-based ultrasound examinations concern the determination of fetal viability, age, number, placental location, and the survey of major fetal structural anomalies.

INDICATION-BASED ULTRASOUND EXAMINATION

Indication-based ultrasound investigations apply to selective – levels 2 and 3 – ultrasound imaging, targeted at women at increased risk of fetal structural anomalies. They entail a more detailed examination of fetal morphology and physiologic function than the screening-based scan. One or several organ systems, depending on the indication, are subjected to scrupulous sonographic investigation. For instance, an indication-based scan of the fetal heart includes not only the visualization of the four chamber view, but also of the ventriculo-arterial outflow, the venous inflow, the aortic arch and the ductus arteriosus. In addition to the extra time spent, these examinations are typically performed by either a sonologist or sonographer with considerable experience and a high level of expertise with ultrasound scanning. Two distinct risk situations can be distinguished for indication-based ultrasound examinations.

Risk factors known prior to pregnancy: Screening is targeted at women at increased risk of fetal structural anomalies because of one or more specific risk factors known *prior* to the index pregnancy, such as a previously affected infant, a parent with a structural anomaly, maternal type 1 diabetes mellitus, maternal use of antiepileptic drugs or certain psychopharmacokinetic drugs (including lithium) which are associated with an increased risk of fetal cardiac anomalies. Agreement seems to exist about the timing of conducting a basic anomaly scan, i.e. 17–20 weeks' gestation, since in most countries pregnancy termination is not legal beyond 24 weeks. The number of routine ultrasound investigations in unselected obstetric populations is limited and may preclude definitive interpretation of abnormal findings. The overall prevalence of major fetal structural anomalies in this high-risk group is 3–4%. Parents in this group often intend to terminate pregnancy when the fetus is structurally abnormal. Lie *et al.* (1994) observed that among women whose first infant has a birth defect, the risk of the same defect in the second infant is 7.6 times higher than expected (95% CI 6.5–8.8), while the risk of a different defect is 1.5 times higher (95% CI 1.3–1.7) than expected.

Risk factors found during pregnancy: Diagnostic investigations for suspected fetal pathology are based on abnormal obstetric findings that become manifest *during* the index pregnancy, such as polyhydramnios, oligohydramnios, severe IUGR and fetal cardiac dysrhythmias. These findings are strongly associated with fetal structural anomalies. Women with pregnancies thus affected are often referred to tertiary centers for diagnostic evaluation by means of detailed ultrasonography and invasive prenatal diagnosis where indicated. The prevalence of fetal structural anomalies in this category approximates 35–40% (Wladimiroff *et al.*, 1988). The anomalies are usually detected after 24 weeks' gestation. In an estimated 20% of cases, more than one organ system is involved. This is often based on the presence of a particular syndrome or chromosome abnormality (Wladimiroff *et al.*, 1988). In advanced pregnancies, swift information on the fetal chromosome pattern is essential for optimal obstetric management. For example, preterm labor is not inhibited and intrauterine hypoxemia not treated by a cesarean delivery if either trisomy 13 or trisomy 18 are diagnosed. Chromosome analysis is preferably performed by obtaining a fetal blood sample where the karyotype should be available within 72 hours (Hollander *et al.*, 1993). Improvement in the level of expertise and the quality of ultrasound equipment has led to the discovery of certain ultrasound markers for chromosome pathology. Examples include nuchal edema (between 10 and 14 weeks of gestation), or atrial or ventricular septal defects as well as duodenal atresia (trisomy 21) (Snijders *et al.*, 1990). When faced with a fetus with a lethal malformation, many parents will opt for termination of pregnancy. In the case of a fetal anomaly compatible with life (for example, intestinal atresia, neural tube defect), the mode (vaginal or cesarean section), timing (preterm or term), and location of the delivery are discussed with the neonatologist and the organ specialist (pediatric surgeon or cardiologist, for example).

The recent introduction of transvaginal sonography has allowed evaluation of fetal anatomy as early as 9–10 weeks' gestation. Though a number of fetal abnormalities have been diagnosed using this technique, a considerable level of expertise is needed before the widescale introduction of this technique. It seems unlikely that transvaginal ultrasound imaging will become an effective tool for the detection of fetal structural anomalies in the near future.

Implications of testing

WHAT DOES AN ABNORMAL TEST RESULT MEAN?

The accuracy of screening-based ultrasound investigations for fetal structural anomalies is determined by the sonographer's level of expertise, the equipment used and the time spent on each examination. Romero (1993) summarized the findings of published studies in which ultrasound was used as a screening method for the detection of anomalies prior to 24 weeks (Table 9.1). The overall sensitivity of ultrasound for the detection of anomalies was 52.9%.

In an hospital-based study Levi *et al.* (1991) examined 16 072 women at low risk of fetal anomalies, who had at least one ultrasound scan during pregnancy. A total of 381 neonates (2.3%) had at least one structural anomaly, benign or undetectable malformations being excluded; in 154 of the 381 affected neonates (40.4%) the anomaly was detected prenatally by means of ultrasound, almost half of these being identified prior to 26

Table 9.1 Comparison of studies evaluating the value of routine ultrasound examinations for the detection of fetal structural anomalies.

REFERENCE	SUBJECTS AND PERIOD	GESTATIONAL AGE (weeks)	PREVALENCE OF ANOMALIES (%)	SENS.	SPEC.	PPV	NPV
Saari-Kemppainen et al. (1990)	4 073 (1986–87)	16–20	0.99	0.40	0.99	0.64	0.99
Levi et al. (1991)	16 072 (1984–89)	12–20	1.61	0.21	1.00	1.00	0.99
Rosendahl and Kivenen (1989)	9 012 (1980–88)	<24	1.03	0.40	—	—	—
Shirley et al. (1992)	6 138 (1989–91)	19	1.36	0.61	0.99	0.98	0.99
Chitty et al. (1991)	8 432 (1988–89)	<24	1.48	0.74	0.99	0.98	1.00
Luck (1992)	8 523 (1990–91)	19	1.95	0.84	0.99	0.99	1.00
Overall	52 295 (1980–91)	<24	—	0.53	0.99	0.96	0.99

NPV, negative predictive value; PPV, positive predictive value; SENS., sensitivity; SPEC., specificity. From Romero (1993), with permission weeks' gestation. While overall sensitivity and specificity were 40% and 99.9% respectively, the results varied markedly according to the organ system being considered. For example, anomaly detection rate ranked highest for the fetal neck (100%) and lowest for fetal facial structures (0%) and fetal cardiovascular system (4%). Hence, reported accuracy estimates of ultrasound investigations for fetal anomalies depend on case definition in terms of the nature and the seriousness of the malformation. On the one hand, the overall sensitivity of an ultrasound examination for the detection of fetal anomalies will be distorted if minor anomalies with a high prevalence that are easily picked up by prenatal ultrasound are included. For example, Luck (1992) evaluated the use of ultrasound at 19 weeks' gestation in a group of 8523 unselected women. Of the 166 newborns with a structural anomaly, 140 were detected prenatally (sensitivity of 84%); 105 (63%) of the 166 newborns had an anomaly of the renal system. The reported favorable sensitivity could be ascribed to the relatively high proportion of minor renal anomalies, which could be easily detected prenatally. On the other hand, a low detection rate for cardiac anomalies was noted by Buskens (personal communication) whose findings were based on the absence or presence of an abnormal four chamber view: the sensitivity for just major cardiac anomalies was 16.7%, while for both minor and major cardiac anomalies it was 4.5%. While the four chamber view is easily obtained, it does not permit the detection of either transposition of the great arteries or coarctation of the aorta. Moreover, smaller ventricular and atrial septal defects may be missed. Based on the four chamber view, only Sharland and Allan (1992) reported a sensitivity as high as 77% for the detection of cardiac abnormalities.

The overall sensitivity of an indication-based ultrasound examination is higher than that of screening-based scanning, with reported values approximating 85%. This is mainly explained by the higher level of scanning expertise in referral centers, better knowledge of genetic syndromes, the availability of superior ultrasound equipment and the availability of pediatric specialists for consultation. Nevertheless, even in experienced hands the reported sensitivity of the detailed cardiac scan remains low, i.e. 65% (Stewart, 1989) in particular as the result of small septal defects being missed. Color-coded Doppler ultrasonography, which permits visualization of blood flow direction, seems to improve the detection of these small defects (Stewart and Wladimiroff, 1993). From the prospect of screening, however, an extended cardiac scan, i.e. including the assessment of venous inflow and arterial outflow, will inevitably be of little value in an obstetric population with a low prevalence of fetal cardiac anomalies (Buskens *et al.* 1995).

The early detection of fetal structural anomalies has the potential to reduce perinatal mortality and morbidity by one of two mechanisms. First, it may reduce mortality by converting neonatal or perinatal deaths to elective terminations of pregnancy. Second, it may reduce morbidity by optimizing the circumstances surrounding the delivery of a fetus with a major but not necessarily lethal anomaly. Several studies have tried to determine the impact of routine ultrasonography on fetal outcome. In the Helsinki trial (Saari-Kemppainen *et al.*, 1990) 9010 pregnant women were randomized either to the group that was offered ultrasound investigation between 16 and 20 weeks' gestation (the screening group) or to the group that had selective ultrasonography, i.e. when medically indicated (the control group). Perinatal mortality was significantly lower in the screening group (4.6 per 1000) compared with the control group (9.0 per 1000). This near 50% reduction in perinatal mortality was mostly due to pregnancy terminations for reasons of fetal structural anomalies. This observation emphasizes the importance of anomaly scanning prior to 22 weeks' gestation. Furthermore, it demonstrates the potential impact of the women's attitudes to pregnancy termination on the efficacy of routine ultrasound examination, in terms of perinatal mortality. In a study involving 13 849 ultrasound scans performed during the second or the third trimester, Hegge *et al.* (1989) examined how often fetal anomalies were identified too late for pregnancy termination; 240

(66%) of the 364 fetuses with at least one anomaly were only identified after 22 weeks' gestation. Two-thirds of the malformed fetuses identified prior to 23 weeks' gestation were aborted or delivered early. Only 34 (14%) of those malformed fetuses identified after 22 weeks were either aborted or delivered early. The study by Hegge *et al.* (1989) illustrates that either some anomalies may not be detectable until after 24 weeks' gestation, or that they may be easily overlooked. From National Institutes of Health consensus meeting in Washington (Consensus Conference, 1984), it was reported that 56% of fetuses with anomalies detected after 22 weeks' gestation had no listed indication for an ultrasound examination.

The reduction in perinatal mortality in women undergoing screening-based ultrasound scanning is mainly determined by the subsequent termination of pregnancies with lethal fetal structural pathology. This was also emphasized in a meta-analysis of the impact of routine ultrasound scanning on pregnancy outcome (Bucher and Schmidt, 1993). In the Routine Antenatal Diagnostic Imaging Ultrasound Study (RADIUS), a randomized controlled trial to determine whether in low-risk women ultrasound screening – conducted at 15–22 weeks and at 31–35 weeks – decreased the frequency of adverse perinatal outcomes, a significantly higher percentage of at least one major fetal structural anomaly was diagnosed in the group undergoing ultrasound screening (34.8%) compared with the group who only had ultrasonography on indication (11.0%) (Ewigman *et al.*, 1993). In the screening group these findings did not result in an increased number of pregnancy terminations, cesarean sections, amniocenteses or prolonged admissions to hospital. The authors concluded that screening ultrasonography did not improve perinatal outcome as compared with the selective use of ultrasonography. The findings of this large trial stimulate two comments. First, the investigators sought to determine whether a diagnostic tool alone could alter outcome. Second, the proportion of fetal structural anomalies detected before 24 weeks' gestation was low, i.e. 16.6% in the screening group compared with 40% in the Helsinki study (Saari-Kemppainen *et al.*, 1990). This raises questions concerning the quality of scanning in the participating centers.

Less clear is the benefit of early detection of nonlethal fetal structural anomalies and the impact of adjustment of obstetric management on perinatal mortality (Buskens *et al.*, 1995). In this respect, some women may be burdened with unwarranted anxiety (Schei, 1992). Larger studies are needed to clarify this issue.

WHAT DOES A NORMAL TEST RESULT MEAN?

Given the high specificity achieved by routine ultrasound examinations and the relatively low prevalence of major fetal structural anomalies, normal findings in low-risk populations are generally reassuring (Table 9.1). High specificity in low-risk populations minimizes the risk of unnecessary interventions as the relative frequency of false positive findings is low (Levi *et al.* 1989).

What is the cost of testing?

Little information is available on the actual costs of routine ultrasound screening. Economic evaluations of ultrasound examinations are complex since these involve many intangible costs of prenatal care which typically pertain to local remuneration structures. Extrapolation of findings is therefore of limited value. Apart from the potential impact on perinatal mortality, economic evaluations should take into account the accuracy of anomaly screening, which varies widely between centers, as accuracy estimates are related to the level of experience of the sonographer, case definition, the number of examinations during pregnancy and the gestational age at which the examination is done. Accuracy estimates are compounded by inadequate ascertainment of newborns with major structural anomalies, especially those anomalies that are not readily apparent at birth (Gomez and Copel, 1993; DeVore, 1994). Moreover, economic evaluations should take into account local policies with respect to pregnancy termination and alteration of obstetric management, and the desires and attitudes of couples, in particular when fetal anomalies are diagnosed. Recently, DeVore compared the cost per detected case of a major fetal structural anomaly in the RADIUS trial to the cost per detected malformed fetus in the California maternal serum alpha-fetoprotein (MSAFP) screening program (DeVore, 1994). Using the data of the RADIUS study, the cost per detected case was $56 008; this was $15 670 (28%) more than the cost per detected case using data from the California MSAFP screening. The authors argue that as the detection rate for malformed fetuses increases, the costs per case identified decreases. If the ultrasound detection rate of malformed fetuses is 5 per 1000 and the cost $200 per ultrasound examination, the cost per case detected would be $40 000 which is similar to the cost of identifying a malformed fetus by universal MSAFP screening (DeVore, 1994).

CONCLUSIONS AND RECOMMENDATIONS

Controversy exists with respect to the impact of routine ultrasonography on perinatal morbidity or mortality. The National Institutes of Health Consensus Conference (1984) speaks against routine obstetric ultrasound examinations, based on concerns of its safety and efficacy in women without specific risk factors. These issues are complex, involving both financial and societal costs, the skill of the ultrasonographers involved in the screening program, and the societal view of severely malformed fetuses. Evaluation of pooled data is further complicated by the varying gestational ages at which ultrasound screening is conducted, the lack of clearly defined end-points for adverse perinatal outcome, the low prevalence of the distinctive fetal anomalies, small sample size, and the incompleteness of follow-up (Gomez and Copel, 1993). However, there is evidence that the policy of routine ultrasound screening significantly improves the detection of fetal structural anomalies when compared with the policy of ultrasonography only for specific medical indications (Saari-Kemppainen et al., 1990; Romero, 1993; Bernaschek et al., 1994). Adequate counseling of the pregnant woman or the couple is essential. The reported overall sensitivity of ultrasound examinations for the detection of fetal structural anomalies prior to 24 weeks' gestation is 53% (Table 9.1), implying that a large proportion of fetal anomalies will be missed. It is emphasized that the level of scanning expertise strongly determines the detection rate of malformed fetuses. Adequate training is a prerequisite to establish a level of ultrasound skills sufficient to have a major impact on detection rate. The arguments in favor of routine anomaly screening in the second trimester in low-risk women are based on the option of pregnancy termination where major fetal structural anomaly is detected, possible early intrauterine treatment, and – perhaps more importantly – the planning of timing, mode, and location of delivery with the objective of prompt neonatal treatment where indicated. The motivation for ultrasound examinations for the detection of fetal structural anomalies in women at increased risk are similar to those for screening in low-risk pregnancies, but there are other arguments as well. Couples who had decided against planning another pregnancy because of a past history of major fetal abnormality might reconsider this decision on the basis of the availability of early anomaly screening and subsequent termination of pregnancy if a major fetal structural anomaly was detected again. Moreover, reassurance is clearly of psychologic benefit to such couples in the case where no fetal structural anomalies are detected. Ultrasound investigation for fetal structural anomalies should preferably be carried out between 17 weeks and 20 weeks of gestation. The impact on perinatal outcome is determined mainly by the percentage of women who intend to terminate the pregnancy if a major fetal structural anomaly is diagnosed prior to 24 weeks' gestation, the gestational age limit for legal abortion in most countries. In populations at increased risk of fetal structural anomaly, the prevalence of a malformation in the present pregnancy will be 3–4%; in the case of abnormal obstetric findings such as polyhydramnios and oligohydramnios, IUGR or fetal cardiac arrhythmias, the prevalence may be as high as 35–40%. In the latter group, multiple structural anomalies will be present in approximately 20%, often as a result of a syndrome or abnormal chromosomal pattern.

SUMMARY

1 WHAT IS THE PROBLEM THAT REQUIRES SCREENING?

FETAL STRUCTURAL ANOMALIES.

a What is the incidence/prevalence of the target condition?

About 2–3% of the newborns have detectable major structural pathology, 20–30% of which result in perinatal death.

b What are the sequelae of the condition which are of interest in clinical medicine?

Fetal malformations are associated with preterm delivery, perinatal death, unnecessary surgery, prolonged postnatal hospitalization, all of which exact emotional, social and financial hardship on the involved families and upon society.

2 THE TEST

a What is the purpose of the test?

The aim of ultrasound investigation performed between 17 weeks and 20 weeks of gestation is to diagnose major structural fetal anomalies.

b The nature of the test

Standard – level 1 – ultrasound examination aimed at the general population (screening-based examination), or selective – levels 2 and 3 – ultrasound examination aimed at women at increased risk of fetal structural anomalies (indication-based examination).

c Implications of testing

1 What does an abnormal test result mean?

Reported positive predictive values of both screening-based and indication-based ultrasound examinations are generally high (0.64–1.00). However, the overall reported sensitivity of screening-based ultrasound examination for the detection of fetal structural anomalies prior to 24 weeks' gestation varies markedly from 0.17 to 0.84. The accuracy of ultrasound examinations for the detection of fetal structural anomalies is determined by the sonographer's level of experience, the equipment used, and the time spent on each examination.

2 What does a normal test result mean?

Routine ultrasound examination for the detection of fetal structural anomalies is associated with high specificity. Normal findings are generally reassuring.

d What is the cost of testing?

Little information is available on the actual costs of ultrasound screening. If the ultrasound detection rate of malformed fetuses is 5 per 1000, the cost at $200 per ultrasound scan would be $40 000 per detected fetus, which is similar to the cost of identifying a malformed fetus by universal maternal serum alpha-fetoprotein screening.

3 CONCLUSIONS AND RECOMMENDATIONS

There is still controversy about the impact of routine ultrasound screening on perinatal mortality and morbidity. There is evidence to suggest that the policy of routine ultrasound screening improves the detection of fetal structural anomalies when compared with the policy of ultrasonography only for specific medical conditions. The impact of routine ultrasound screening for the detection of fetal structural anomalies on perinatal mortality is mainly determined by the proportion of women who intend to terminate pregnancy when a major fetal malformation is identified prior to 24 weeks' gestation, the gestational age limit for legal abortion in most industrialized countries. The efficacy of intervention strategies for nonlethal fetal structural anomalies is still questionable. It is argued that adequate training is a prerequisite to establish a level of ultrasound skills sufficient to have a major impact on detection rates.

REFERENCES

Bernaschek G, Stuempflen I & Deutinger J (1994) The value of sonographic diagnosis of fetal malformations: different results between indication-based and screening-based investigations. *Prenat Diagn* **14:** 807–812.

Bucher HC & Schmidt JG (1993) Does routine ultrasound scanning improve in pregnancy? Meta-analysis of various outcome measures. *Br Med J* **307:** 13–16.

Buskens E, Grobbee DE Hess J & Wladimiroff JW (1985) Prenatal diagnosis of congenital heart disease; prospects and problems. *Eur J Obstet Gynecol Reprod Biol* **60:** 5–11.

Chitty LS Hunt GH Moore J & Lobb MO (1991) Effectiveness of routine ultrasonography in detecting fetal structural anomalies in a low risk population. *Br Med J* **303:** 1165–1169.

Consensus Conference (1984) The use of diagnostic ultrasound imaging during pregnancy. *JAMA* **252:** 669–672.

DeVore GR (1994) The routine antenatal diagnostic imaging with ultrasound study: another perspective. *Obstet Gynecol* **84:** 622–626.

Ewigman BG, Crane JP Frigoletto FD *et al.* (1993) A randomized trial of prenatal ultrasound screening in a low risk population: impact on perinatal outcome. *N Engl J Med* **329:** 821–827.

Gomez KJ & Copel JA (1993) Ultrasound for fetal structural anomalies. *Curr Opin Obstet Gynecol***5:** 204–210.

Hegge FN, Franklin RW, Watson PT, & Calhoun BC (1989) An evaluation of the time of discovery of fetal malformation by an indication-based system for ordering obstetrical ultrasound. *Obstet Gynecol* **74:** 21–24.

Hollander NS den, Stewart PA Cohen-Overbeek TE *et al.* (1992) Cordocentese en structurele afwijkingen bij de foetus. *Ned Tijdschr Obstet Gynecol* **105:** 343–345.

Levi S, Crouzet P Schaaps JP *et al.* (1989) Ultrasound screening for fetal malformations. *Lancet* **i:** 678.

Levi S, Hyjazi Y Schaaps JP Defoort P Coulon R & Buekens P (1991) Sensitivity and specificity of routine antenatal screening for congenital anomalies by ultrasound: the Belgian multicentric study. *Ultrasound Obstet Gynecol* **1**: 102–10.

Lie RT, Wilcox AJ & Skjaerven R (1994) A population based study of the risk of recurrence of birth defects. *N. Engl J Med* **331**: 1–4.

Luck CA (1992) Value of routine ultrasound scanning at 19 weeks: a four year study of 8,849 deliveries. *Br Med J* **304**: 1474–78.

Morrison I (1985) Perinatal mortality: basic considerations. *Semin Perinatol* **9**: 144–150.

Romero R (1993) Routine obstetric ultrasound (editorial). *Ultrasound Obstet Gynecol* **3**: 303–7.

Rosendahl H & Kivenen S (1989) Antenatal detection of congenital malformations by routine ultrasonography. *Obstet Gynecol* **73**: 947–51.

Saari-Kemppainen A Karjalainen O Ylostalo P & Heinonen OP (1990) Ultrasound screening and perinatal mortality: controlled trial of systematic one-stage screening in pregnancy. The Helsinki Ultrasound Trial. *Lancet* **i**: 387–91.

Schei B (1992) The routine use of ultrasound in antenatal care: is there a hidden agenda? *Issues Reprod Genet Eng* **5**: 13–20.

Sharland GK & Allan LDS (1992) Screening for congenital heart disease prenatally: results of a 2½-year study in the South East Thames region. *Br J Obstet Gynaecol* **99**: 220–25.

Shirley IM Bottomly F & Robinson VP (1992) Routine radiographer screening for fetal abnormalities by ultrasound in a unselected population. *Br J Radiol* **65**: 564–9.

Stewart PA (1989) *Fetal echocardiography*. Thesis, Erasmus University: Rotterdam.

Stewart PA & Wladimiroff JW (1993) Fetal echocardiography and color Doppler flow imaging: the Rotterdam experience. *Ultrasound Obstet Gynecol* **3**: 168–175.

Wladimiroff JW Sachs ES Reuss A Stewart PA Pijpers L & Niermeijer MF (1988) Prenatal diagnosis of chromosome abnormalities in the presence of fetal structural defects. *Am J Med Genet* **29**: 289–291.

10

Doppler Velocimetry for the Detection of Intrauterine Growth Restriction

Sicco Scherjon

WHAT IS THE PROBLEM THAT REQUIRES SCREENING?

INTRAUTERINE GROWTH RESTRICTION (IUGR).

Intrauterine growth restriction is a major clinical problem. While the phrases 'IUGR' and 'small for gestational age' (SGA) are often used interchangeably, they are not the same. The phrase IUGR denotes a fetus who has experienced intrauterine nutritional deficiency which has resulted in a reduction of fetal growth velocity. When severe, the fetus also has hypoxemia. Only half of SGA infants are also growth restricted.

What is the incidence/prevalence of the target condition?

Several definitions based on birthweight (less than 2.3rd, 5th or 10th percentile) are commonly used to define both IUGR and SGA. A birthweight below the 10th percentile means that 10% of newborns in the population are by definition SGA. Growth curves should be based on the population served and take into account maternal height, parity, and fetal sex. Definitions of IUGR such as the ponderal index or skinfold thickness more accurately identify the IUGR fetus (Villar *et al.*, 1990), but are more complicated to perform than the measurement of birthweight. An alternative to birthweight alone is the calculation of the difference between actual birthweight and predicted birthweight based on several physiological determinants (Sanderson *et al.*, 1994). The major problem with any single physical measurement as a definition of IUGR is that there are many causes of an SGA fetus other than IUGR.

What are the sequelae of the condition which are of interest in clinical medicine?

More than a third of structurally normal singletons who die in utero are IUGR. The condition is also associated with an increased risk of perinatal complications such as fetal distress and depression at birth (Kramer *et al.*, 1990; Sanderson *et al.*, 1994). The ponderal index is an independent predictor of neonatal morbidity whether the newborn is above or below the 10th centile of the growth curve (Villar *et al.*, 1990). Newborns with IUGR are at increased risk of compromised neurodevelopment. Both minor neurologic dysfunction and lower developmental scores are more common in IUGR infants (Hadders-Algra and Touwen, 1990; Martikainen, 1992; Ounsted *et al.*, 1984; Teberg *et al.*, 1988).

THE TEST

What is the purpose of the test?

To detect IUGR. A major problem in screening for IUGR is the absence of a 'gold standard'.

The nature of the test

Doppler ultrasonography allows the noninvasive measurement of blood flow velocity which is in turn a reflection of resistance to flow. Since the measurement of velocity is dependent on the angle of insonation, a variety of angle-independent indices are used that combine both systolic and diastolic velocities (Figure 10.1).

Two basic types of Doppler technology are used in obstetrics. Continuous wave (CW) has the advantage of requiring less expensive and less complicated equipment. It can be used when simultaneous visualization of the targeted vessel is unnecessary (e.g. the umbilical artery and uterine arteries). Pulsed Doppler (PD) is obligatory when the vessel of interest must be visualized (e.g. the fetal aorta and cerebral circulation). The indices measured by CW and PD instrumentation are comparable. Color PD imaging facilitates the examination by shortening the time needed to identify the targeted vessel. As a result, the success rate is increased (Noordam *et al.*, 1994). A ratio of the umbilical and cerebral artery indices (U/C ratio) (Wladimiroff *et al.*, 1987) can be used to illustrate the hemodynamic redistribution of blood flow to the brain associated with IUGR.

RELIABILITY AND TECHNOLOGY ASSESSMENT

The location of the vessel insonated affects the Doppler measurement (Maulik *et al.*, 1989; Mehalek *et al.*, 1989). For example, resistance to flow through the uterine artery is lower on the placental side of the uterus compared with the nonplacental side. Thus, it is common practice to take the mean of the measurements from the two uterine arteries. The resistance to flow in the umbilical artery is lowest at the placental and highest

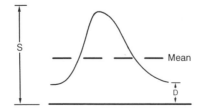

Figure 10.1   Flow velocity waveform. The waveform is characterized by three different indices as proposed by three different authors: $\frac{S}{D}$ = S/D ratio (Stuart *et al.*, 1980); $\frac{S-D}{S}$ = Resistance index (Pourcelot, 1974); $\frac{S-D}{\text{mean}}$ = Pulsatility index (Gosling and King, 1975).

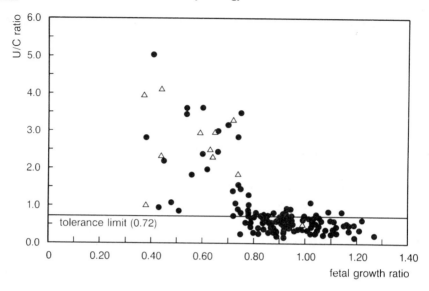

Figure 10.2 The relation between Umbilical/Cerebral (U/C) ratio and fetal growth. In cases of moderate/severe growth restriction (i.e. a fetal growth ratio below 80%) a tendency of a rising U/C ratio is seen. In all cases of intrauterine fetal death (open triangle), except in one case, the U/C ratio appeared to be above the tolerance limit. Filled circles show liveborn infants. U/C ratio, Umbilical Pulsatility Index/Cerebral Pulsatility Index ratio.

at the fetal cord origin. As a result, it is customary to measure the umbilical artery resistance in a free-floating midsegment of the cord. Fetal breathing and movement also affects the Doppler index. Measurements should be performed during fetal apnoe and in the absence of fetal movements. The reliability is improved if the mean from three to six waveforms is used (Spencer and Price, 1989; Spencer *et al.*, 1991). Examiner experience and equipment variation have only minor impact on reproducibility (Nienhuis *et al.*, 1988; Tessler *et al.*, 1990; Scherjon *et al.*, 1993a).

Implications of testing

WHAT DOES AN ABNORMAL TEST RESULT MEAN?

The most characteristic change of the flow velocity waveform (FVW) in the umbilical artery and the descending aorta of the IUGR fetus is a reduction and even loss or reversal of the end-diastolic velocities. As a result, the Doppler resistance indices are increased. Several gestational age-dependent normative curves (Arduini *et al.*, 1987; Wladimiroff *et al.*, 1987; Woo *et al.*, 1987; Pearce *et al.*, 1988; McCowan *et al.*, 1988; Cameron *et al.*, 1989) have been published: indices either above the 95th centile (van Vught 1991), or 2 standard deviations above the mean (Newnham *et al.*, 1990) are typically considered abnormal. Both the umbilical and uterine artery resistance indices are inversely proportional to the fetal P_{O_2} (Weiner, 1990). Diastolic velocities should be considered as a continuum. As the index rises, both the severity of the growth restriction and hypoxemia increase (Divon *et al.*, 1989; Weiner, 1990; Scherjon *et al.*, 1993b) (Figure 10.2). Reversal of the umbilical artery end-diastolic flow is the most extreme waveform abnormality.

The value of Doppler velocimetry as a test for IUGR can be expressed in terms of likelihood ratios. Likelihood ratios (Table 10.1) are combined with the prevalence to calculate the post-test probabilities (Table 10.2) (as described in Chapter 1). Table 10.2 ranks the vessels according to the test performance. In studies where the prevalence of IUGR exceeds 5%, uteroplacental artery Doppler performs the worst as a screen for IUGR, whereas the fetal cerebral artery – especially the U/C ratio – performs the best. There are no substantial differences among likelihood ratios in studies where the prevalence of IUGR is below 5%. Use of the Ponderal Index rather than birthweight to diagnose IUGR does not alter test performance (Sijmons et al., 1989). The ultrasonic estimate of fetal weight is superior to Doppler for the diagnosis of low birthweight (Chang et al., 1993).

Doppler indices may be elevated weeks or even months before IUGR is clinically detectable. The placentas of newborns with abnormal FVWs often show obliteration of tertiary stem villi which is consistent with a failure of trophoblastic invasion (Giles et al., 1985; Arabin et al., 1988). Growth-restricted fetuses with absent end-diastolic velocity (AEDV) are consistently hypoxemic and/or acidemic compared with gestational age-corrected norms for the fetuses of nonlaboring patients (Hackett et al., 1987; Nicolaides et al., 1988; Al-Ghazali et al., 1990; Weiner, 1990; Pardi et al., 1993). The same cannot be said when diastolic flow is still present. While several studies report the reappearance of diastolic velocities (up to 30%), this is rare in the setting of severe IUGR if diastolic flow is absent in all sections of the umbilical cord and there is decreased middle cerebral artery resistance. There is no physiologic explanation for a decrease in resistance known in the absence of either resolving placentitis or pharmacologic therapy. Nevertheless, Doppler studies should probably not be used as a definite argument for the immediate delivery of a preterm fetus (Johnstone et al., 1988; Wenstrom et al., 1991; Bell et al., 1992).

Hypoxemia/acidemia in the umbilical cord blood at delivery is less common when the elevated umbilical artery pulsatility index (PI) of an SGA pregnancy is associated with normal fetal heart rate testing (4%). The likelihood of hypoxemia being present at delivery increases to over 60% if the fetal heart rate pattern is abnormal (Pardi et al., 1993). Flow velocity waveform abnormalities occur earlier than abnormalities in fetal heart rate variability (Pattinson et al., 1991; Soothill et al., 1993). A low cerebral artery PI may precede an abnormal fetal heart rate pattern by weeks or even months (Arduini et al., 1992). Decreased cerebral resistance is often associated with an elevated resistance in the descending aorta and the umbilical artery (Wladimiroff et al., 1986). This 'brain sparing', defined as a raised U/C ratio, identifies the fetus whose IUGR is likely to be based on uteroplacental dysfunction severe enough to impede oxygen delivery. In some studies of SGA fetuses, umbilical artery velocimetry was a better predictor of perinatal distress than either the abdominal circumference measurement or the biophysical profile score (James et al., 1992).

Though the application of Doppler velocimetry has in some observational studies been associated with a decrease in the number of labor inductions and operative deliveries for fetal distress in pregnancies with an SGA fetus (Almstrom et al., 1992; Pattinson et al., 1994), this is not true in randomized control trials (RCT) (Johnstone et al., 1993).

The published RCTs of routine Doppler ultrasound in either general obstetric populations or in high-risk pregnancies are summarized in Table 10.3 and the potential effects on pregnancy outcome in Table 10.4.

Screening studies: The routine use of Doppler has no effect on gestational age at delivery, the rates of either labor induction or cesarean section including elective sections. Neither neonatal intensive care nor medium care nursery admissions are altered (Trudinger et al., 1987; Tyrrell et al., 1990; Newnham et al., 1991; Davies et al., 1992; Omzigt et al., 1994; Whittle et al., 1994).

Table 10.1 Test characteristics of maternal and fetal vessels in the prediction of IUGR.

ARTERY	STUDIES	n	PREV. (%)	SENS. (%)	SPEC. (%)	LR(pos)	LR(neg)	PPV (%)	NPV (%)
uteroplacental	11	2422	32.9	49.5	77.0	2.3	0.64	47.9	74.3
umbilical	39	6545	37.0	59.1	83.4	5.0	0.49	63.8	77.4
aorta	7	1294	46.1	49.1	78.4	4.7	0.67	71.2	59.4
cerebral	10	1367	40.6	50.9	89.0	12.9	0.55	79.2	71.8
U/C ratio	9	1124	41.2	69.2	89.2	17.3	0.34	78.3	75.7

IUGR, intrauterine growth restriction; n, total number of patients included in the studies; PREV., prevalence of IUGR in the studies; SENS., sensitivity of the test to predict IUGR; SPEC., specificity of the test to predict IUGR; LR(pos), likelihood ratio for a positive test result; LR(neg), likelihood ratio for a negative test result; PPV, positive predictive value of the test; NPV, negative predictive value of the test; U/C ratio, ratio of umbilical pulsatility index to cerebral pulsatility index

Table 10.2 Post-test probabilities of IUGR according to test result.

ARTERY	LR$^{(pos)}$	LR$^{(neg)}$	PREVALENCE (%)	POST-TEST PROBABILITY	
				POSITIVE TEST (%)	NEGATIVE TEST (%)
uteroplacental	2.3	0.64	10 40	20 61	7 30
aorta	4.7	0.67	10 40	34 76	7 31
umbilical	5.0	0.49	10 40	36 77	5 25
cerebral	12.9	0.55	10 40	59 90	6 27
U/C ratio	17.3	0.34	10 40	66 92	4 19

Table 10.3 Evaluation of screening for IUGR using Doppler velocimetry.

SCREENING		
Study	**Risk population**	**Outcome**
Trudinger et al. (1987)	high risk	no effect on interventions; less fetal distress in labor; no effect on neonatal morbidity
Newnham (1993)	high risk	no effect on neonatal morbidity or obstetric management
Omzigt et al. (1994)	university population	no effect on antenatal and neonatal admissions; no obstetric management effect; PM halved
Davies et al. (1992)	general obstetric population	higher PM in study group; no reduction in antenatal admissions
Tyrell et al. (1990)	high risk	lower gestational age at delivery; lower incidence of low Apgar scores; no increase in obstetric interventions
Whittle et al. (1994)	unselected population	no difference in antenatal and neonatal admissions, and neonatal morbidity
Almstrom et al. (1992)	SGA pregnancies	less monitoring, fewer antenatal admissions, fewer inductions, and fewer emergency cesarean sections
Pattinson et al. (1994)	high-risk pregnancies	AEDV in control group showed more stillbirths; Doppler group had fewer antenatal and neonatal admissions
Johnstone et al. (1993)	high-risk pregnancies	no reduction in admissions, FHR testing, interventions; no reduction in PM

AEDV, absent end-diastolic velocity; FHR, fetal heart rate; IUGR, intrauterine growth restriction; PM, perinatal mortality; SGA, small for gestational age

Studies of both high-risk and low-risk pregnancies have failed to show any improvement in perinatal outcome with the addition of Doppler velocimetry (Trudinger et al., 1987; Newnham et al., 1991; Davies et al., 1992). Surprisingly, the perinatal mortality rate for the Doppler group was four times higher in the low-risk population of normally formed fetuses compared with the control group where no Doppler ultrasound was used (Davies et al., 1992). Newnham et al. (1991) also observed an increase in the incidence of low Apgar scores in a Doppler screened group. It may be that normal Doppler findings provide false reassurance to clinicians and pregnant women (Bewley et al., 1991). In other studies of high-risk pregnancies, the routine use of Doppler screening was associated with a reduction in the frequency of low Apgar scores and a reduction in serious neonatal morbidity (Tyrrell et al., 1990). Excluding congenital malformations, perinatal mortality was reduced to a third of the control group, mainly because there were fewer stillbirths (Omzigt et al., 1994; Whittle et al., 1994). These inconsistent findings should not be a surprise considering the diverse pathologies being sought by a single test.

Hospital admission in IUGR: In some countries, the woman whose fetus is suspected of being growth retarded is routinely hospitalized for bed rest. Thus, the ability to predict

Table 10.4   The effects of Aspirin or hospital admission on pregnancy outcome with abnormal Doppler findings.

STUDY	RISK POPULATION	INTERVENTION	OUTCOME
Trudinger et al. (1988)	raised umbilical artery SD	aspirin (150 mg/day)	increased BW in study group
McParland et al. (1990)	abnormal utero-placental Doppler	aspirin (75 mg/day)	less proteinuric PIH
Nienhuis et al. (1990)	university population	Doppler indication for antenatal admission	reduction of admissions; no effect on neonatal outcome
Omzigt (1993)	university population	Doppler indication for antenatal admission	no reduction in antenatal or neonatal admissions

BW, birthweight; PIH, pregnancy-induced hypertension

accurately the absence of IUGR could theoretically lead to more selective maternal hospitalization and a reduction in unnecessary fetal monitoring and interventions (Nienhuis et al., 1994). Several uncontrolled studies suggested this might be true (Ruissen et al., 1991; Almstrom et al., 1992). However, this conclusion is not supported by RCTs (Davies et al., 1992; Omzigt et al., 1994; Nienhuis, 1995).

Bed rest: The return of end-diastolic velocities after they were initially recorded as absent is associated with a better pregnancy outcome than pregnancies where they do not return. One possible explanation for the apparently better outcome is a gain in pregnancy duration. However, the incidence of IUGR (defined as a birthweight below the 10th centile) is also lower (Brar and Platt, 1989; Bell et al., 1992). This suggests that the initial assessment of absent diastolic flow was erroneous. There are no physiologic explanations for a sudden improvement in flow in the absence of resolving placentitis or pharmacologic therapy. Some note a decrease in umbilical artery resistance in half the women with bed rest. This decline in resistance is associated with both an increase in birthweight and a decrease in the risk of fetal distress and perinatal death (Sengupta et al., 1991). A lack of improvement after the initiation of bed rest is thought by some to identify a patient group which might benefit from more intensive surveillance.

Aspirin: Trudinger et al. (1988) observed in a small RCT that aspirin (150 mg per day) increased birthweight and placental weight of fetuses with an elevated umbilical artery S/D ratio. Unfortunately, their sample was very small. Another trial by Newnham et al. (1995) was unable to demonstrate a benefit of aspirin (100 mg per day) in IUGR fetuses with an elevated umbilical artery resistance index.

Fetal distress: Antepartum identification of the pregnancy at increased risk of an adverse perinatal outcome remains an obstetric challenge. While some Doppler screening studies report or suggest a decrease in perinatal mortality (especially the stillbirth rate) in the Doppler group, none reveal the expected, concomitant effect on obstetric management or reduction in interventions (Trudinger et al., 1987; Omzigt et al., 1994; Pattinson et al., 1994; Whittle et al., 1994). In one study, the apparent benefit of Doppler measurements on perinatal mortality is no longer present after correcting for congenital abnormalities and birthweights less than 1000 grams (Omzigt et al., 1994). Pattinson et al. (1994) reported that the actions triggered by Doppler studies are associated with a reduction in both hospital days (antenatal and neonatal) and the risk of fetal distress in fetuses considered SGA. The knowledge of AEDV has also been associated with an improvement in fetal survival. In high-risk pregnancies, umbilical Doppler studies are predictive of fetal distress (Maulik *et al.*, 1990), although the nonstress test (NST) may be superior (Devoe *et al.*, 1990). One should consider explanations for a nonreactive NST other than fetal distress when the Doppler studies are normal, such as a prolonged quiet sleep or the maternal ingestion of a drug acting on the nervous system.

In one observational study, fetuses with abnormal uteroplacental FVWs and normal birthweights were more likely to develop perinatal complications (Bower *et al.*, 1993). In another, abnormal Doppler velocimetry was associated with a poor fetal or neonatal outcome when the intrapartum fetal heart rate tracing suggested fetal distress (Ogunyemi *et al.*, 1992). However, the use of intrapartum Doppler velocimetry in low-risk pregnancies as a screening test in the latent phase of labor failed to predict subsequent fetal distress (Sarno *et al.*, 1989). This may be because of the high frequency of cord compression as a cause of fetal distress in labor.

WHAT DOES A NORMAL TEST RESULT MEAN?

A normal umbilical artery Doppler indicates normal trophoblastic invasion and conversion of the maternal spiral arteries to low resistance vessels. Diastolic flow rises with advancing gestational age in both the maternal and fetal arteries. Normal umbilical artery velocimetry is not associated with an abnormal biophysical profile. Doppler ultrasound can also be used to exclude IUGR secondary to uteroplacental dysfunction (Table 10.2). This is perhaps its greatest value. Fetuses who are SGA with normal umbilical artery velocimetry are at no greater risk of developing fetal distress than are appropriately grown fetuses (Pattinson *et al.*, 1991).

What is the cost of testing?

Doppler studies can be conducted for little additional cost if an ultrasound examination is already being performed. The charge for the umbilical artery velocimetry is currently about US $25 per test. The cost of a Doppler measurement as part of a screening program can be estimated at around $50. If screening is performed in a low-risk population with an IUGR prevalence below 10%, the cost of identifying one IUGR fetus is over 10 times more than if the same technique is used in a high-risk population (IUGR prevalence of 30%) (Tables 10.5 and 10.6).

The potential harm of routine Doppler ultrasound screening includes both false reassurance and overtreatment. The need for further testing is only increased in the abnormal Doppler group (e.g. biophysical testing) (Tyrrell *et al.*, 1990). Doppler screening does not decrease the use of fetal heart rate testing, ultrasound examinations or fetal blood sampling during labor (Newnham *et al.*, 1991; Davies *et al.*, 1992). In high-risk pregnancies, Doppler screening has been associated with increased fetal monitoring (Johnstone *et al.*, 1993). It is possible that the finding of a normal umbilical artery resistance index could lead to a more conservative management program and actually reduce the need for intervention in some SGA pregnancies (Burke *et al.*, 1990). In addition, while only an impression of a change in the cascade of fetal testing has been observed after the introduction of Doppler velocimetry by some investigators, most note an increase in the use of other testing modalities.

Table 10.5 Economic evaluations of Doppler screening programs for IUGR.

SCREENING PRORAM	TOTAL COST (10 000 SCREENED) ($)	COST PER PATIENT SCREENED ($)	COST PER POSITIVE SCREENED FETUS ($)	COST PER IUGR FETUS IDENTIFIED ($)
Prevalence < 10%	500 000	50	545	3 163
Prevalence > 10%	500 000	50	166	287
Mixed risk population[a]	337 033	25	151	266

[a] As defined by Omzigt et al. (1994) using a risk classification

Table 10.6 The composition of a mixed risk population is supposed to be the same as given in the study by Omzigt et al. (1994). The percentage of patients tested and the number of Doppler measurements per patient are also extracted from this study.

PREGNANCY RISK (% OF THE POPULATION)	PATIENTS TESTED (%)	MEASUREMENTS PER PATIENT TESTED	IUGR (%)
high (40%)	69	3.8	40
medium (30%)	30	1.8	15
low (30%)	29	1.7	6

CONCLUSIONS AND RECOMMENDATIONS

Doppler measurement of fetal and maternal arterial resistances is rapid and noninvasive. Thus it is attractive as a potential screening test for IUGR secondary to uteroplacental dysfunction. Unfortunately, the benefits of routine Doppler ultrasound screening in practice have been limited in terms of improving perinatal outcome measures. Doppler is not useful as a screening test for IUGR in low-risk populations but might be of value in a high-risk population. The current best application of Doppler velocimetry to obstetrics is as part of the overall testing process to aid the identification of the SGA fetus, small because of uteroplacental dysfunction and thus at high risk for hypoxemia/acidemia. It may be appropriate to reassess the application of Doppler ultrasound to the screening of IUGR fetuses should there be further development of management options.

Doppler analysis of fetal hemodynamics allows caregivers to shift their focus from the fetus whose SGA status is clinically unimportant and only statistically defined to the fetus who has fetoplacental dysfunction and hypoxemia. The U/C ratio is a better criterion of placental dysfunction than ultrasound biometric measurements (Bilardo *et al.*, 1990). Doppler studies of fetal vessels may thus provide useful information for the supervision of high-risk pregnancies complicated by IUGR.

SUMMARY

1

WHAT IS THE PROBLEM THAT REQUIRES SCREENING?

INTRAUTERINE GROWTH RESTRICTION (IUGR).

a What is the incidence/prevalence of the target condition?

Most definitions are unfortunately based on a birthweight centile. Definitions of IUGR such as the Ponderal Index or skinfold thickness are more accurate in their identification of IUGR, but more complicated to perform than the measurement of birthweight. A major problem with any single physical measurement as a definition of IUGR is that there are many causes of an SGA fetus other than IUGR.

b What are the sequelae of the condition which are of interest in clinical medicine?

Fetal distress, depression at birth, compromised neurodevelopment, and perinatal death.

2

THE TEST

a What is the purpose of the test?

To detect IUGR.

b The nature of the test

Doppler velocimetry of maternal and/or fetal arteries.
Continuous wave (CW) can be used when simultaneous visualization of the targeted vessel is unnecessary; CW has the advantage of requiring less expensive and less complicated equip-

ment. Pulsed wave Doppler (PD) is obligatory when the vessel of interest must be visualized. The indices measured by CW and PD instrumentation are comparable.

c Implications of testing

1 What does an abnormal test result mean?

An elevated Doppler resistance index in the setting of sonographic parameters consistent with SGA is consistent with uteroplacental dysfunction. There is an inverse relationship between the resistance index in either the umbilical or uterine arteries and the fetal Po_2. Unfortunately, randomized controlled trials of Doppler screening for IUGR have failed to change outcome beneficially.

2 What does a normal test result mean?

Normal umbilical artery velocimetry is not associated with an abnormal biophysical profile. Doppler ultrasound can also be used to exclude IUGR secondary to uteroplacental dysfunction. Fetuses who are SGA with normal umbilical artery velocimetry are at no greater risk of developing fetal distress than are appropriately grown fetuses.

d What is the cost of testing?

The cost per case identified of Doppler screening for IUGR depends on the prevalence of IUGR in the population screened. In most RCTs, Doppler screening has led to the increased use of other fetal surveillance tests independent of the population studied, without an improvement in outcome.

3 CONCLUSIONS AND RECOMMENDATIONS

Doppler measurement of fetal and maternal arterial resistances is rapid and noninvasive; thus it is attractive as a potential screening test for IUGR secondary to uteroplacental dysfunction. Unfortunately, the benefits of routine Doppler ultrasound screening in practice have been at best limited. Doppler is not useful as a screening test for IUGR in low-risk pregnancies. It might be of use in high-risk pregnancies. The current best application of Doppler velocimetry in obstetrics is as part of the overall testing process to aid the identification of the SGA fetus, small because of uteroplacental dysfunction.

REFERENCES

Al-Ghazali WH, Chapman MG, Rissik JM & Allan LD (1990) The significance of absent end-diastolic flow in the umbilical artery combined with reduced fetal cardiac output estimation in pregnancies at high risk for placental insufficiency. *J Obstet Gynecol* **10:** 271–275.

Almstrom H, Axelson O, Cnattingius S et al. (1992) Comparison of umbilical artery velocimetry and cardiotocography for surveillance of small-for-gestational-age fetus. *Lancet* **340:** 936–940.

Arabin B, Siebert M, Jimenez E & Saling E (1988) Obstetrical characteristics of a loss of end-diastolic velocities in the fetal aorta and/or umbilical artery using Doppler ultrasound. *Gynecol Obstet Invest* **25:** 173–180.

Arduini D, Rizzo G, Mancuso S & Romanini C (1987) Longitudinal assessment of blood flow velocity waveforms in the healthy human fetus. *Prenat Diagn* **7:** 613–617.

Arduini D, Rizzo G & Romanini C (1992) Changes of Pulsatility Index from fetal vessels preceding the onset of late decelerations in growth-retarded fetus. *Obstet Gynecol* **79:** 605–610.

Bell JG, Ludomirsky A, Bottalico J & Weiner S (1992) The effect of improvement of umbilical artery absent end-diastolic velocity on perinatal outcome. *Am J Obstet Gynecol* **167**: 1015–1020.

Bewley S, Cooper D & Campbell S (1991) Doppler investigation of uteroplacental blood flow resistance in the second trimester: a screening study for pre-eclampsia and intrauterine growth retardation. *Br J Obstet Gynaecol* **98**: 871–879.

Bilardo CM, Nicolaides KH & Campbell S (1990) Doppler measurements of fetal and uteroplacental circulations: relationship with venous blood gases measured at cordocentesis. *Am J Obstet Gynecol* **162**: 115–120.

Bower S, Schuchter K & Campbell S (1993) Doppler ultrasound screening as part of routine antenatal screening: prediction of pre-eclampsia and intrauterine growth retardation. *Br J Obstet Gynaecol* **100**: 989–994.

Brar HS & Platt LD (1989) Antepartum improvement of abnormal umbilical artery velocimetry: does it occur? *Am J Obstet Gynecol* **160**: 36–39.

Burke G, Stuart B, Crowley P, Ni Scanaill S & Drumm J (1990) Is intrauterine growth retardation with normal umbilical artery blood flow a benign condition? *Br Med J* **300**: 1044–1045.

Cameron A, Nicholson S, Nimrod C et al. (1989) Duplex ultrasonography of the fetal aorta, umbilical artery, and placental arcuate artery throughout normal human pregnancy. *J Can Assoc Radiol* **40**: 145–149.

Chang TC, Robson SC, Spencer JAD & Gallivan S (1993) Identification of fetal growth retardation: comparison of Doppler waveform indices and serial ultrasound measurements of abdominal circumference and fetal weight. *Obstet Gynecol* **82**: 230–236.

Davies JA, Gallivan S & Spencer JAD (1992) Randomised controlled trial of Doppler ultrasound screening of placental perfusion during pregnancy. *Lancet* **340**: 1299–1303.

Devoe LD, Gardner P, Dear C & Castillo RA (1990) The diagnostic values of concurrent nonstress testing, amniotic fluid measurment, and Doppler velocimetry in screening a general high risk population. *Am J Obstet Gynecol* **163**: 1040–1048.

Divon MY, Girz BA, Lieblich R & Langer O (1989) Clinical management of the fetus with markedly diminished umbilical artery end-diastolic flow. *Am J Obstet Gynecol* **161**: 1523–1527.

Giles WB, Trudinger BJ & Cook CM (1985) Fetal umbilical artery flow velocity-time waveforms in twin pregnancies. *Br J Obstet Gynaecol* **92**: 490–497.

Gosling RG & King DH (1975) Ultrasound angiology. In Marcus AW & Adamson L (eds). Arteries and Veins. Edinburgh: Churchill Livingstone, pp 61–98.

Hackett GA, Campbell S, Gamsu H, Cohen-Overbeek T & Pearce JMF (1987) Doppler studies in the growth retarded fetus and prediction of necrotising enterocolitis, haemorrhage and neonatal morbidity. *Br Med J* **294**: 13–16.

Hadders-Algra M & Touwen BCL (1990) Body measurements, neurological and behavioral development in six-year-old children born preterm and/or small-for-gestational. *Early Human Develop* **22**: 1–13.

James DK, Parker MJ & Smoleniec JS (1992) Comprehensive fetal assessment with three ultrasonographic characteristics. *Am J Obstet Gynecol* **166**: 1486–1495.

Johnstone FD, Haddad NG, Hoskins P, McDicken W, Chambers S & Muir B (1988) Umbilical artery Doppler flow velocity waveform: the outcome of pregnancies with absent end diastolic flow. *Eur J Obstet Gynecol Reprod Biol* **28**: 171–178.

Johnstone FD, Prescott R, Hoskins P, Greer IA, McGlew T & Compton M (1993) The effect of the introduction of umbilical artery Doppler recordings to obstetric practice. *Br J Obstet Gynaecol* **100**: 733–741.

Kramer MS, Olivier M, McLean FH, Willis DM & Usher RH (1990) Impact of intrauterine growth retardation and body proportionality on fetal and neonatal outcome. *Pediatrics* **86**: 707–713.

Martikainen MA (1992) Effects of intrauterine growth retardation and its subtypes on the development of the preterm infant. *Early Human Develop* **28**: 7–17.

Maulik D, Yarlagadda AP, Youngblood JP & Willoughby L (1989) Components of variability of umbilical arterial Doppler velocimetry – a prospective analysis. *Am J Obstet Gynecol* **160**: 1406–1412.

Maulik D, Yarlagadda P, Youngblood JP & Ciston P (1990) The diagnostic efficacy of the umbilical arterial systolic/diastolic ratio as a screening tool: a prospective blinded study. *Am J Obstet Gynecol* **162**: 1518–1525.

McCowan LM, Ritchie K, Mo LY, Bascom PA & Sherret H (1988) Uterine artery flow velocity waveforms in normal and growth retarded pregnancies. *Am J Obstet Gynecol* **158**: 499–504.

McParland P, Pearce JM & Chamberlain GVP (1990) Doppler ultrasound and aspirin in recognition and prevention of pregnancy-induced hypertension. *Lancet* **335**: 1552–1555.

Mehalek KE, Rosenberg J, Berkowitz GS, Chitkara U & Berkowitz RL (1989) Umbilical and uterine artery flow velocity waveforms. Effect of sampling site on Doppler ratios. *J Ultrasound Med* **8**: 171–176.

Newnham JP, Patterson LL, James IR, Diepeveen DA & Reid SE (1990) An evaluation of the efficacy of Doppler flow velocity waveform analysis as a screening test in pregnancy. *Am J Obstet Gynecol* **162**: 403–410.

Newnham JP, O'Dea MRA, Reid KP & Diepeveen DA (1991) Doppler flow velocity waveform analysis in high risk pregnancies: a randomized controlled trial. *Br J Obstet Gynaecol* **98**: 956–963.

Newnham JP, Godfrey M, Walters B, Phillips J & Evans S (1995) Low dose aspirin for the treatment of fetal growth restriction: a randomized controlled trial. *Proceedings of the Combined New Zealand and Australian Perinatal Society*, Auckland, abstract 87.

Nicolaides KH, Bilardo CM, Soothill PW & Campbell S (1988) Absence of end diastolic frequencies in the umbilical artery: a sign of fetal hypoxia and acidosis. *Br Med J* 297: 1026–1027.

Nienhuis SJ (1995) Costs and effects of Doppler ultrasound measurements in suspected intrauterine growth retardation – a randomised clinical trial. Thesis Maastricht. Maastricht: Universitaire Pers Maastricht.

Nienhuis SJ, vanVught JMG, Hoogland HJ, Ruissen CJ & deHaan J (1988) Interexaminer variability study of fetal velocity waveforms. *Gynecol Obstet Invest* 25: 152–157.

Nienhuis SJ, Zusterzeel NMAJ & Hoogland HJ (1994) Routine clinical policy and application of Doppler measurements in suspect intrauterine growth retardation in university hospitals in The Netherlands. *Eur J Obstet Gynecol Reprod Biol* 56: 31–36.

Noordam MJ, Heydanus R, Hop WCJ, Hoekstra FME & Wladimiroff JW (1994) Doppler colour flow imaging of fetal intracerebral arteries and umbilical artery in the small for gestational age fetus. *Br J Obstet Gynaecol.* 101: 504–508.

Ogunyemi D, Stanley R, Lynch R, Edwards D & Fukushima T (1992) Umbilical artery velocimetry in predicting perinatal outcome with intrapartum fetal distress. *Obstet Gynecol* 80: 377–380.

Omzigt AWJ, Reuwer PJHM & Bruinse HW (1994) A randomized controlled trial on the clinical value of umbilical Doppler velocimetry in antenatal care. *Am J Obstet Gynecol* 170: 625–634.

Ounsted MK, Moar VA & Scott A (1984) Children of deviant birthweight at the age of seven years: health, handicap, size and developmental status. *Early Human Develop* 9: 323–340.

Pardi G, Cetin I, Marconi AM *et al.* (1993) Diagnostic value of blood sampling in fetuses with growth retardation. *N Engl J Med* 328: 692–696.

Pattinson R, Dawes G, Jennings J & Redman C (1991) Umbilical artery resistance index as a screening test for fetal well being. I: Prospective revealed evaluation. *Obstet Gynecol* 78: 353–358.

Pattinson RC, Norman K & Odendaal HJ (1994) The role of Doppler velocimetry in the management of high risk pregnancies. *Br J Obstet Gynaecol.* 101: 114–120.

Pearce JM, Campbell S, Cohen-Overbeek T, Hackett G, Hernmandez J & Royston JP (1988) References ranges and sources of variation for indices of pulsed Doppler flow velocimetry waveforms from the uteroplacental and fetal circulation. *Br J Obstet Gynaecol* 95: 248–256.

Pourcelot L (1974) Applications cliniques de l'examen Doppler transcutané. In Peronneau P (ed) Vélocimétrie ultrasonoré Doppler. Paris: Séminaire INSERM, pp. 213–240.

Ruissen CJ, Nienhuis SJ, Hoogland HJ, Vles J, Gerver JW & deHaan J (1991) Cost effectiveness of a Doppler based policy of intrauterine growth retardation – a randomized controlled trial. *J Matern Fetal Invest* 1: 126.

Sanderson DA, Wilcox MA & Johnson IR (1994) The individualised birthweight ratio: a new method of identifying intrauterine growth retardation. *Br J Obstet Gynaecol* 101: 310–314.

Sarno AP, Brar HS, Phelan JP & Platt LD (1989) Intrapartum Doppler velocimetry, amniotic fluid volume, and fetal heart rate as predictors of subsequent fetal distress. *Am J Obstet Gynecol* 161: 1508–1514.

Scherjon SA, Kok JH, Oosting H & Zondervan HA (1993a) Intra-observer and inter-observer reliability of the pulsatility index calculated from pulsed Doppler flow velocity waveforms in three fetal vessels. *Br J Obstet Gynaecol* 100: 134–138.

Scherjon SA, Smolders-deHaas H, Kok JH, Oosting H & Zondervan HA (1993b) The 'brain-sparing' effect: antenatal cerebral Doppler findings in relation to neurologic outcome in very preterm infants. *Am J Obstet Gynecol* 169: 169–175.

Sengupta S, Harrigan JT, Rosenberg JC, Davis E & Knuppel RA (1991) Perinatal outcome following improvement of abnormal umbilical artery velocimetry. *Obstet Gynecol* 78: 1062–1066.

Sijmons EA, Reuwer PJHM, VanBeek E & Bruinse HW (1989) The validity of screening for small for gestational age and low weight for length infants by Doppler ultrasound. *Br J Obstet Gynaecol* 96: 557–561.

Soothill PW, Ajayi RA, Campbell S & Nicolaides KH (1993) Prediction of morbidity in small and normally grown fetuses by fetal heart rate variability, biophysical profile score and umbilical artery Doppler studies. *Br J Obstet Gynaecol* 100: 742–745.

Spencer JAD & Price J (1989) Intraobserver variation in Doppler ultrasound indices of placental perfusion derived from different numbers of waveforms. *J Ultrasound Med* 8: 197–199.

Spencer JAD, Price J & Lee A (1991) Influence of fetal breathing and movements on variability of umbilical Doppler indices using different numbers of waveforms. *J Ultrasound Med* 10: 37–41.

Stuart B, Drumm J, Fitzgerald DE & Duignan NM (1980) Fetal blood velocity waveforms in normal pregnancy. *Br J Obstet Gynaecol* 87: 780–785.

Teberg AJ, Walther FJ & Pena IC (1988) Mortality, morbidity and outcome of the small for gestational age infant. *Semin Perinatol* 12: 84–94.

Tessler FN, Kimme-Smith C, Sutherland ML, Schiller VL, Perrella RR & Grant EG (1990) Inter and intra observer variability of Doppler peak velocity measurements: an in vitro study. *Ultrasound Med Biol* 16: 653–657.

Trudinger BJ, Giles WB, Cook CM, Connelly A & Thompson RS (1987) Umbilical artery flow velocity waveforms in high-risk pregnancy. Randomised clinical trial. *Lancet* i: 188–190.

Trudinger BJ, Cook CM, Thompson RS, Giles WB & Connelly A (1988) Low-dose aspirin therapy improves fetal weight in umbilical placental insuffuciency. *Am J Obstet Gynecol* **159**: 681–685.

Tyrrell SN, Lilford RJ, MacDonald HN, Nelson EJ, Porter J & Gupta JK (1990) Randomized comparison of routine vs highly selective use of Doppler ultrasound and biophysical scoring to investigate high risk pregnancies. *Br J Obstet Gynaecol* **97**: 909–916.

van Vught JMG (1991) Validity of umbilical artery blood velocimetry in the prediction of intrauterine growth retardation and fetal compromise. *J Perinat Med* **19**: 15–20.

Villar J, deOnis M, Kestler E, Bolanos F, Cerezo R & Bernedes H (1990) The differential neonatal morbidity of the intrauterine growth retardation syndrome. *Am J Obstet Gynecol* **163**: 151–157.

Weiner, CP (1990) The relationship between the umbilical artery systolic:diastolic ratio and umbilical blood gas measurements in specimens obtained by cordocentesis. *Am J Obstet Gynecol* **162**: 1198–1202.

Wenstrom KD, Weiner CP & Williamson RA (1991) Diverse maternal and fetal pathology associated with absent diastolic flow in the umbilical artery of high-risk fetuses. *Obstet Gynecol* **77**: 374–378.

Whittle MJ, Hanretty KP, Primrose MH & Neilson JP (1994) Screening for the compromised fetus: a randomized trial of umbilical artery velocimetry in unselected pregnancies. *Am J Obstet Gynecol* **170**: 555–559.

Wladimiroff JW, Tonge HM, Stewart PA & Reuss A (1986) Severe intrauterine growth retardation; assessment of its origin from fetal arterial flow velocity waveforms. *Eur J Obstet Gynecol Reprod Biol* **22**: 23–28.

Wladimiroff JW, Vanden Wijngaard JAGW, Degani S, Noordam MJ, VanEyck J & Tonge HM (1987) Cerebral and umbilical arterial blood flow velocity waveforms in normal and growth-retarded pregnancies. *Obstet Gynecol* **69**: 705–709.

Woo JSK, Liang ST, Lo RLS & Chan FY (1987) Middle cerebral artery Doppler flow velocity waveforms. *Obstet Gynecol* **70**: 613–616.

11

Fundal Height Measurement

Cynthia J. Berg & Jeanne C. McDermott

WHAT IS THE PROBLEM THAT REQUIRES SCREENING?

A SIZE FOR DATE DISCREPANCY IN THE SIZE OF THE UTERINE FUNDUS DURING PREGNANCY.

The height of the uterine fundus is routinely measured to detect a discrepancy between the size and the estimated duration of gestation. A size for date discrepancy is one of the most common problems encountered in obstetrics and can result from a variety of abnormalities. In some cases, the discrepancy is detectable with a single measurement; in other cases, serial measurements are required. This chapter examines the use of fundal height measurement as a screening tool for the five most common causes of a size for dates discrepancy: intrauterine growth restriction (IUGR), multifetal pregnancies, hydramnios, molar pregnancy, and errors in estimating gestational age.

What is the incidence/prevalence of the target condition?

The prevalence of *IUGR* when defined as birthweight for gestational age below specified percentiles ranges from 2.5% to 10% of births (Seeds, 1984). The prevalence of *multifetal pregnancy* ranges from a low of 0.43% of pregnancies in Japan through about 1.2% in the USA and Scotland to 5.72% in Nigeria (Wenstrom and Gall, 1988). *Hydramnios* complicates 0.2–1.6% of pregnancies (Cardwell, 1987). A *molar pregnancy* occurs in 0.05–0.1% of pregnancies in the industrialized nations. It approaches 1% in areas of Asia (Goldstein and Berkowitz, 1986).

The first day of the last menstrual period is traditionally used to establish the duration of gestation, though this method is fraught with potential errors. Gestational age estimates based on the last menstrual period agree within 1 week of the best obstetric estimate (using all modalities including ultrasound) in only 60% of patients (Goldenberg *et al.*, 1989a). Even among women with 'certain' dates, the range of error compared with ultrasonography is up to 54 days (Geirsson and Busby-Earle, 1991). Among women referred for an ultrasound examination because of suspected IUGR, over one-third have their expected date of confinement recalculated (Whetham *et al.*, 1976). Since the follicular phase of a cycle can be significantly longer than 14 days but not shorter than 6–7 days, the majority of dating errors overestimate rather than underestimate the true gestational age.

What are the sequelae of the condition which are of interest in clinical medicine?

Intrauterine growth restriction is associated with a perinatal mortality rate 4–8 times greater than that for the appropriately grown infant. Morbid events include fetal distress requiring cesarean delivery and neonatal hypoglycemia, hypocalcemia, hypothermia, polycythemia, and longterm neurobehavioral problems (Seeds, 1984).

Both the mother and the fetuses are subject to increased morbidity and mortality in multifetal pregnancies. Perinatal (Kiely, 1990) and neonatal (Kleinman *et al.*, 1991) mortality are 4–5 times higher for twins than singletons. The increased rate of death is due to all causes (Kleinman *et al.*, 1991). Maternal complications which are more common in women with multifetal pregnancies include hyperemesis, preeclampsia, hydramnios, preterm rupture of membranes, preterm labor and delivery, cesarean delivery and postpartum hemorrhage (Wenstrom and Gall, 1988).

The sequelae of hydramnios also affect both the mother and fetus. Hydramnios is often associated with fetal malformation. Depending on the presence or absence of associated conditions, the perinatal mortality rates range from 2.4% to over 60% when hydramnios is present (Desmedt *et al.*, 1990). Maternal complications include an increased risk of preeclampsia, respiratory embarrassment, cesarean delivery, preterm delivery, and postpartum hemorrhage (Cardwell, 1987).

The most serious sequela of molar pregnancy is the development of persistent gestational trophoblastic neoplasia which occurs in 15% to 20% of such pregnancies. Other serious complications include hyperemesis gravidarum, preeclampsia, pulmonary embolization of trophoblastic tissue, and disseminated intravascular coagulation (Kohorn, 1984).

Erroneous dating of the pregnancy may also lead to serious problems. Term fetuses misclassified as post-term may be subjected to unnecessary and costly interventions such as antepartum fetal surveillance, induction of labor, and cesarean delivery for a failed induction. Preterm fetuses who are misclassified as term may be delivered without optimal management. Term pregnancies misclassified as preterm may be subjected to unnecessary tocolysis. A post-term fetus misclassified as term may continue in utero without appropriate monitoring and result in a stillbirth.

THE TEST

What is the purpose of the test?

Though fundal height measurement has been used to estimate fetal age and weight, its main use as a screening tool is to determine whether the uterine size is appropriate for the estimated dates. A fundal height measurement smaller than expected may indicate either IUGR or an error in the estimated gestational age. A large fundal height measurement may indicate macrosomia, multifetal pregnancies, hydramnios, molar pregnancy, an error in dating uterine fibroids, or a full bladder. In addition, large variation in the growth of biologically normal fetuses may cause size for dates discrepancies.

A number of countries have adopted a policy of one or two ultrasound examinations as part of routine antenatal care (Holzgreve, 1990). In other countries such as the USA, the majority of women undergo one or more 'indicated' ultrasound examinations during pregnancy (Ewigman *et al.*, 1993). Yet a role still exists for the routine measurement of fundal height during each antenatal visit. While the detection rates of multifetal pregnancies, molar pregnancies and dating errors approach 100% using a mid-second trimester ultrasound examination, serial fundal height measurements are still necessary to identify conditions that develop later in pregnancy such as IUGR and hydramnios.

The nature of the test

Measurement issues: The measurement of fundal height is subject to many sources of variation. Though the current practice is to measure in centimeters above the symphysis pubis, the measurement was originally made in relation to several landmarks on the maternal abdomen. In addition to the normal, random variation inherent to any measurement, the conditions of fundal height measurement are usually not standardized. The measurement is affected by such factors as maternal position (Engstrom et al., 1993b), whether a tape measure or a pair of calipers is used (Beazley and Underhill, 1970; Engstrom et al., 1993a), whether the measurement is from the superior or inferior aspect of the pubic symphysis, whether the tape is curved around the uterus or held horizontally (Engstrom et al., 1993a), whether the measurement is made in the midline or to the superior fetal pole, and whether the bladder is full (Engstrom et al., 1989). Finally, the measurements should be graphed to aid the identification of any patterns, as many problems become evident only after repeated screening (Belizan et al., 1990).

Criteria for an abnormal test: There is no consensus. Many criteria have been used to define a size for dates discrepancy: below the 10th or above the 90th centile; more than 2 cm or 3 cm below or above the mean; 1 or 2 standard deviations (SD) below or above the mean for gestation. In addition, a single abnormal measurement, two consecutive abnormal measurements, any three abnormal measurements, the percentage of all measurements that are abnormal (20%, 30%, or 40%), and the lack of growth for three successive measurements have all been used to define an abnormal fundal height. One practical rule of thumb is that the fundal height in centimeters is approximately equal to the gestational age in weeks between 20 and 31–36 weeks' gestation. Thereafter, most norms indicate that the rate of fundal height growth slows.

Several normal curves for fundal height have been developed (Westin, 1977; Belizan et al., 1978; Quaranta et al., 1981; Calvert et al., 1982; Cox et al., 1983; Jimenez et al., 1983; Rogers and Needham, 1985; Persson et al., 1986; Pearce and Campbell, 1987; Azziz et al., 1988). The populations used to derive these norms tend to exclude women with pregnancy complications or who deliver small for gestational age infants. Opinion differs as to whether a single norm should be used for all populations (Kiserud, 1986), whether separate norms should be used for developing countries (Pattinson, 1988) rather than those used for developed countries (Calvert et al., 1982), or whether individual norms are needed for each local or institutional population (Azziz et al., 1988).

The cut-off chosen to define abnormal fundal height growth, along with the prevalence of IUGR in the population screened, will have an effect on the sensitivity, specificity, and positive and negative predictive values of the test (Goldenberg et al., 1989b). Thus, the caregiver may want to set the cut-off at a level that provides an acceptable false negative rate and a false positive rate that does not overwhelm the clinical resources available to follow up women with a positive screen (Calvert et al., 1982).

Sensitivity, specificity and predictive value of the test: Most studies that have formally evaluated fundal height measurement have used IUGR as the outcome of interest. Studies of the relationship between fundal height measurement and other conditions of interest are extremely limited. Over 25 studies published since 1977 have attempted to evaluate fundal height measurement as a screening tool for IUGR (Table 11.1). Although a wide range of sensitivities are reported (partly the result of inconsistent definitions of

Table 11.1 Fundal height measurement as a screening tool for intrauterine growth restriction.

REFERENCE	IUGR DEFINITION/ PREVALENCE	POPULATION STUDIED	DEFINITION OF POSITIVE TEST	SENSITIVITY (%)	SPECIFICITY (%)	PPV (%)	NPV (%)
Westin (1977)	BW > 1 SD below mean prevalence 11%	Sweden N = 428	A ≥ 3 cm below mean B static/falling FHM	A 68 B 52 A or B 75	A 89 B 95	A 44 B 54	A 96 B 95
Belizan et al. (1978)	BW < 10th percentile prevalence 32%	Guatemala N = 139	< 10th percentile × ≥ 1	86	89	79	93
Quaranta et al. (1981)	BW < 10th percentile prevalence 30%	England N = 138	2 consecutive/3 isolated FHM < 10th percentile	73	79	60	88
Wallin et al. (1981)	BW ≥ 2 SD below mean prevalence not stated	Sweden N = 812 Neonatal ward newborns	> 3 cm below mean × ≥ 3 or 3 static, consecutive FHM	62	88	42	94
Rosenberg et al. (1982)	BW < 10th percentile prevalence 6.6%	Scotland n = 761	A 2 consecutive/3 isolated FHM < 10th percentile B 20%, or C 30%, or D 40% FHM < 10th percentile	A 56 B 61 C 52 D 48	A 85 B 79 C 92 D 92	A 21 B 17 C 31 D 30	A 96 B 97 C 96 D 96
Calvert et al. (1982)	BW < 5th percentile prevalence 6.6% BW < 10th percentile prevalence 12%	England n = 381	Applied: A Westin criteria B Belizan criteria C Quaranta criteria	< 5th A 72 B 60 C 36 < 10th A 76 B 64 C 36	< 5th A 58 B 76 C 92 < 10th A 60 B 79 C 94	< 5th A 11 B 15 C 24 < 10th A 20 B 29 C 43	< 5th A 97 B 96 C 94 < 10th A 95 B 94 C 92

	BW definition	Country / N	FHM definition	< 5th / < 10th	< 5th / < 10th	< 5th / < 10th	< 5th / < 10th
Cox et al. (1983)	BW < 5th percentile prevalence 30% BW ≤ 10th percentile prevalence 48%	Ireland N = 123	≥ 2 FHM below 10th percentile	70 58	87 95	70 92	87 71
Chattingius et al. (1984)	BW ≥ 2 SD below mean prevalence 2.7%	Sweden N = 527 Women with IUGR risk factors	low (L) – last FHM ≥ 3 cm below the mean static (S) – last 3 FHM same but no FHM > 2 cm below mean catch-up (C) – one FHM > 3 cm below mean, but last < 3 cm below mean	L 50 S 7 C 29 L + C 79 L + C + S 86	L 98 S 87 C 94 L+C 92 L+C + S 79	L 39 S 1 C 12 L+C 21 L+C+S 10	L 99 S 97 C 98 L+C 99 L+C+S 99.5
Rogers and Needham (1985)	BW < 10th percentile prevalence 10.4%	England N = 250	Westin definition	73	92	51	97
Tjon et al. (1985)	Lubchenko reference prevalence 8%	Lesotho N = 122 Hospital deliveries	(A) first FHM < 10th percentile Belizan (B), Quaranta (C), Westin (D)	A 40 B 70 C 56 D 100	A 96 B 84 C 93 D 49	A 50 B 28 C 45 D 16	A 95 B 97 C 95 D 100
Linasmita (1985)	BW < 10th percentile prevalence 7%	Thailand N = 257	2 consecutive/3 isolated FHM < 10th percentile	61	96	55	97
Persson et al. (1986)	BW < 10th percentile prevalence 9%	Sweden N = 2941	FHM > 2 SD below mean	27	88	18	92
Garde (1986)	BW < 10th percentile prevalence 32%	South Africa N = 92	slope of FHM less than norm	85	93	87	94
Linasmita (1986)	BW < 10th percentile prevalence 7%	Thailand N = 483	2 consecutive/3 isolated FHM < 10th percentile	65	96	58	97

Table 11.1 (contd.)

REFERENCE	IUGR DEFINITION/ PREVALENCE	POPULATION STUDIED	DEFINITION OF POSITIVE TEST	SENSITIVITY (%)	SPECIFICITY (%)	PPV (%)	NPV (%)
Okonofua et al. (1986)	BW < 10th percentile prevalence 7%	London N = 100	2 consecutive FHM < 10th percentile	71	85	31	98
Pearce and Campbell (1987)	BW < 10th percentile prevalence 14.3%	England n = 200	FHM < 10th percentile	76	79	36	95
Mathai et al. (1987)	BW > 1 SD below mean prevalence – at risk 27% – low risk 9%	India at risk, N = 150 low risk, N = 208	< 1 SD below mean	78	88	70	92
Fescina et al. (1987)	BW < 10th percentile prevalence 38%	Uruguay high risk, N = 100	FHM < 10th percentile	56	91	80	77
Mathai (1988)	probably same as Mathai et al. (1987) prevalence 12.2%	India low risk, N = 253	> 3 cm below mean	77	79	33	96
Azziz et al. (1988)	BW < 10th percentile prevalence 14.6%	USA N = 192	A 1 FHM $\geq$ 1 SD below mean B 2 FHM $\geq$ 1 SD below mean C 3 FHM $\geq$ 1 SD below mean	A 86 B 75 C 61	A 89 B 95 C 98	A 57 B 72 C 81	A 97 B 96 C 95
Pattinson (1988)	BW < 10th percentile prevalence 14.4%	South Africa N = 97	2 consecutive FHM < 10th percentile, or 3 consecutive static FHM Belizan (B), Quaranta (Q), Calvert (C) charts	B 86 Q 93 C 93	B 89 Q 51 C 75	B 57 Q 24 C 38	B 97 Q 98 C 98

Stuart et al. (1989)	BW < 10th percentile prevalence: A General population 7.6% B Women having ≥ 4 FHMs 7.2%	England A, N = 1139 B, N = 319	FHM < 10th percentile	A 51 B 65	A 88 B 88	A 26 B 21	A 96 B 97
Norton (1989)	BW < 10th percentile prevalence 26%	Australia/NZ N = 34	FHM < 10th percentile	86	85	60	96
Pattinson (1989)	criteria not stated prevalence: A 14.1% B 9.5%	South Africa A, N = 97 B, N = 126	2 consecutive/3 isolated FHM < 10th percentile	A 86 B 42	A 89 B 92	A 57 B 36	A 97 B 94
Lindhard et al. (1990) RCT	BW < 10th percentile prevalence: A 7.6% (w/ FHM) B 5.7% (w/o FHM)	Denmark A, N = 804 B, N = 835	< 10th percentile × ≥ 2 FHMs, or ≥ 2 consecutive FHM > 20% fall, or 3 static consecutive FHMs	A 28 B 48	A 97 B 97	A 41 B 47	A 94 B 97
Grover et al. (1991)	BW > 1 SD below mean prevalence 26%	India n = 400	FHM > 1 SD below mean	81	93	84	92
Cronje et al. (1993)	Dunn reference prevalence 13.7%	South Africa n = 314	≥ 2 successive/3 isolated FHM < 10th percentile or 3 static consecutive FHM	42	83	28	90

BW, birthweight; FHM, fundal height measurement; IUGR, intrauterine growth restriction; n, number of patients; NPV, negative predictive value; PPV, positive predictive value; SD, standard deviation abnormal), the sensitivity has centered around 65% and specificity around 90%. Since the prevalence of IUGR differed in the populations studied, the positive predictive value varied, as would be expected. The sensitivity of fundal height measurement to detect IUGR improves when the measurements are made by only one or two caregivers rather than by several different people (86% versus 42%), although this factor does not improve specificity or predictive power (Pattinson and Theron, 1989).

The only randomized controlled trial of fundal height measurement compared pregnancies with and without quantitative fundal height measurements (Lindhard et al., 1990). There were no differences found between the groups regarding the prediction of IUGR infants, the use of interventions or additional diagnostic procedures, or the condition of the newborn. However, other sophisticated screening tools such as ultrasonography were routinely used.

A few authors have specifically evaluated fundal height measurement as a screening tool for multifetal pregnancies. Most studies reported very high sensitivity of a 'high' fundal height measurement (99–100%) (Westin, 1977; Linasmita, 1986; Neilson et al., 1988; Engstrom and Work, 1992), although Smibert (1962) and Persson et al. (1986) reported lower sensitivities of 50% and 76%, respectively.

While no published studies have specifically evaluated the detection of hydramnios by the measurement of fundal height, authors typically refer to increased uterine size as a characteristic of hydramnios (Cardwell, 1987) and report a definite relationship between excessive amniotic fluid and fundal height (Cabrol et al., 1987). Where mentioned, all cases of hydramnios had a fundal height measurement that was over 2 cm or 2 SD above the mean (Westin, 1977; Linasmita, 1986). Several authors reported that increased uterine size in women with an IUGR fetus was due to hydramnios (Westin, 1977; Wallin et al., 1981; Linasmita, 1986).

Although review of the literature revealed no formal evaluation of the ability of fundal height measurement to ascertain molar pregnancies, authors reported that in 38–50% of molar pregnancies, the uterine size is approximately 4 weeks larger than dates (Kohorn, 1984).

No studies were identified that evaluated fundal height measurement as a screening tool for dating errors.

Validity: Although it is not possible to directly measure the uterus, several investigators have compared tape measurements of the palpated fundal height with ultrasound measurements of the uterine fundus and/or fetus. Bagger et al. (1985) observed a correlation of 0.86 between ultrasound and tape estimates of fundal height. The mean difference for five observers ranged from +0.49 to −1.97 cm. Engstrom et al. (1993c) found a mean absolute error of 1.25 cm, with a maximum error of 8.6 cm. Fifty-eight per cent of the tape measurements were within 1 cm and 79% were within 2 cm of the ultrasound estimates. Tape measurements of fundal height are affected by fetal presentation and uterine wall thickness. They are unaffected by maternal height, weight, body mass index, abdominal subcutaneous fat, parity and fetal gestational age.

Reliability and reproducibility. Both intraobserver and interobserver problems with either reliability or reproducibility are described. Mean intraobserver differences of fundal height measurement range from 0.4 cm to 2.0 cm, with a maximum difference of 8.0 cm, whereas intraobserver standard deviations for repeated measures range from 0.8 cm to 1.35 cm, and coefficients of variation from 2.2% to 4.8% (Beazley and Underhill, Calvert et al. 1982; Pschera and Soderberg, 1983; Bagger et al. 1985; Rogers and Needham, 1985; Engstrom et al., 1993a). These are large enough to be clinically relevant.

Interobserver variation of fundal height measurement tends to be larger than intraobserver variation. The mean difference in fundal height measurement between observers ranges from 0.5 cm to 4.0 cm, with a maximum difference of 13 cm. The standard deviation of interobserver variation ranges from 0.7 cm to 3.6 cm, with reported coefficients of variation from 6.4% to 7.8% (Beazley and Underhill, 1970; Calvert *et al.*, 1982; Pschera and Soderberg, 1983; Bagger *et al.*, 1985; Belizan *et al.*, 1987; Bailey *et al.*, 1989; Crosby and Engstrom, 1989; Engstrom *et al.*, 1993a). Beazley and Underhill found that 85% of measurements were within 1.3 cm of those made by other observers, but Crosby and Engstrom found that only 14–45% were within 2 cm.

The majority of studies use tape measures only. Investigators report no difference in reliability among providers with different levels of training (Calvert *et al.*, 1982; Rogers and Needham, 1985), nor is there any effect of gestational age on the reliability of the fundal height measurement (Bagger *et al.*, 1985). The few studies that compared tape measurements with those obtained using pelvimetry calipers observed that the caliper measurements are slightly more reproducible and give a smaller measurement (Beazley and Underhill, 1970; Engstrom *et al.*, 1993a).

Implications of testing

WHAT DOES AN ABNORMAL TEST RESULT MEAN?

A discrepancy between uterine size and dates should trigger an ultrasound examination in locales where ultrasonography is available. Depending on the underlying cause, appropriate follow-up and clinical care for IUGR, multifetal pregnancy, hydramnios or molar pregnancy should be undertaken. In areas where ultrasonography is not readily available, a size for dates discrepancy can be evaluated using other techniques such as X-ray imaging, amniography, and physical examination to detect more than one fetus or excess amniotic fluid, or by monitoring maternal weight gain and fetal movement.

WHAT DOES A NORMAL TEST RESULT MEAN?

Normal fundal height measurements are reassuring, especially when graphed and found to be increasing along the lines of normal growth curves. However, a normal fundal height measurement is not definitive evidence of fetal and maternal wellbeing. The caregiver must still use clinical judgment and continue to assess the pregnancy using those modalities accepted as appropriate care.

What is the cost of testing?

Fundal height measurement is among the least expensive tools in antenatal care. The simple supplies required include a tape measure, a chart or, preferably, a fundal height graph to record the information, and knowledge of gestational age. The training required is minimal and the measurement itself takes less than a minute.

When a large size for dates discrepancy of unknown etiology is discovered, the first step is an ultrasound examination to document fetal biometry for gestational age and fetal growth, the number of fetuses, amniotic fluid volume, and fetal and placental abnormalities. The total charge for such an ultrasound examination ranges from US $150 to $200 (see Chapter 8 for more detailed information on ultrasound costs). The number of ultrasound examinations ordered as a result of fundal height measurement screening will depend on the prevalence and timing of ultrasound use in the population. Early, routine ultrasound examination will usually diagnose multifetal pregnancies, molar pregnancies and resolve date discrepancies. Even without routine ultrasonography, approximately 60% of women are candidates for an indicated ultrasound examination (Ewigman *et al.*, 1993).

The most prevalent condition identified by serial fundal height measurements is IUGR. If we assume an IUGR prevalence of 10%, a prevalence of hydramnios of 1%, a sensitivity of fundal height measurement for the diagnosis of IUGR of 60%, a sensitivity of fundal height measurement for the diagnosis of hydramnios of 100%, and a predictive value of a positive test of 50%, then approximately 13% of the population would be referred for ultrasound examination to evaluate fetal growth as a result of fundal height screening. At an average charge of $200 per ultrasound examination, $2600 would be spent per 100 women screened with fundal height measurement to identify six of the ten cases of IUGR and the one case of hydramnios. This would be $26 per woman screened and about $370 per positive detected. Once a definitive diagnosis is made, subsequent costs depend on the particular condition found (for example IUGR, multifetal pregnancies).

CONCLUSIONS AND RECOMMENDATIONS

Fundal height measurement should be a routine part of antenatal care (US Public Health Service, 1989). It is one of the least expensive and simplest procedures in the obstetric armamentarium. The increased use of ultrasound as a screening test in developed countries may alter the role of fundal height measurement. However, it remains an important and appropriate test in countries without universally available ultrasonography and other advanced technology.

Fundal height measurement can effectively identify a size for dates discrepancy secondary to a variety of causes, with a sensitivity that ranges from about 65% (IUGR) to nearly 100% (twins and hydramnios). The cause of the discrepancy can be further evaluated using other tests. The initial costs of fundal height measurement are exceptionally low, and there are no reported risks. However, the charge for the follow-up ultrasound examination would average $26 per woman or about $370 per positive detected.

The effect of the diagnosis of a size for dates discrepancy on clinical management depends on the condition identified. Molar pregnancies should be terminated and the patient followed with serial beta-human chorionic gonadotropin measurements to search for persistent trophoblastic disease. A diagnosis of IUGR or hydramnios allows the possibility of close monitoring, treatment and early delivery to minimize fetal and maternal compromise. Antenatal diagnosis of multi fetal pregnancy allows the woman and her care provider to plan an optimal antenatal and delivery strategy. Accurate dating of pregnancy prevents unnecessary intervention in falsely labeled preterm and, particularly, post-term pregnancies. Moreover, true preterm and post-term fetuses are more likely to receive appropriate management.

Even those who advocate routine antenatal ultrasound screening rarely recommend its use at every antenatal visit due to its labor-intensive nature and the high skill level required (Editorial, 1989). Clinicians must rely on clinical suspicion, raised mainly by a size for dates discrepancy identified by fundal height measurement, to appropriately order subsequent ultrasound tests. However, as the use of routine ultrasound becomes more widespread, researchers may wish to re-evaluate the costs and benefits of the procedures.

SUMMARY

WHAT IS THE PROBLEM THAT REQUIRES SCREENING?

A SIZE FOR DATES DISCREPANCY IN THE SIZE OF THE UTERINE FUNDUS DURING PREGNANCY.

a What is the incidence/prevalence of the target condition?
IUGR – 2.5% to 10% of births
Multiple fetal pregnancy – 0.43% to 5.72% of births.
Hydramnios – 0.2% to 1.6% of pregnancies.
Molar pregnancy – 0.05% to 0.1% of pregnancies in the West, 1% in areas of Asia.
Erroneous date – only 40% are within 1 week.

b What are the sequelae of the condition which are of interest in clinical medicine?
Increased maternal and perinatal morbidity and mortality.

THE TEST

a What is the purpose of the test?
To detect a size for dates discrepancy

b The nature of the test
The measurement of the uterine fundus height.

c Implications of testing

1 What does an abnormal test result mean?

An ultrasound examination is required to determine the cause.

2 What does a normal test result mean?

Normal fundal height measurements are reassuring, especially when increasing along the lines of normal growth curves.

d What is the cost of testing?
The cost of fundal height measurement itself is minimal. For follow-up of abnormal test, an average charge of US $200 per ultrasound scan, $2600 would be spent per 100 women screened with fundal height measurement to identify six of the ten cases of IUGR and the one case of hydramnios. This would be $26 per woman screened and about $370 per positive detected.

3 CONCLUSIONS AND RECOMMENDATIONS

The uterine fundus should be measured at each antenatal visit to screen for size for dates discrepancy even if an ultrasound examination has been performed.

The technique used for fundal height measurement should be as consistent as possible to improve the reproducibility and reliability of the test, using as few care providers per woman as possible.

Measurements should be routinely graphed and a definition of what is abnormal selected.

Research should be undertaken to identify the most appropriate definition of an abnormal test, whether population-based curves are necessary, and the role of fundal height measurement in settings where ultrasound scans are routinely performed.

REFERENCES

Azziz R, Smith S & Fabro S (1988) The development and use of a standard symphysial-fundal height growth curve in the prediction of small for gestational age neonates. *Int J Gynecol Obstet* **26:** 81–87.

Bagger PV, Eriksen PS, Secher NJ, Thisted J & Westergaad L (1985) The precision and accuracy of symphysis-fundus distance measurements during pregnancy. *Acta Obstet Gynecol Scand* **64:** 371–374.

Bailey SM, Sarmandal P & Grant JM (1989) A comparison of three methods of assessing interobserver variation applied to measurement of the symphysis-fundal height. *Br J Obstet Gynaecol* **96:** 1266–1271.

Beazley JM & Underhill RA (1970) Fallacy of the fundal height. *Br Med J* **4:** 404–406.

Belizan JM, Villar J Nardin JC, Malamud J & De Vicuna LS (1978) Diagnosis of intrauterine growth retardation by a simple clinical method: measurement of uterine height. *Am J Obstet Gynecol* **131:** 643–646.

Belizan JM, Villar J & Nardin JC (1990) Poor predictive value of symphysial-fundal height when misused in clinical practice. *Am J Obstet Gynecol* **162** (5): 1348–1349.

Cabrol D, Landesman R, Muller J, Uzan M, Sureau C & Saxena BB (1987) Treatment of polyhydramnios with prostaglandin synthetase inhibitor (indomethacin). *Am J Obstet Gynecol* **157:** 422–6

Calvert JP, Crean EE, Newcombe RG & Pearson JF (1982) Antenatal screening by measurement of symphysis-fundus height. *Br Med J* **285:** 846–9.

Cardwell MS (1987) Polyhydramnios: A Review. *Obstet Gynecol Surv* **42:** 612–7.

Cnattingius S, Axelsson O & Lindmar G (1984) Symphysis-fundus measurements and intrauterine growth retardation. *Acta Obstet Gynecol Scand* **63:** 335–340.

Cox G, Walsh P, Stack J & Murphy H (1983) The value of fundal height measurement in prediction of fetal growth retardation. *Irish Med J* **76:** 95–6.

Cronje HS, Bam RH & Muir A (1993) Validity of symphysis fundus growth measurements. *Int J Gynecol Obstet* **43:** 157–161.

Crosby ME & Engstrom JL (1989) Inter-examiner reliability in fundal height measurement. *Midwives Chron Nurs Notes* **102:** 254–6.

Desmedt EJ, Henry OA & Beischer N (1990) Polyhydramnios and associated maternal and fetal complications in singleton pregnancies. *Br J Obstet Gynaecol* **97:** 1115–1122.

Engstrom JL & Work BA (1992) Prenatal prediction of small and large-for-gestational age neonates. *J Obstet Gynecol Neonatal Nurs* **21:** 486–495.

Engstrom JL, Ostrenga KG, Plass RV & Work BA (1989) The effect of maternal bladder volume on fundal height measurements. *Br J Obstet Gynaecol* **96:** 987–91.

Engstrom JL, McFarlin BL & Sittler CP (1993a) Fundal height measurement. Part 2 – Intra- and interexaminer reliability of three measurement techniques. *J Nurs Midwifery* **38:** 17–22.

Engstrom JL, Piscioneri LA, Low LK, McShane H & McFarlin B (1993b) Fundal height measurement. Part 3 – The effect of maternal position on fundal height measurements. *J Nurs Midwifery* **38:** 23–27.

Engstrom JL, McFarlin BL & Sampson MB (1993c) Fundal height measurement. Part 4 – Accuracy of clinicians' identification of the uterine fundus during pregnancy. *J Nurs Midwifery* **38:** 318–23.

Ewigman BG, Crane JP, Frigoletto FD *et al.* (1993) Effect of prenatal ultrasound screening on perinatal outcome. *N Engl J Med* **329:** 821–7.

Fescina RH, Martell M, Martinez G, Lastra L & Schwarcz R (1987) Small for dates: evaluation of different diagnostic methods. *Acta Obstet Gynecol Scand* **66:** 221–226.

Garde PM (1986) Growth rate score to screen for intrauterine growth retardation. *Trop Doctor* **15:** 71–74.

Geirsson RT & Busby-Earle RMC (1991) Certain dates may not provide a reliable estimate of gestational age. *Br J Obstet Gynaecol* **98:** 108–9.

Goldenberg RL, Davis RO, Cutter GR, Hoffman HJ & Brumfield CG (1989a) Prematurity, postdates, and growth retardation: the influence of use of ultrasonography on reported gestational age. *Am J Obstet Gynecol* **160:** 462–70.

Goldenberg RL, Cutter GR, Hoffman HJ, Foster JM, Nelson KG & Hauth JC (1989b) Intrauterine growth retardation: standard for diagnosis. *Am J Obstet Gynecol* **161:** 271–277.

Goldstein DP & Berkowitz RS (1986) The management of molar pregnancy and gestational trophoblastic tumors. In Kistner RW (ed.) *Gynecology Principles and Practice*. Chicago: Year Book Medical Publishers.

Grover V, Usha R, Lalra S & Sachdeva S (1991) Altered fetal growth: antenatal diagnosis by symphysis-fundal height in India and comparison with western charts. *Int J Gynecol Obstet* **35:** 231–234.

Holzgreve W. (1990) Sonographic screening for anatomic defects. *Semin Perinatol* **14:** 504–13.

Jimenez JM, Tyson JE & Reisch JS (1983) Clinical measures of gestational age in normal pregnancies. *Obstet Gynecol* **61:** 438–43.

Editorial (1989) *Br Med J* **298:** 618.

Kiely JL (1990) The epidemiology of perinatal mortality in multiple births. *Bull NY Acad Med* **66:** 618–637.

Kiserud T. (1986) Fundal height growth in rural Africa. *Acta Obstet Gynaecol Scand* **65:** 713–15.

Kleinman JC, Fowler MG & Kessel SS (1991) Comparison of infant mortality among twins and singletons: United States 1960 and 1983. *Am J Epidemiol* **133:** 133–43.

Kohorn EI (1984) Molar pregnancy: presentation and diagnosis. *Clin Obstet Gynecol* **27:** 181–91.

Linasmita V (1985) Antenatal screening of small-for-gestational age infants by symphysial-fundal height measurement. *J Med Assoc Thailand* **68:** 587–91.

Linasmita V (1986) Serial symphysis-fundal height measurement of abnormal fetal growth. *J Med Assoc Thailand* **69:** 585–8.

Lindhard A, Nielsen PV, Mouritsen LA, Zachariassen A, Sorensen HU & Rosesno H (1990) The implications of introducing the symphyseal-fundal height-measurement. A prospective randomized controlled trial. *Br J Obstet Gynaecol* **97:** 675–80.

Mathai M, Jairaj P & Muthurathnam S (1987) Screening for light-for-gestational age infants: a comparison of three simple measurements. *Br J Obstet Gynaecol* **94:** 217–21.

Mathai M (1988) Prediction of small-for-gestational-age infants using a specially calibrated tape measure. *Br J Obstet Gynaecol* **95:** 313–4.

Neilson JP, Verkuyl DAA & Bannerman C (1988) Tape measurement of symphysis-fundal height in twin pregnancies. *Br J Obstet Gynaecol* **95:** 1054–59.

Norton R (1989) The prediction of intrauterine growth retardation in remote area aboriginal women using serial fundal-symphysial height measurements. *Aust NZ J Obstet Gynaecol* **29:** 306–7.

Okonofua FE, Ayangade SO, Chan RCW & O'Brien PMS (1986) A prospective comparison of clinical and ultrasonic methods of predicting normal and abnormal fetal growth. *Int J Gynecol Obstet* **24:** 447–451.

Pattinson RC (1988) Antenatal detection of small-for-gestational-age babies: choice of a symphysis-fundal growth curve. *S African Med J* **74:** 282–283.

Pattinson RC & Theron GB (1989) Inter-observer variation in symphysis-fundus measurements. *S African Med J* **76:** 6212.

Pearce JM & Campbell S (1987) A comparison of symphysis-fundal height and ultrasound as screening tests for light-for-gestational age infants. *Br J Obstet Gynaecol* **94:** 100–104.

Persson B, Stangenberg M, Lunell NO, Brodin U, Holmberg NG & Vaclavinkova V (1986) Prediction of size of infants at birth by measurement of symphysis fundus height. *Br J Obstet Gynaecol* **93:** 206–11.

Pschera H & Söderberg G (1983) Estimation of fetal weight by external abdominal measurements. *Acta Obstet Gynaecol Scand* **62:** 175–179.

Quaranta P, Currell R & Redman CWG (1981) Prediction of small-for-dates infants by measurement of symphysial-fundal-height. *Br J Obstet Gynaecol* **88:** 115–19.

Rogers MS & Needham PG (1985) Evaluation of fundal height measurement in antenatal care. *Aust NZ J Obstet Gynaecol* **25:** 87–90.

Rosenberg K, Grant JM, Tweedie I, Aitchison T & Gallagher F (1982) Measurement of fundal height as a screening test for fetal growth retardation. *Br J Obstet Gynaecol* **89:** 447–50.

Seeds JW (1984) Impaired fetal growth: definition and clinical diagnosis. *Obstet Gynecol* **64:** 303–10.

Smibert J (1962) Some observations on the height of the fundus uteri in pregnancy. *Aust NZ J Obstet Gynaecol* **8:** 125–131.

Stuart JM, Healy TJG, Sutton M & Swingler GR (1989) Symphysis-fundus measurements in screening for small-for-dates infants: a community based study in Gloucestershire. *J R Coll Gen Pract* **39:** 45–48.

Tjon A, Ten WE, Kusin JA & De With C (1985) Fundal height measurement as an antenatal screening method. *J Trop Pediat* **31:** 249–52.

US Public Health Service (1989) Expert Panel on the Content of Prenatal Care. *Caring For Our Future: The Content of Prenatal Care*. Washington, DC: Public Health Service, DHHS.

Wallin A, Gyllenswärd A & Westin B (1981) Symphysis-fundus measurement in prediction of fetal growth disturbances. *Acta Obstet Gynaecol Scand* **60:** 317–323.

Wenstrom KD & Gall SA (1988) Incidence, morbidity and mortality, and diagnosis of twin gestations. *Clin Perinatol* **15:** 1–11.

Westin B (1977) Gravidogram and fetal growth. *Acta Obstet Gynecol Scand* **56:** 273–82.

Whetham JCG, Muggah H & Davidson S (1976) Assessment of intrauterine growth retardation by diagnostic ultrasound. *Am J Obstet Gynecol* **125:** 577–80.

12

Screening for Preterm Delivery & Low Birthweight Using Maternal Height & Weight

Lambert H. Lumey

WHAT IS THE PROBLEM THAT REQUIRES SCREENING?

PRETERM DELIVERY (< 37 WEEKS) AND LOW BIRTHWEIGHT (< 2500 g).

What is the incidence/prevalence of the target condition?

The prevalence of preterm delivery ranges from 5% to 15% and that of low birthweight from 5% to 10% in selected populations. The rate varies considerably by geographic region and by race, which is likely to be due in part to biological differences and in part to the difficulties associated with obtaining representative samples from well-defined populations. For the present analysis, two data sources are utilized. The first is from Amsterdam (Doornbos and Nordbeck, 1985) and the second from California (Van den Berg and Oechsli, 1984). Both populations are relatively well-defined and include adequate numbers of white, black and Asian subjects.

For the Netherlands, all women delivering in three Amsterdam hospitals participating in the Gemeenschappelijke Verloskundige Registratie obstetric database (1972–1982) with pertinent information on the variables of interest were included. Data were obtained from published reports (Doornbos and Nordbeck, 1985). This population comprises Dutch women, black women mainly from Surinam and the Dutch Antilles, and Asian women mainly of Indian, Chinese or Indonesian origin. In the Netherlands, about 30% of births are planned home deliveries, and hospital births generally reflect a selection of at-risk pregnancies. There is universal health coverage in the Netherlands and the selected population represents an urban population with a wide variety of economic and social characteristics deficient only in the extremes.

For the USA, women with pertinent information from the Child Health and Development Study (CHDS) (1959–1967) were included. A data tape was kindly provided by R. E. Christianson of the CHDS for secondary analyses. This population from the San Francisco East Bay area of California comprises white, black and Asian women who were members of the Kaiser Foundation Health Plan. In this prepaid medical insurance plan, comprehensive medical care is provided to members and their families who also form an urban population with a wide variety of economic and social characteristics deficient only in the extremes.

What are the sequelae of the condition which are of interest in clinical medicine?

Perinatal mortality (PNM) and morbidity are markedly increased among preterm delivery and low birthweight infants. In Amsterdam, 75% of PNM occurs in preterm delivery infants who comprise only 7.2% of all births, and 80% of PNM occurs in low birthweight infants who comprise only 7.8% of all births. In California, these figures are 59% and 8.5% for preterm delivery infants, and 65% and 6% for low birthweight infants, respectively.

THE TESTS

What is the purpose of the tests?

To identify a subgroup of women at increased risk of preterm delivery or low birthweight.

What is the nature of the tests?

Measurements of height and weight are commonly made during prenatal visits. These measurements are valid, accurate, and reliable when appropriate equipment is used. They have been used to identify women with an increased risk of delivering preterm delivery or low birthweight infants since there is evidence that women of low height or weight are, on average, at an increased risk for such adverse outcomes. However, while it is often useful to describe a subpopulation by its mean height and weight, the effectiveness of prenatal tests to predict accurately for a given individual an increased risk of preterm delivery and/or low birthweight has not been satisfactory in the past (Creasy et al., 1980; Fortney and Whitehorne, 1982; Van den Berg and Oechsli, 1984). Thus the data of the Amsterdam and California populations were examined to test the performance of these tests with a relatively extreme cut-off point: a very low height (< 150 cm or 59 inches) or a very low weight (< 50 kg or 110 lb) in predicting these adverse outcomes. Test performances were examined separately for women of different ethnicity.

TEST PERFORMANCE AMONG AMSTERDAM AND CALIFORNIA
WOMEN OF DIFFERENT ETHNICITY

Results of screening for preterm delivery and low birthweight using tests for low maternal height and weight are given in Tables 12.1–12.4. The number of subjects in the study groups is given first, and then the prevalence of a preterm delivery and low birthweight pregnancy outcome and of the presumed risk factor (low height or weight) are given as percentages thereof. Also as percentages, the sensitivity, specificity, and the positive and negative predictive values are given, together with likelihood ratios associated with positive and negative test results. All these performance statistics are presented for the three ethnic groups, first separately, and then combined in the form of a weighted

Table 12.1　Screening for *preterm delivery* (PTD) using very low maternal height (< 150 cm).

POPULATION	WHITES		BLACKS		ASIANS		ALL
	NL	US	NL	US	NL	US	
number	15 754	10 422	1 086	3 795	1 416	629	33 102
prevalence of PTD (%)	6	6	11	15	8	8	7
prevalence of height < 150 cm	0.4	2	2	2	11	15	2
sens. (%)	1	4	2	3	15	19	3
spec. (%)	100	98	98	98	89	86	98
LR$^{(pos)}$	—	2.0	1.0	1.5	1.4	1.4	1.5
LR$^{(neg)}$	1.0	1.0	1.0	1.0	1.0	0.9	1.0
PPV (%)	9	10	9	19	11	11	11
npv (%)	94	94	89	85	93	92	93

LR $^{(pos)}$, likelihood ratio of a positive test result; LR $^{(neg)}$, likelihood ratio of a negative test result; NL, the Netherlands; NPV, negative predictive value; PPV, positive predictive value; sens., sensitivity; spec., specificity; US, USA

average. These analyses were repeated in a population of pregnant women severely malnourished during the Dutch famine of 1944–1945, using weight loss in pregnancy as the test criterion. In this population (Lumey *et al.*, 1993) even weight loss in pregnancy performed no better than low maternal weight in predicting an adverse pregnancy outcome (data not shown).

Implications of testing maternal height as a screening test for (a) preterm delivery

WHAT DOES AN ABNORMAL TEST RESULT MEAN?

As the overall sensitivity and positive predictive value of low maternal height as a screening test for *preterm delivery* are low (3% and 11%, respectively), the test has little implication for clinical practice (Table 12.1). Despite a likelihood ratio of 1.5 for a positive test result, the test would miss nearly all women with an adverse outcome and the probability of an adverse outcome among women with a positive test is very low. Sensitivity is highest among Asian women (15% and 19%).

WHAT DOES A NORMAL TEST RESULT MEAN?

The specificity of a negative test is high in all subgroups and the weighted average across all populations is 98%. The probability of *preterm delivery* after a normal test result is 7%. However, the prevalence of preterm delivery in the untested population

Table 12.2   Screening for low birthweight (LBW) using low maternal height.

POPULATION	WHITES		BLACKS		ASIANS		ALL
	NL	US	NL	US	NL	US	
number	17 435	10 422	1 405	3 795	1 670	629	35 356
prevalence of LBW	7	5	9	10	10	7	7
prevalence of height < 150 cm	0.4	2	2	2	11	15	2
sens. (%)	1	5	5	5	16	17	4
spec. (%)	100	98	98	98	89	86	98
LR$^{(pos)}$	—	2.5	2.5	2.5	1.5	1.2	2.0
LR$^{(neg)}$	1.0	1.0	1.0	1.0	0.9	1.0	1.0
PPV (%)	14	11	23	19	14	8	14
npv (%)	93	95	91	90	91	93	93

See footnote to Table 12.1 for key

is the same, as would be expected given a LR$^{(neg)}$ of approximately 1. Thus, in this sense too, the measurement of maternal height is of little value as a screening test for *preterm delivery*.

(b) Low birthweight

WHAT DOES AN ABNORMAL TEST RESULT MEAN?

As the overall sensitivity and positive predictive value of low maternal height as a screening test for *low birthweight* are very low (4% and 14% respectively), the test has little implications for clinical practice (Table 12.2). The sensitivity is highest among Asian women (17%), but the positive predictive value is highest in black women (about 20%). The likelihood ratio of a positive test result across all populations is 2.0.

WHAT DOES A NORMAL TEST RESULT MEAN?

The specificity of a negative test is relatively high in all subgroups and the weighted average across all populations is 98%. The probability of *low birthweight* after a normal test result is 7%. The prevalence of *low birthweight* in the untested population is the same; however, LR^{neg} is approximately equal to 1.

Table 12.3 Screening for *preterm delivery* (PTD) using low maternal weight (< 50 kg).

POPULATION	WHITES		BLACKS		ASIANS		ALL
	NL	US	NL	US	NL	US	
number	16 599	11 730	1 047	4 083	1 329	699	35 487
prevalence of PTD	6	6	11	15	8	8	7
prevalence of weight < 50 kg	2	7	7	5	28	40	6
sens. (%)	3	9	9	4	41	43	8
spec. (%)	98	93	93	95	73	61	94
LR$^{(pos)}$	1.5	1.3	1.3	0.8	1.5	1.1	1.3
LR$^{(neg)}$	1.0	1.0	1.0	1.0	0.8	0.9	1.0
PPV (%)	9	8	13	13	11	10	9
NPV (%)	94	94	89	85	94	92	93

See Table 12.1 for key

Implications of testing maternal weight as a screening test for (a) preterm delivery

WHAT DOES AN ABNORMAL TEST RESULT MEAN?

Since the overall sensitivity and positive predictive value of *low maternal weight* as a screening test for *preterm delivery* are low (8% and 9%, respectively), the measurement has little implication for clinical practice (Table 12.3). Its sensitivity is highest among Asian women, exceeding 40%; unfortunately the positive predictive value in this group did not exceed 11%. The LR^{pos} is 1.3 overall.

WHAT DOES A NORMAL TEST RESULT MEAN?

The specificity of a negative test is relatively high in all subgroups and the weighted average across all populations is 94%. Specificity was lowest among Asian women. The probability of preterm delivery after a normal test result is 7%. Unfortunately, again the prevalence of preterm delivery in the untested population is the same (LR$^{(neg)}$ close to 1).

(b) Low birthweight

WHAT DOES AN ABNORMAL TEST RESULT MEAN?

As the overall sensitivity and positive predictive value of low maternal weight as a screening test for a *low birthweight* neonate are low (11% and 16%), the measurement has

Table 12.4 Screening for *low birthweight* (LBW) using low maternal weight (< 50 kg).

POPULATION	WHITES		BLACKS		ASIANS		ALL
	NL	**US**	**NL**	**US**	**NL**	**US**	
number	18 151	11 730	1 295	4 083	1 544	699	37 502
prevalence of LBW	7	5	10	10	10	7	7
prevalence of weight < 50 kg	2	7	7	5	28	40	6
sens. (%)	6	13	9	9	48	54	11
spec. (%)	98	94	93	96	74	61	95
LR$^{(pos)}$	3.0	2.2	1.3	1.5	1.9	1.4	2.2
LR$^{(neg)}$	1.0	0.9	1.0	0.9	0.7	0.8	0.9
PPV (%)	19	10	12	18	17	10	16
NPV (%)	93	95	90	91	93	95	93

See Table 12.1 for key

few, if any, uses as a screening tool in clinical practice (Table 12.4). Sensitivity is highest among Asian women (50%), but the positive predictive value does not exceed 19% in any of the subgroups. The LR$^{(pos)}$ across all populations is 2.2.

WHAT DOES A NORMAL TEST RESULT MEAN?

The specificity of a negative test is relatively high in all subgroups and the weighted average across all populations is 95%. The probability of *low birthweight* after a normal test is 7%, which is the same as the prevalence of *low birthweight* in the untested population (LR$^{(neg)}$ is approximately 1).

What is the cost of testing?

The direct costs of height and weight measurements per antenatal visit are negligible given that measuring equipment is purchased once and used for many years. Other costs include patient and staff time for measurement (maybe 30 seconds per visit) and waiting time (which can be considerable).

CONCLUSIONS AND RECOMMENDATIONS

Screening for preterm delivery or low birthweight cannot be achieved successfully with either very low maternal height or low maternal weight as test criteria. The predictive values of a positive test for preterm delivery are 11% and 9%, and for low birthweight are 14% and 16%, respectively. This means, for example, that only one out of six to seven women with low height or weight actually delivers a low birthweight infant. Given the relatively low prevalence of preterm delivery and low birthweight, even a doubling in risk (at the aggregate level) after positive testing for low birthweight does not provide useful additional information for clinical practice.

Normal test results do not provide useful information either, as the probability of an adverse outcome after a normal test is the same as the average prevalence of preterm delivery and low birthweight (about 7%) in unscreened populations; all the LR^{neg} values were close to 1.

Whereas the combined effect of low prepregnancy maternal weight and low weight gain in pregnancy on low birthweight may seem dramatic (Eastman and Jackson 1968), the predictive value of having both characteristics with respect to low birthweight among term births in their study was only 6% in white women and 16% in black women. This is no higher than the positive predictive value of low maternal weight alone in our populations.

In the light of the evidence presented here, and because of other evidence which shows no benefit of weight measurements for individual screening and prediction of these or other adverse conditions (Chalmers *et al.* 1989), measuring maternal weight (or height) routinely during pregnancy should be abandoned. In order to document height and weight distributions in various subgroups of the clinic population it is still important to measure maternal height and weight at least once, preferably early in pregnancy.

SUMMARY

1 WHAT IS THE PROBLEM THAT REQUIRES SCREENING?

PRETERM DELIVERY AND LOW BIRTHWEIGHT.

a What is the incidence/prevalence of the target condition?

The prevalence of preterm delivery ranges from 5% to 15% and of low birthweight from 5% to 10% in selected populations.

b What are the sequelae of the condition which are of interest in clinical medicine?

Perinatal mortality and morbidity is markedly increased among preterm delivery and low birthweight infants.

2 THE TESTS

a What is the purpose of the tests?

To detect patients at risk for either preterm delivery or a low birthweight infant.

b The nature of the tests

Measurement of maternal height and weight.

c Implications of testing

1 What does an abnormal test result mean?

Only one out of six to seven women with low height or weight actually delivers preterm or has a low birthweight infant.

2 What does a normal test result mean?

Normal test results do not provide useful information since the probability of an adverse outcome after a normal test is the same as the prevalence of preterm delivery and low birthweight in unscreened populations.

d What is the cost of testing?

The marginal costs are negligible.

3 CONCLUSIONS AND RECOMMENDATIONS

Screening for preterm delivery or low birthweight cannot be achieved successfully with either very low maternal height or low maternal weight as test criteria.

REFERENCES

Chalmers I, Enkin M & Keirse MJNC (eds) (1989) *Effective Care in Pregnancy and Childbirth*. Oxford University Press.
Creasy RK, Gummer BA & Liggins GC (1980) System for predicting spontaneous preterm birth. *Obstet Gynecol* **55:** 692–695.
Doornbos JPR & Nordbeck HJ (1985) *Perinatal mortality. Obstetric risk factors in a community of mixed ethnic origin in Amsterdam*. Thesis, University of Amsterdam.
Eastman NJ & Jackson E (1968) Weight relationships in pregnancy. I. The bearing of maternal weight gain and pre-pregnant weight on birth weight in full term pregnancies. *Obst Gyn Survey* **23:** 1003–1025.
Fletcher RH, Fletcher SW & Wagner EH (1988) *Clinical Epidemiology: The Essentials*, 2nd edn. Baltimore: Williams & Wilkins.
Fortney JA & Whitehorne EW (1982) The development of an index of high risk pregnancy. *Am J Obstet Gynecol* **143:** 501–508.
Lumey LH, Ravelli ACJ, Wiessing LG, Koppe JG, Treffers PE & Stein ZA (1993) The Dutch famine birth cohort study: design, validation of exposure, and selected characteristics of subjects after 43 years follow-up. *Paed Perinat Epidemiol* **7:** 354–367.
Van den Berg BJ & Oechsli FW (1984) Prematurity. In Bracken MB (ed). *Perinatal Epidemiology*. Oxford: Oxford University Press.

13

Blood Pressure Measurement in Antenatal Care

Gustaaf A. Dekker

PREGNANCY-ASSOCIATED HYPERTENSION.

The phrase 'preeclampsia-eclampsia syndrome' is defined as hypertension new to pregnancy manifesting after 20 weeks' gestation that is associated with new onset of proteinuria which resolves after delivery. The phrase 'gestational hypertension' is used to denote hypertension new to pregnancy that resolves after delivery but is not associated with proteinuria. Chronic hypertension is hypertension that predates pregnancy or appears prior to 20 weeks' gestation.

What is the incidence/prevalence of the target condition?

The application of epidemiologic methods is bedeviled by the protean nature of the disease and the plethora of diagnostic classifications (Davies and Dunlop, 1983). The true prevalence of pregnancy-associated hypertension cannot be stated given the variable diagnostic criteria. The reported prevalence is influenced by the availability and use of health care services, the interests and awareness of medical attendants and the accuracy with which measurements are made and recorded.

The reported prevalence of pregnancy-associated hypertension ranges from 2% to 35% depending on the diagnostic criteria used and the population studied (Campbell *et al.*, 1985; Long and Oats, 1987; Sibai, 1990). Chronic hypertension accounts for approximately 30% of pregnancy-associated hypertension (Working Group on High Blood Pressure in Pregnancy, 1990). In the remaining 70%, the hypertension resolves after delivery and is presumably caused in some manner by pregnancy. The prevalence of pregnancy-associated hypertension is two to three times higher in nulliparas than in multiparas. Data from the National Hospital Discharge Survey in the USA (Saftlas *et al.*, 1990) indicate that the syndrome of preeclampsia complicates 2.6% of all births.

What are the sequelae of the condition which are of interest in clinical medicine?

Hypertension during pregnancy poses risk to both mother and fetus. Preeclampsia is associated with an increase in perinatal mortality and morbidity (Naeye and Friedman,

1979; Working Group on High Blood Pressure in Pregnancy, 1990). On the other hand, gestational hypertension in industrialized countries is associated neither with an increase in perinatal mortality or morbidity, nor with a decrease in birthweight.

Maternal sequelae: Hypertension is not a disease but a reflection of the maternal response to an underlying disease. The primary pathology is not known but is apparently localized within the gravid uterus. It is associated with impaired endovascular trophoblast invasion, acute atherosis and endothelial dysfunction. Secondary pathology includes the signs that define preeclampsia: hypertension and proteinuria. Peripheral disturbances of preeclampsia can become so severe that they initiate new or tertiary pathology. Significant tertiary complications include eclampsia, cerebral hemorrhage, hepatic rupture, hemolysis, thrombocytopenia and elevated levels of hepatic enzymes (Redman, 1987, 1989).

The overall maternal mortality has declined dramatically in industrialized countries over the last 60 years. Hypertension and its sequelae account for the largest proportion (12–60%) (Kaunitz et al., 1985; Rochat et al., 1988; Department of Health, 1991; Schuitemaker et al., 1991). In the UK, 56% of deaths in women with pregnancy-associated hypertension are attributed to eclampsia, and 81% are judged to reflect substandard care (Department of Health, 1991). In nonindustrialized countries which have maternal mortality rates 100–200 times higher than Europe and North America, it is estimated that 15% of maternal deaths are associated with hypertensive disorders of pregnancy, and that 10% are associated with eclampsia (Duley, 1992).

Perinatal sequelae: Perinatal risk rises progressively with the diastolic blood pressure irrespective of gestational age, though there is controversy as to whether that rise begins at 90 mmHg or 110 mmHg in the absence of proteinuria. There is general agreement that the risk rises when the diastolic pressure exceeds 90 mmHg if proteinuria is present (Page and Christianson, 1976; Friedman and Neff, 1977; Naeye and Friedman, 1979). Hypertensive disorders of pregnancy increase the risk of intrauterine growth restriction (IUGR) almost 15 times compared with a normotensive pregnancy (Harvey, 1987). Hypertension is present in about 60% of pregnancies complicated by IUGR that end in fetal death and/or preterm delivery (Visser et al., 1986).

THE TEST

What is the purpose of the test?

To allow the diagnosis and correct classification of hypertension in pregnancy.

The most important consideration in the classification of hypertension during pregnancy is its differentiation into hypertension that predates pregnancy and pregnancy-associated hypertension.

The nature of the test

METHODOLOGICAL ASPECTS

Three groups of variables affect the diagnosis of hypertension: (1) the intrinsic physiologic variation of systemic pressure, (2) the way blood pressure is measured, and (3) the cut-off point used to divide normal from abnormal (Davies and Dunlop, 1983). There is wide variation in the blood pressure values of both nonpregnant and pregnant women. Studies of the general pregnant population have found that 50% of women with a hypertensive measurement are normotensive on subsequent follow-up (Walker, 1991).

Blood pressure is not an absolute value. Thus, the definition of hypertension is fairly arbitrary and a rigid cut-off point should be avoided (Walker, 1991). Blood pressure normally falls during the first and second trimesters before rising again towards term to a level similar to the value in the nonpregnant population.

Hypertension is considered a defining characteristic of preeclampsia even though it is a secondary feature. There are two general problems in using hypertension in this way. First, the concept of hypertension is artificial. An arbitrary cut-off is employed to divide a continuous variable. Second, the rise in peripheral resistance is a more fundamental feature of the disorder. It is only because cardiac output is usually maintained that the change in peripheral resistance can be discerned by measuring the blood pressure (Redman, 1987).

The hypertension of preeclampsia is categorized either by an absolute cut-off or by an incremental increase over a baseline in the first half of pregnancy. The conventional dividing line is 140/90 mmHg. The use of a diastolic blood pressure of at least 90 mmHg or more throughout pregnancy (Nelson, 1955) has two main advantages: firstly, in the first trimester of pregnancy it is 3 standard deviations above the mean and in the third trimester it is 2 standard deviations above the mean (MacGillivray et al., 1969), and secondly, it corresponds with the point of inflexion of the curve relating diastolic blood pressure to perinatal mortality. Unfortunately from the standpoint of a screening tool, at least 20% of pregnant women have a blood pressure of 140/90 mmHg or higher at least once in the second half of pregnancy (Redman, 1987).

The Committee on Terminology of the American College of Obstetricians and Gynecologists defines hypertension as either a *systolic* pressure – of 140 mmHg or more, or an increment of 30 mmHg or more from a baseline value established in the first half of pregnancy – or a *diastolic* pressure – of a value of 90 mmHg or more, or an increment of 15 mmHg or more above baseline. The absolute blood pressure level or threshold increments in pressures must be observed on at least two occasions 6 hours apart (Working Group on High Blood Pressure in Pregnancy, 1990). However, the rise in blood pressure is unreliable since a gradual increase in blood pressure from the second to the third trimester is normal. MacGillivray et al. (1969) reported that 73% of primigravid women with normotensive pregnancies demonstrated an increase in diastolic blood pressure of more than 15 mmHg at some stage during the course of their pregnancies. Redman and Jefferies (1988) applied several cut-offs in 16 211 singleton pregnancies to determine the best means of diagnosing preeclampsia. They proposed that the definition of preeclampsia should include a first-trimester diastolic blood pressure below 90 mmHg, a subsequent increase of at least 25 mmHg and a maximum reading of at least 90 mmHg.

Blood pressure measurement prior to 20 weeks' gestation is an essential part of antenatal care. It provides baseline blood pressure levels from which all increases will be judged, and helps the caregiver diagnose chronic hypertension. Women with chronic hypertension have a 25% increase in the risk of developing superimposed preeclampsia (Working Group on High Blood Pressure in Pregnancy, 1990). Incidentially, many women with well-established chronic hypertension become normotensive by 10–13 weeks' gestation when antenatal care is often initiated. If it is not possible to differentiate between chronic hypertension and preeclampsia, the patient should be managed as having preeclampsia as the risks are greater for this condition.

Maternal mortality is associated with poor or no antenatal care (Sibai, 1990; Odum and Akinkugbe, 1991). The management of pregnancy-associated hypertension is founded on comprehensive antenatal care, early diagnosis and admission to hospital for rest and observation, and a well-timed delivery to preempt complications. Most patients with pregnancy-associated hypertension have no clinical symptoms. It can be reliably detected only by repetitive searches for the early signs and symptoms in the second half of pregnancy.

Screening for preeclampsia begins at 20 weeks. The standard pattern of antenatal care (monthly visits at 20, 24, and 28 weeks) leaves intervals where severe, early-onset preeclampsia can evolve undetected. In the Oxford region of England, 50% of antenatal eclampsia occurs before 28 weeks. To identify all cases of preeclampsia, women would need to be screened weekly after 20 weeks. This is not feasible. The individual's risk for preeclampsia should be assessed at the end of the first trimester (Redman, 1989). Some of the factors that predispose to preeclampsia are nulliparity, extremes of age, previous history of preeclampsia, family history of preeclampsia, chronic hypertension and/or renal disease, migraine, diabetes, collagen diseases, multiple fetal pregnancy, placental hydrops, and hydrops fetalis. Based on the presence or absence of these risk factors, antenatal care can be individualized.

TECHNIQUES

The most widely used technique for the measurement of systemic blood pressure by an indirect method employs the mercury sphygmomanometer. The anaeroid gauge is subject to many more potential errors and should not be used for the screening of pregnant women (Murnaghan, 1987). Automated, noninvasive devices for the measurement of blood pressure have gained popularity because of their relatively low cost, reasonable accuracy, and capacity for frequent measurements (Shennan et al., 1993; Brown et al., 1994). Oscillometry is an indirect method based on the measurement of manometric oscillations induced by arterial pulsations during cuff deflation. Oscillometric techniques are increasingly used in clinical obstetrics. The oscillation of pressure in a sphygmomanometer cuff begins above systolic pressure and continues below diastolic pressure, so that systolic and diastolic pressures are estimated indirectly according to an empirically derived algorithm. The point of maximum oscillation corresponds to the mean intra-arterial pressure. The method works reasonably well, but in some women it may be seriously in error. Ultrasound techniques use a transmitter and receiver placed over the brachial artery under a sphygmomanometer cuff. Though the test is reasonably accurate, serious errors have been reported (Quinn, 1991; Franx et al., 1994).

The most important advantages of automated devices are absence of observer bias, digit preference and threshold avoidance. Despite these theoretical advantages, there is no automatic blood pressure recording device available that is universally reliable. Overall, automated blood pressure recorders tend to overestimate the systolic and underestimate the diastolic blood pressure. Each time such a device is used, it should be calibrated against a mercury sphygmomanometer (Australian Society for the Study of Hypertension in Pregnancy, 1991).

At present, the auscultatory technique based on the Korotkoff sounds remains the standard method for recording blood pressure. Phase I defines the systolic pressure. In nonpregnant women, phase V (extinction of Korotkoff sounds) is recommended as the diastolic end-point rather than phase IV (muffling). Gallery et al. (1994) compared Korotkoff phases IV and V in a large series of normotensive, chronic hypertensive and preeclamptic women in the second and third trimesters. They concluded that (1) phase IV–V differences, although statistically significant, are small in the majority of pregnant women, particularly in those with preeclampsia, and (2) both phase IV and V are reproducible measurements. A consensus report from the USA recommended that both phase IV and V be recorded throughout pregnancy (Working Group on High Blood Pressure in Pregnancy, 1990).

It is essential that the technique and conditions for measurement be standardized. Measuring blood pressure with the cuff on the superior arm of a patient in a lateral recumbent position will result in a decrease in diastolic blood pressure of approximately 10–14 mmHg due to a decrease in hydrostatic pressure relative to the level of the heart. The same mechanism explains the pressor response during a roll-over test (Wichman *et al.*, 1984; Dekker *et al.*, 1990). However, the roll-over test is of little or no value in predicting preeclampsia. If blood pressure is measured in the supine position, decreased venous return secondary to compression of the vena cava may cause supine hypotension. During pregnancy, blood pressure should be measured with the woman in a sitting or semireclining position. The right arm should be used, placed in a horizontal position to the heart level. The size of the cuff relative to the diameter of the arm is critical. The cuff should be a minimum of 40% of the arm circumference. In general, error can be reduced by using a large, adult-sized cuff for all but the thinnest arms (Pickering and Blank, 1990).

Implications of testing

WHAT DOES AN ABNORMAL TEST RESULT MEAN?

An elevated blood pressure is consistent with the diagnosis of hypertension. The presence of more than 300 mg protein per 24 hours and hypertension new to pregnancy is sufficient for the diagnosis of preeclampsia.

High blood pressure resulting from an increase in systemic peripheral resistance can be the first sign of circulatory maladaption. The timely diagnosis of preeclampsia remains the pivotal function of antenatal care. Despite many potential screening tests, only a few appear promising (Chesley and Sibai, 1988; Dekker and Sibai, 1991). Both the evaluation of incremental changes in blood pressure during pregnancy and the mean arterial blood pressure in the second trimester (MAP-2) are poor predictors of preeclampsia (Villar and Sibai, 1989). This is due to a variety of factors: (1) the absolute blood pressure may still lie within the accepted reference range; (2) blood pressure fluctuates over short periods; (3) a response to the stress of being in medical setting; (4) measurement errors. Though these tests are poor predictors of preeclampsia, their negative predictive values are high. A pregnant woman who has a diastolic blood pressure of about 70 mmHg or lower at the end of the second trimester, or a MAP-2 of 80 mmHg or lower, runs a low risk of developing preeclampsia.

Although the predictive value of a single blood pressure determination at any time in pregnancy, or a MAP-2, is limited, it is emphasized that a rise in blood pressure in the second trimester is abnormal. Although the clinical signs and symptoms of preeclampsia may not yet be present, such women deserve careful observation. This is especially true of women who have chronic hypertension (August and Lindheimer, 1991). A timely diagnosis of hypertension allows the obstetician to intensify antenatal surveillance. Such surveillance may include laboratory tests to differentiate between preeclampsia and chronic hypertension, and to determine the severity of the illness. If preeclampsia is suspected or confirmed, hospitalization and bed rest is the most common 'treatment' prior to delivery. Crowther and Chalmers (1989) reviewed the literature on the effects of hospitalization and bed rest, and concluded that hospitalization of women with non-proteinuric hypertension may reduce the incidence of severe hypertension (diastolic pressure 110 mmHg or more), and that bed rest appears to promote diuresis and decrease edema. However, the effect of bed rest on the development of proteinuria is inconsistent, and there are no data providing any evidence for a beneficial effect on perinatal outcome. Thus, the main reason to hospitalize women with pregnancy-associated hypertension is the need for a thorough evaluation and frequent maternal and fetal surveillance to detect deterioration. Whether the hospitalization should be linked with strict bed rest is less clear. Outpatient management may be considered in gestationally hypertensive patients with apparently mild and stable disease free of proteinuria. Outpatient management can only be a safe substitute for hospitalization if it includes blood pressure monitoring, patient instruction, structured bed rest, daily urine dipstick measurements of proteinuria, and fetal monitoring.

Low-dose aspirin has been used in an attempt to prevent preeclampsia. According to the available evidence, women at high risk for early-onset (before 32 weeks' gestation) preeclampsia are most likely to benefit from low-dose aspirin. Since early-onset preeclampsia may begin at any time after 20 weeks, it is necessary to initiate low-dose aspirin therapy early in pregnancy, preferably at 10–14 weeks. It is too late to initiate therapy (CLASP, 1994; Dekker, 1995) after the recognition of hypertension.

WHAT DOES A NORMAL TEST RESULT MEAN?

Though a 'normal' blood pressure is no guarantee of the absence of preeclampsia, it is reassuring. Most obstetric textbooks suggest that the clinical course of the preeclampsia is characterized by a chronic, gradual evolution that begins with weight gain followed by hypertension and proteinuria. However, one retrospective study of a black population in the southern USA found that prior to the onset of eclamptic convulsions, 23% had minimal or absent hypertension, 19% had no proteinuria, and in 32% there was no edema (Sibai, 1990).

What is the cost of testing?

One could argue that the cost of measuring blood pressure is negligible. However, antenatal care is governed by instruments to identify preeclampsia – i.e., blood pressure devices, weighing scales and dipsticks. Unfortunately, the development of proteinuria is a late feature. Thus, the routine use of dipsticks in a normotensive population is probably as ineffective as measuring maternal weight gain (see Chapter 12). If these tests were unnecessary, the number of antenatal visits could be reduced. Thus, if the number of antenatal visits is in great part dictated by the goal of early detection of preeclampsia, then the cost of screening is considerable.

CONCLUSIONS AND RECOMMENDATIONS

Measuring blood pressure before 20 weeks' gestation (preferably in the first trimester) is an essential part of antenatal care because it provides baseline blood pressure levels and facilitates the diagnosis of chronic hypertension. Reliable and standardized blood pressure measurements are important. Pregnant woman should be assessed at booking and again prior to 20 weeks' gestation for evidence of hypertension. Antenatal care and the frequency of visits can then be individualized. In pregnant women with an above-average risk of the development of preeclampsia, the intervals between antenatal visits should be shorter, especially during the second trimester. Prediction remains an elusive goal. However, every patient with an elevated blood pressure requires further testing.

The diagnosis of pregnancy-associated hypertension should lead to early hospital admission and a well-timed delivery to preempt complications.

Gestational hypertension and preeclampsia may well be two different diseases. Second-trimester increments in diastolic or systolic blood pressure MAP-2 values do not predict preeclampsia. However, normal values appear to be reassuring. It is abnormal for blood pressure to rise during the second trimester. Although it may be too early in pregnancy to diagnose preeclampsia, such women deserve careful observation.

SUMMARY

1 WHAT IS THE PROBLEM THAT REQUIRES SCREENING?

PREGNANCY-ASSOCIATED HYPERTENSION.

a What is the incidence/prevalence of the target condition?

The reported incidence ranges from 2% to 35% depending on the diagnostic criteria used and the population studied. The prevalence is two to three times higher in nulliparas compared with multiparas. Chronic hypertension accounts for about 30% of hypertension during pregnancy. Preeclampsia complicates 2–4% of all births.

b What are the sequelae of the condition which are of interest in clinical medicine?

Preeclampsia is associated with a marked increase in maternal and perinatal mortality and morbidity. Gestational hypertension, on the other hand, in industrialized countries is associated neither with an increase in maternal and perinatal mortality or morbidity, nor with a decrease in birthweight.

2 THE TEST

a What is the purpose of the test?

To enable the diagnosis and correct classification of hypertension in pregnancy.

b The nature of the test

The most widely used and reliable technique for the measurement of blood pressure by the indirect method involves the use of the mercury sphygmomanometer. The anaeroid gauge is subject to many more potential errors than the simple mercury manometer, and should not be used for the screening of pregnant women.

c Implications of testing

I What does an abnormal test result mean?

An elevated blood pressure is consistent with the diagnosis of hypertension. The presence of significant proteinuria with hypertension new to pregnancy is sufficient for the diagnosis of preeclampsia. Prediction remains an elusive goal.

2 What does a normal test result mean?

Though a 'normal' blood pressure is no guarantee of the absence of preeclampsia, it is reassuring.

d **What is the cost of testing?**

Antenatal visits are dominated by elements whose main purpose is to identify preeclampsia. If the number of antenatal visits is in great part dictated by the goal of early detection of preeclampsia, then the cost of screening is considerable.

3 CONCLUSIONS AND RECOMMENDATIONS

The measurement of systemic blood pressure is an important part of antenatal care. Antenatal care and the frequency of the visits can then be individualized. Every woman presenting with an elevated blood pressure deserves further laboratory testing and fetal evaluation. The diagnosis of pregnancy-associated hypertension should lead to early admission to hospital and a well-timed delivery to preempt complications.

REFERENCES

August P & Lindheimer MD (1991) Preeclampsia revisited. *Curr Obstet Med* **1:** 249–273.

Australian Society for the Study of Hypertension in Pregnancy (1994) Management of Hypertension in Pregnancy. *Consensus Statement.*

Brown MA, Reiter L, Buddle ML *et al.* (1994) Auscultatory and ambulatory blood pressure monitoring in pregnancy (Abstract 51, IXth ISSHP World Congress, March 1994, Sydney). *Hypertension in Pregnancy* **13:** 338.

Campbell DM, MacGillivray I & Carr-Hill R (1985) Pre-eclampsia in second pregnancy. *Br J Obstet Gynaecol* **92:** 131–140.

Chesley LC & Sibai BM (1988) Clinical significance of elevated mean arterial pressure in the second trimester. *Am J Obstet Gynecol* **159:** 275–279.

CLASP Collaborative Group (1994) A randomized trial of low dose aspirin for the prevention and treatment of pre-eclampsia among 9364 pregnant woman. *Lancet* **343:** 619–629.

Crowther C & Chalmers I (1989) Bed rest and hospitalization during pregnancy. In Chalmers I, Enkin M & Keirse MJNC (eds) *Effective Care in Pregnancy and Childbirth*, pp 624–632. Oxford University Press.

Davies AM & Dunlop W (1983) Hypertension in pregnancy. In Barron SL & Thomson AM (eds) *Obstetrical Epidemiology*, pp 167–208. London: Academic Press.

Dekker GA (1995) The pharmacologic prevention of preeclampsia. *Clin Obstet Gynecol* **9:** 509–528.

Dekker GA & Sibai BM (1991) Early detection of preeclampsia. *Am J Obstet Gynecol* **165:** 160–172.

Dekker GA, Makovitz JW & Wallenburg HCS (1990) Prediction of pregnancy-induced hypertensive disorders by angiotensin II sensitivity and supine pressor test. *Br J Obstet Gynaecol* **97:** 817–821.

Department of Health (1991) Department of Health, Welsh Office, Scottish Home and Health Department, DHSS Northern Ireland, *Report on Confidential Enquiries into Maternal Death in the United Kingdom 1985–1987.* London: HMSO.

Duley L (1992) Maternal mortality associated with hypertensive disorders of pregnancy in Africa, Asia, Latin America and the Caribbean. *Br J Obstet Gynaecol* **99:** 547–553.

Franx A, van der Post JAM, Elfering IM, *et al.* (1994) Validation of automated blood pressure recording in pregnancy. *Br J Obstet Gynaecol* **101:** 66–69.

Friedman EA & Neff RK (1977) *Pregnancy Hypertension. A Systematic Evaluation of Clinical Diagnostic Criteria*, 258 pp. Littleton, Mass: PSG Publishing.

Gallery EDM, Brown MA, Ross MR *et al.* (1994) Diastolic blood pressure in pregnancy: phase IV or phase V Korotkoff sounds. *Hypertension in Pregnancy* **13:** 285–292.

Harvey D (1987) The management of the newborn baby of the hypertensive mother. In: Sharp F, Symonds EM (eds) *Hypertension in Pregnancy*, pp 327–339. Ithaca, NY: Perinatology Press.

Kaunitz AM, Hughes JM, Grimes DA, *et al.* (1985) Causes of maternal mortality in the United States. *Obstet Gynecol* **65:** 605–612.

Long P & Oats J (1987) Preeclampsia in twin pregnancy-severity and pathogenesis. *Aust NZ J Obstet Gynaecol* 27: 1–5.

MacGillivray I, Rose GA & Rowe B (1969) Blood pressure survey in pregnancy. *Clin Sci* 37: 395–407.

Murnaghan GA (1987) Methods of measuring blood pressure and blood pressure variability. In Sharp F, Symonds EM (eds) *Hypertension in Pregnancy*, pp 19–28. Ithaca, NY: Perinatology Press

Naeye RL & Friedman CA (1979) Causes of perinatal death associated with gestational hypertension and proteinuria. *Am J Obstet Gynecol* 133: 8–10.

Nelson TR (1955) A clinical study of pre-eclampsia. *J Obstet Gynaecol Br Commonw* 62: 48–57.

Odum CU & Akinkugbe A (1991) The causes of maternal deaths in eclampsia in Lagos, Nigeria. *W African J Med* 10: 371–376.

Page EW & Christianson R (1976) Influence of blood pressure with and without proteinuria upon outcome of pregnancy. *Am J Obstet Gynecol* 126: 821–833.

Pickering TG & Blank SG (1990) Blood pressure measurement and ambulatory blood pressure monitoring; evaluation of available equipment. In Laragh JH and Brenner BM (eds) *Hypertension: Pathophysiology, Diagnosis, and Management*, pp. 1429–1441. New York: Raven Press.

Quinn MJ (1991) Blood pressure measurement in pregnancy (letter). *Lancet* 338: 130.

Quinn M (1994) Automated blood pressure measurement devices: a potential source of morbidity in preeclampsia? *Am J Obstet Gynecol* 170: 1303–1307.

Redman CWG (1987) The definition of pre-eclampsia. In Sharp F and Symonds EM (eds), *Hypertension in Pregnancy*, pp 3–17. Ithaca, NY: Perinatology Press.

Redman CWG (1989) Hypertension in pregnancy. In Turnbull A and Chamberlain G (eds) *Obstetrics*, pp 515–541. Edinburgh: Churchill Livingstone.

Redman CWG & Jefferies M (1988) Revised definition of pre-eclampsia. *Lancet* i: 809–812.

Rochat RW, Koonin LM, Atrash HK & Jewett JF (1988) Maternal mortality in the United States – report from the Maternal Mortality Collaborative. *Obstet Gynecol* 72: 91–97.

Saftlas AF, Olson DR, Franks AL, Atrash HK & Pokras R (1990) Epidemiology of preeclampsia and eclampsia in the United States, 1979–1986. *Am J Obstet Gynecol* 163: 460–465.

Schuitemaker NWE, Bennebroek Gravenhorst J, van Geijn HP, et al. (1991) Maternal mortality and its prevention. *Eur J Obstet Gynecol Reprod Biol* 42: S31-S35.

Shennan AH, Kissane J & De Swiet M (1993) Validation of the SpaceLabs 90207 ambulatory blood pressure monitor for use in pregnancy. *Br J Obstet Gynaecol* 100: 904–908.

Sibai BM (1990) Preeclampsia-eclampsia. *Curr Probl Obstet Gynecol Fertil* 13: 3–45.

Villar MA & Sibai BM (1989) Clinical significance of elevated mean arterial blood pressure in second trimester and threshold increase in systolic or diastolic blood pressure during third trimester. *Am J Obstet Gynecol* 160: 419–423.

Visser GH, Huisman A, Saathof PW & Sinnige HA (1986) Early fetal growth retardation: obstetric background and recurrence rate. *Obstet Gynecol* 67: 40–43.

Walker JJ (1991) Hypertensive drugs in pregnancy: antihypertensive therapy in pregnancy, preeclampsia, and eclampsia. *Clin Perinatol* 18: 845–873.

Wichman K, Ryden G & Wichman M (1984) The influence of different positions and Korotkoff sounds on the blood pressure measurements in pregnancy. *Acta Obstet Gynecol Scand* 118: 25–28.

Working Group on High Blood Pressure in Pregnancy (1990) National High Blood Pressure Education Program Working Group Report on High Blood Pressure in Pregnancy – Consensus Report. *Am J Obstet Gynecol* 163: 1689–1712.

14

Asymptomatic Bacteriuria in Pregnancy

Dwight J. Rouse

WHAT IS THE PROBLEM THAT REQUIRES SCREENING?

ASYMPTOMATIC BACTERIURIA LEADING TO SYMPTOMATIC UPPER
AND/OR LOWER URINARY TRACT INFECTION.

What is the incidence/prevalence of the target condition?

Asymptomatic bacteriuria (ASB) is defined as more than 100 000 bacteria per ml of urine
in a patient without symptoms of urinary tract infection. The condition is present in 2–
10% of gravidas at their first antenatal visit (Whalley, 1967; Norden and Kass, 1968).
Pregnancy does not predispose to the acquisition of ASB as only 1% of initially screen
negative gravidas develop ASB during pregnancy (Savage et al., 1967; Stenqvist et al.,
1989). The likelihood of ASB varies inversely with socioeconomic status and directly
with certain maternal conditions such as sickle cell trait (Andriole and Patterson, 1991).

What are the sequelae of the condition which are of interest in clinical medicine?

Asymptomatic bacteriuria in nongravid women poses little or no significant health risk
(Pels et al., 1989). This is not the case during pregnancy. Thirty per cent of gravid women
with untreated asymptomatic bacteriuria develop symptomatic urinary tract infection in
pregnancy (Whalley, 1967). Many of these acute infections can be classified as pyelonephritis on the basis of fever and flank pain. Conversely, only 0.2–2.0% of gravidas
who are screened early in gestation and found not to have bacteriuria will subsequently
develop symptomatic urinary tract infection during pregnancy (Norden and Kass, 1968;
Bachman et al., 1993). Pyelonephritis can be life-threatening during pregnancy: both
adult respiratory distress syndrome and septic shock can occur (Cunningham et al., 1984;
Hankins and Whalley, 1985). Asymptomatic bacteriuria is associated with an increased
risk of preterm delivery, but whether it plays a causative role is controversial (Andriole
and Patterson, 1991; Smaill, 1993a).

THE TESTS

What is the purpose of the tests?

To identify women with ASB because such women are at high risk for symptomatic urinary tract infection during pregnancy.

The nature of the tests

Urine culture remains the standard against which all other tests are judged for detection of asymptomatic bacteriuria. As originally defined, two consecutive clean voided urine specimens with more than 100 000 bacteria per ml of the same organism or one specimen with more than 100 000 bacteria per ml obtained by catheterization were required to diagnose ASB (Kass, 1962a, b). More recent studies have utilized one clean voided specimen with more than 100 000 bacteria per ml for diagnosis (Bachman *et al.*, 1993). In order to decrease the cost and shorten the time required for screening, other tests have been evaluated. These include urinalysis, urine dipstick studies for leukocyte esterase and/or nitrites, and Gram staining. Table 14.1 (adapted from Bachman *et al.*, 1993) summarizes the results of a comprehensive evaluation of screening methods for asymptomatic bacteriuria of pregnancy.

The sensitivities and specificities in Table 14.1 are, for the most part, in accordance with the results from multiple previous investigations (Pels *et al.*, 1989). However, better results have been reported for combined leukocyte esterase and nitrite testing in pregnancy. Defining a positive result as one in which either test was positive, sensitivity and specificity for ASB were 92% and 95% respectively in one investigation (Robertson and Duff, 1988) and 73% and 86% respectively in another (Etherington and James, 1993).

Implications of testing

WHAT DOES AN ABNORMAL TEST RESULT MEAN?

Either a positive urine culture or one combination of tests listed in Table 14.1 suggests that the patient has ASB. A 7-day course of oral antibiotics will sterilize the urine in 65–90% of patients with ASB and prevent 80% of the cases of pyelonephritis (Gordon and Hankins, 1989; Andriole and Patterson, 1991; Smaill, 1993b). Because *Escherichia coli* accounts for the majority of cases of ASB, the antibiotic chosen should have activity against this organism (Gordon and Hankins, 1989). Single-dose oral therapy is promising but less extensively evaluated (Gordon and Hankins, 1989; Andriole and Patterson, 1991; Smaill, 1993b). Follow-up urine cultures and retreatment if the bacteriuria persists are recommended (Gordon and Hankins, 1989; Andriole and Patterson, 1991).

Given the relatively high sensitivity and specificity reported by some but not all investigators for several of the nonculture methods of ASB screening (e.g. combined leukocyte esterase and nitrite testing), it might be reasonable to forego urine culture and rely on a nonculture method for screening and treatment. With high sensitivity, most cases of ASB will be detected, and with good specificity the number of false positive tests (and the number of patients unnecessarily treated) should be acceptable. However, a sensitivity of 40–50% would be too low for clinical applicability. In certain settings, e.g. where urine culture is unavailable or inconvenient, dipstick testing for leukocyte esterase and nitrites and foregoing culture may be considered.

Table 14.1 Test results of urine samples obtained on initial visit from 1047 pregnant women.

TEST	NUMBER OF POSITIVE SAMPLES	NUMBER POSITIVE BY CULTURE	SENSITIVITY (%)	SPECIFICITY (%)	PPV (%)
urine dipstick					
leukocyte esterase activity	33	4	16.7	97.2	12.1
nitrites present	14	11	45.8	99.7	78.6
leukocyte activity or nitrites present	44	12	50.0	96.9	27.3
leukocyte activity and nitrites present	3	3	12.5	100	100
Gram stain					
borderline or positive	133	22	91.7	89.2	16.5
positive	72	20	83.3	94.9	27.8
urinalysis					
> 10 leukocytes	16	6	25.0	99.0	37.5
> 50 leukocytes	5	2	8.3	99.7	40.0
bacteria present	432	18	75.0	59.7	4.2
bacteria present or leukocytes > 20	440	20	83.3	58.9	4.5
urine culture positive	24	24			

PPV, positive predictive value

WHAT DOES A NORMAL TEST RESULT MEAN?

Only 0.2–2.0% of gravidas will develop a symptomatic urinary tract infection during pregnancy after a negative culture for asymptomatic bacteriuria (Norden and Kass, 1968; Bachman *et al.*, 1993). No follow-up urine infection screening is recommended for these patients. However, as a result of lower test sensitivity, gravidas screened only by noncul-ture methods can be expected to have higher rates of symptomatic urinary tract infection during pregnancy. The optimal follow-up of women screened for ASB by nonculture methods has not been established.

What is the cost of testing?

The cost-effectiveness of ASB screening during pregnancy has been comprehensively evaluated. Bachman *et al.* (1993) analyzed ASB detection techniques using the following cost estimates (US $, 1993):

> dipstick urine test $1
> Gram stain $15
> urinalysis $15
> urine culture $25

These investigators assumed that a urine culture would be performed for each screen posi-tive. Making the assumption that only one specific screening test would be used, these investigators concluded that testing for nitrites was the most cost-effective approach ($127 per case of ASB detected) (Table 14.2). However, more than half of the cases of ASB would not be detected by only measuring nitrites. Several other methods detected more cases, but at greater incremental cost, which was calculated as the average cost of detecting an additional positive culture not detected by a positive nitrite test alone. Note that if the com-bination of leukocyte esterase and nitrite testing is assumed to be more sensitive than in Table 14.1 (Robertson and Duff, 1988; Etherington and James, 1993), such testing would detect the majority of cases of ASB in a very cost-effective manner. For example, using the data of Bachman *et al.* (1993) but substituting 80% sensitivity for their 50% sensitivity, the combination of leukocyte esterase and nitrite testing would detect 19 of the 24 cases of ASB. If the positive patients were immediately treated with oral antibiotics rather than subjected to a confirmatory culture, the cost per case of ASB detected using Bachman and colleagues' cost estimates would be US $50 (1993).

Wadland and Plante (1989) conducted a cost-benefit analysis of screening for ASB in preg-nancy using a decision analysis model. They concluded that screening (and treatment) for ASB using a culture-based method results in cost savings of $28.85 (US, 1989) per patient screened as compared with no screening. Their analysis was robust: screening remained cost-saving over a wide range of assumptions. Since leukocyte esterase and nitrite screening is a more cost-effective approach to ASB detection than culture (i.e. the incremental cost of detecting an additional positive culture is less for leukocyte esterase and nitrite testing than for urine culture), screening and treatment based on a dipstick test for leukocyte esterase and nitrites should also decrease costs.

CONCLUSIONS AND RECOMMENDATIONS

From 2% to 10% of pregnant women have ASB; 30% of these will develop acute and often serious urinary tract infection in pregnancy. The diagnosis and treatment of ASB by any of the aforementioned methods prevents the progression of ASB to symptomatic infection and is cost-saving. Therefore, all pregnant women should be screened for ASB at their first antenatal visit. Screening can be cost-effectively accomplished either by culture or with

Table 14.2 Cost effectiveness of screening tests for asymptomatic bacteriuria in initial evaluation of 1047 pregnant women.

TEST	NUMBER OF POSITIVE SAMPLES	TOTAL COST[a] ($)	INCREMENTAL COST PER ADDITIONAL POSITIVE CULTURE ($)	NO. OF MISSED CULTURES
urine dipstick				
leukocyte esterase activity	33	1 872	b	20
nitrites present	14	1 397	c	13
leukocyte activity or nitrites present	44	2 147	750	12
leukocyte activity and nitrites present	3	1 122	b	21
Gram stain				
borderline or positive	133	19 030	1 603	2
positive	72	17 505	1 790	4
urinalysis				
> 20 leukocytes	16	16 105	b	18
> 50 leukocytes	5	15 830	b	22
bacteria present	432	26 505	3 587	6
bacteria present or leukocytes > 20	440	26 705	3 615	4
urine culture positive	24	26 175	1 906	0

[a] US$ 1993. Total costs are based on the assumption that only one specific screening test is used and positive screens are assessed with urine culture. For example, if all cases with positive leukocyte activity undergo urine culture, this results in a cost of (1047 × $1) + (33 × $25) = 1872; [b] This approach detects fewer positive cultures than the least costly method; [c] Most cost-effective approach ($127 per case identified)

dipstick testing for leukocyte esterase and nitrites (with the presence of either substance defining a positive test). Individual practice situations will influence the optimal method of screening.

Patients with a positive screen should be treated with a 7-day course of oral antibiotics with activity against *E. coli*. After completion of therapy, the urine should be reassessed to document cure. Single-dose or short-course antibiotic therapy, while promising, requires further study. Finally, certain gravidas at high risk of urinary tract infection (e.g. those with insulin-dependent diabetes mellitus, sickle cell trait, nephrolithiasis, a history of frequent urinary tract infections or a known urinary tract abnormality) may benefit from periodic screening for ASB throughout their pregnancy, although the optimal timing and frequency of assessment have not been established by controlled investigations.

SUMMARY

1 WHAT IS THE PROBLEM THAT REQUIRES SCREENING?

ASYMPTOMATIC BACTERIURIA LEADING TO SYMPTOMATIC UPPER AND/OR LOWER URINARY TRACT INFECTION.

a What is the incidence/prevalence of the target condition?

Asymptomatic bacteriuria is present in 2–10% of gravidas at their first antenatal visit.

b What are the sequelae of the condition which are of interest in clinical medicine?

Thirty per cent of gravid women with untreated asymptomatic bacteriuria develop symptomatic urinary tract infection. Only 0.2–2.0% of gravidas who are screened early in gestation and found not to have bacteriuria will subsequently develop symptomatic urinary tract infection during pregnancy. Pyelonephritis can be life-threatening during pregnancy: both adult respiratory distress syndrome and septic shock can occur. Asymptomatic bacteriuria is associated with an increased risk of preterm delivery, but whether it plays a causative role is controversial.

2 THE TESTS

a What is the purpose of the tests?

To identify women with ASB during pregnancy who are at high risk for symptomatic urinary tract infection.

b The nature of the tests

Urine culture remains the standard against which all other tests are judged for detection of asymptomatic bacteriuria. Other tests which have been evaluated include urinalysis, urine dipstick studies for leukocyte esterase and/or nitrites, and Gram staining.

c Implications of testing

1 What does an abnormal test result mean?

Either a positive urine culture or one combination of tests listed in Table 14.1 suggests that the patient has ASB. A 7-day course of oral antibiotics will sterilize the urine in 65–90% of patients with ASB and prevent 80% of the cases of pyelonephritis.

2 What does a normal test result mean?

Only 0.2–2.0% of gravidas will develop a symptomatic urinary tract infection during pregnancy after a negative culture for asymptomatic bacteriuria.

d What is the cost of testing?

Most screening modalities are predicted to be cost-beneficial from the standpoint of preventing pyelonephritis.

3 CONCLUSIONS AND RECOMMENDATIONS

About 2–10% of pregnant women have ASB; 30% will develop acute and often serious urinary tract infection in pregnancy. The diagnosis and treatment of ASB by any of the methods listed above prevents the development of symptomatic infection and is cost-saving. All pregnant women should be screened for ASB at their first antenatal visit.

REFERENCES

Andriole VT & Patterson TF (1991) Epidemiology, natural history, and management of urinary tract infections in pregnancy. *Med Clin North Am* **75:** 359–373.

Bachman JW, Heise RH, Naessens JM & Timmerman MG (1993) A study of various tests to detect asymptomatic urinary tract infections in an obstetric population. *JAMA* **270:** 1971–1974.

Cunningham FG, Leveno KJ, Hankins GDV & Whalley PJ (1984) Respiratory insufficiency associated with pyelonephritis during pregnancy. *Obstet Gynecol* **63:** 121–125.

Etherington IJ & James DK (1993) Reagent strip testing of antenatal urine specimens for infection. *Br J Obstet Gynaecol* **100:** 806–808.

Gordon MC & Hankins GDV (1989) Urinary tract infections and pregnancy. *Comp Ther* **15:** 52–58.

Hankins GDV & Whalley PJ (1985) Acute urinary tract infections in pregnancy. *Clin Obstet Gynecol* **28:** 266–278.

Kass EH (1962a) Pyelonephritis and bacteriuria. A major problem in preventive medicine. *Ann Int Med* **56:** 46–53.

Kass EH (1962b) Maternal urinary tract infection. *NY State J Med* **62:** 2822–6.

Norden CW & Kass EH (1968) Bacteriuria of pregnancy – a critical appraisal. *Am Rev Med* **19:** 431–70.

Pels RJ, Bor DH, Woolhandler S, Himmelstein DU & Lawrence RS (1989) Dipstick urinalysis screening of asymptomatic adults for urinary tract disorders. *JAMA* **262:** 1220–4.

Robertson AW & Duff P (1988) The nitrite and leukocyte esterase tests for the evaluation of asymptomatic bacteriuria in obstetric patients. *Obstet Gynecol* **71:** 878–81.

Savage WE, Hajj SN & Kass EH (1967) Demographic and prognostic characteristics of bacteriuria in pregnancy. *Medicine* **46:** 385–407.

Smaill F (1993a) Antibiotic vs. no treatment for asymptomatic bacteriuria. In Enkin MW, Keirse MJNC, Renfrew MJ & Neilson JP (eds) *Pregnancy and Childbirth Module*, from the Cochrane Database of Systematic Reviews, 03170, 2 April 1992, Disk Issue 2. Oxford: Update Software.

Smaill F (1993b) Single dose vs. 4–7 day antibiotic for bacteriuria. In Enkin MW, Keirse MJNC, Renfrew MJ, Neilson JP (eds) *Pregnancy and Childbirth Module*, from the Cochrane Database of Systematic Reviews, 03171. Oxford: Update Software, Disk Issue 2.

Stenqvist K, Dahlen-Nilsson I, Lidin-Janson G *et al.* (1989) Bacteriuria in pregnancy: frequency and risk of acquisition. *Am J Epidemiol* **129:** 372–9.

Wadland WC & Plante DA (1989) Screening for asymptomatic bacteriuria in pregnancy. *J Fam Pract* **29:** 372–6.

Whalley PJ (1967) Bacteriuria of pregnancy. *J Obstet Gynecol* **97:** 723–38.

15

Random Blood Glucose, Glucose Tolerance, 'Postprandial Glucose' & Urine Glucose Tests

Stephen K. Hunter

WHAT IS THE PROBLEM THAT REQUIRES SCREENING?

GESTATIONAL DIABETES MELLITUS.

What is the incidence/prevalence of the target condition?

Gestational diabetes mellitus is defined as 'carbohydrate intolerance of variable severity with onset or first recognition during the present pregnancy' (Second International Workshop, 1985). By definition, clinical gestational diabetes excludes patients with previously known diabetes. The reported prevalence of gestational diabetes varies widely, due in large part to differences in the screening criteria and testing procedures. The prevalence of gestational diabetes is also dependent on such factors as ethnicity and geographic location (Hadden, 1985; Green et al., 1990; Dornhorst et al., 1992; Nahum and Huffaker, 1993; Kirshon and Wait, 1990) as well as maternal age (Coustan et al., 1989). Based on the 100 g, 3-hour oral glucose tolerance test (OGTT), the prevalence of gestational diabetes in the USA ranges between 2% (Coustan et al., 1989) and 6% (Amankwah et al., 1977). Using diagnostic criteria suggested by the National Diabetes Data Group (NDDG), the prevalence rate varies widely around the world ranging from 4% in Israel and Mexico (Friedman et al., 1985; Forsbach et al., 1988) to 15% in Florence, Italy (Mell. et al., 1989). Some investigators have suggested defining gestational diabetes by setting population-specific standards for each region (Green et al., 1990; Nahum and Huffaker, 1993). The incidence of gestational diabetes seems to vary among populations similar to the variation observed for type 1 and type 2 diabetes. However, these apparent differences are confounded by the use of different screening and diagnostic criteria (Magee et al., 1993). For example, Li et al. (1987) retested 216 women diagnosed with gestational diabetes based on a 100 g OGTT and NDDG criteria, using the 75 g OGTT and World Health Organization (WHO) criteria. The prevalence of gestational diabetes was almost halved using the latter definition.

What are the sequelae of the condition which are of interest in clinical medicine?

There is little question that women who develop gestational diabetes are at increased risk of health problems later in life. The pioneering studies of O'Sullivan and Mahan (1964) were based on the concept that gestational diabetes is a risk factor for the subsequent development of diabetes. The progression of gestational diabetes to type 2 diabetes later in life has been well documented (O'Sullivan, 1991), though the risk varies widely owing in part to differing diagnostic criteria. Two studies (Damm et al., 1989; O'Sullivan, 1989) which did include a control group observed a 6-fold to 18-fold increase in the likelihood of developing diabetes (18% versus 0%, and 36.4% versus 5.5%) by 28 years after the pregnancy complicated by gestational diabetes. Women who have had gestational diabetes also have a higher prevalence of obesity, hyperlipidemia, atherosclerotic vascular disease, increased systolic blood pressure, and mortality (O'Sullivan, 1988). In addition to the increase in longterm maternal morbidity, short-term morbidity during pregnancy (hydramnios, hypertension, and cesarean section) has been reported to be increased in some (Cousins et al., 1987) but not all series (Weiner, 1988).

It is unclear whether gestational diabetes is associated with increased perinatal mortality in modern obstetrics. O'Sullivan et al. (1973a) reported an increased perinatal mortality in untreated gestational diabetes pregnancies compared with controls (6.4% versus 1.5%). Pettit et al. (1980) also showed an increase in the perinatal mortality rate among untreated Pima Indians who had elevated 2-hour glucose levels after receiving a 75 g glucose challenge in the third trimester. However, it is possible that these differences are explained by other prognostic factors which were not taken into account. These patients were studied at a time when obstetricians focused primarily on maternal outcome. Since then, their focus has become more balanced between mother and fetus. There has been no increase in the perinatal mortality rate of women with gestational diabetes reported in any recently published series. Whether this is due to increased screening and surveillance of gestational diabetes-complicated pregnancies, a general improvement in obstetric care, or a true lack of an association is impossible to discern.

The association between gestational diabetes and neonatal morbidity is better established. Perinatal morbidity commonly reported to be increased with gestational diabetes includes an increased risk of macrosomia, birth trauma, neonatal hypoglycemia, hyperbilirubinemia, hypocalcemia, and polycythemia (Oh, 1988). The macrosomic offspring of women with gestational diabetes are at increased risk for childhood obesity (Pettit et al., 1985; Freinkel, 1989). The prevalence of type 2 diabetes is also increased during childhood and later in life in the offspring of mothers with gestational diabetes (Pettit et al., 1985). It is unknown whether this is a reflection of the intrauterine environment or genetics. One animal study reported subclinical islet cell injury in fetuses and offspring when exposed to conditions of chronic hyperglycemia (Freinkel et al., 1986), further suggesting the potential for longterm morbidity. It has not been determined whether treatment of gestational diabetes eliminates these potential sequelae.

THE TESTS

What is the purpose of the tests?

The purpose of testing is to identify pregnant women with gestational diabetes, as assessed by the oral glucose tolerance test. It is assumed but unproven that treatment and surveillance will reduce both short-term and longterm maternal and perinatal morbidity.

The nature of the tests

SCREENING TESTS

Several methods have been used to identify high-risk women who should undergo formal testing in the hope of curtailing cost and improving efficiency. The taking of a patient history focusing on presumed specific risk factors such as a family history of diabetes, a previous perinatal loss, or macrosomic infant would be the simplest screening test. Unfortunately, history is insensitive, identifying only half of those women who develop gestational diabetes, and leads to large numbers of unnecessary OGTTs since specificity is only 56% (O'Sullivan et al., 1973a). Thus, some laboratory test is required.

Oral glucose challenge test: A 50 g glucose challenge test is administered between 24 weeks and 28 weeks of gestation. Some investigators (Super et al., 1991; Dong et al., 1993) suggest screening during the first trimester women who are thought to be at high risk for gestational diabetes. Typically, a 1-hour blood glucose level is determined. The 1-hour period is more efficient to administer in an outpatient setting than a later determination, but one author has suggested that a 2-hour blood sample may improve test specificity (Weiner et al., 1986).

There is disagreement on the most appropriate 50 g 1-hour glucose value to use as a threshold for the performance of a diagnostic glucose tolerance test. The ideal evaluation of a screening test would subject each individual to both the screening test and standard diagnostic tests. Only the study by O'Sullivan and Mahan (1964) fulfils this criterion. In a follow-up study, O'Sullivan et al. (1973b) showed that the sensitivity and specificity of a 50 g glucose screening test for gestational diabetes were 79% and 87% respectively, using a 130 mg/dl cut-off by the Somogyi–Nelson technique on whole blood. Most current cut-off recommendations are based on this work and take into account the change in sample material from whole blood to plasma or serum. The glucose concentration measured in plasma or serum is approximately 14% higher than in whole blood. A cut-off of 140 mg/dl (7.8 mmol/l) is most commonly used. If a cut-off of 140 mg/dl is used, approximately 14% of the population will require an OGTT and the diagnosis of gestational diabetes will be missed in approximately 10% of the affected population (Coustan et al., 1989; Dooley et al., 1989). If a cut-off of 130 mg/dl (7.2 mmol/l) were used, virtually all cases of gestational diabetes would be identified, but 23% of the pregnant population would require an OGTT (Cousins et al., 1991). One study (Nahum and Huffaker, 1993) looked at racial differences and concluded that race-specific glucose thresholds were warranted. The choice of a cut-off will depend on the levels of sensitivity and specificity that would be acceptable.

Though the test is usually administered without regard to fasting status, recent studies indicate that (a) the fasting interval does affect the insulin response during a glucose challenge test; (b) the effect of fasting on insulin response may affect screening results (Berkus et al., 1990); and (c) these effects can be of sufficient magnitude to alter the operating characteristics of the test, i.e. produce important changes to the sensitivity and specificity (Lewis et al., 1993). In one study examining the reproducibility of the 50 g 1-hour glucose challenge (Monteros et al., 1993), 80 pregnant women were tested on two consecutive days. The daily reproducibility for normal results was 90% and 83% for abnormal results at 28 weeks' gestation.

Some groups (Second International Workshop, 1985; American Diabetes Association, 1986) recommend universal screening. However, because the prevalence of gestational diabetes increases with maternal age, others (American College of Obstetricians and Gynecologists, 1986) recommend screening only those gravidas aged 30 years or more, and younger women with presumed high-risk factors for gestational diabetes. If the goal is to identify as many women with gestational diabetes as possible, this approach will fail since more than 50% of women with gestational diabetes are under 30 years old (Weiner *et al.*, 1986; Coustan *et al.*, 1989).

Random glucose testing: Several authors have suggested that a random blood glucose sample be used as a screening test for gestational diabetes. Stangenberg *et al.* (1985) measured random capillary blood glucose values in 1500 pregnant women. Surprisingly, the value was not influenced by the time of day the sample was obtained or the trimester of pregnancy. They suggested a value of 6.5 mmol/l or greater be used to define the need for an OGTT. Unfortunately, the usefulness of this screening technique was not determined. Lind (1985) measured a random venous blood glucose level in 2400 consecutive antenatal women between 28 weeks and 32 weeks of gestation and calculated the 99th centile for women who had eaten within 2 hours, or more than 2 hours from the time of testing. They suggested a cut-off value of 115 mg/dl (6.4 mmol/l) if testing is done within 2 hours of a meal and 104 mg/dl (5.8 mmol/l) if it is done more than 2 hours after a meal. Four patients with previously unsuspected diabetes mellitus were identified and an additional 4 patients with gestational diabetes were diagnosed. Though these authors concluded that random blood glucose screening is useful and convenient, their analyses were incomplete.

Urine glucose: The renal tubular reabsorption of glucose is less efficient during pregnancy (Davison and Hytten, 1975) and urine glucose excretion can be intermittent (Lind and Hytten, 1972). Watson (1990) measured random urine glucose levels in 500 consecutive pregnant women on each prenatal visit and compared it with the result of their 1-hour 50 g glucose challenge performed at 28 weeks. Twenty-two patients were identified as having gestational diabetes. Only 6 (27%) of these 22 women with gestational diabetes had glucosuria. As a screening test for gestational diabetes, glucosuria has a 27% sensitivity and a positive predictive value of only 7.1%. The determination of urinary glucose is therefore not recommended as a screening test for gestational diabetes.

STANDARD REFERENCE TESTS

The 100 g OGTT is administered after 72 hours of carbohydrate loading to pregnant women who exceeded a specified blood glucose value on a screening test. As with the screening tests, controversy exists as to what plasma glucose cut-off value should be used to make the diagnosis of gestational diabetes. Glucose measurements in the O'Sullivan studies were on whole blood. Since the glucose concentration measured in plasma or serum is approximately 14% higher than whole blood, the NDDG proposed increasing the cut-off when plasma or serum is used (Table 15.1). Since the enzymatic methods used today are more specific for glucose and about 5 mg/dl lower than the Somogyi-Nelson method used by O'Sullivan, it has been suggested by one group that the cut-offs be further reduced (Carpenter and Coustan, 1982) (Table 15.1). Two additional studies (Neiger and Coustan, 1991; Sacks *et al.*, 1989) lend support to this proposal.

Whatever the criteria selected, the diagnosis of gestational diabetes is made when values at two or more time points are abnormal. Some authors recommend repeating the OGTT later in pregnancy for women who have one, but not two, elevated values. Neiger and Coustan (1991b) reported that 34% of women who had one abnormal glucose value on their initial OGTT had two abnormal values on a repeat test 1 month later. Harlass *et al.* (1991a) found that the overall reproducibility of an OGTT was 78% when administered 1–2 weeks apart under similar conditions.

In an attempt to standardize glucose tolerance testing, the World Health Organization (WHO) recommended that the same 75 g, 2-hour OGTT used for the testing of nonpregnant patients be applied during pregnancy (WHO, 1980). Glucose intolerance would be

Table 15.1   Currently recommended cut-off values in plasma or serum for the diagnosis of gestational diabetes.

NATIONAL DIABETES DATA GROUP VALUES	
Fasting	105 mg/dl (5.8 mmol/l)
1 hour	190 mg/dl (10.6 mmol/l)
2 hour	165 mg/dl (9.2 mmol/l)
3 hour	145 mg/dl (8.1 mmol/l)
Suggested modification of the recommended cut-off-values to account for the more specific glucose testing methods	
Fasting	95 mg/dl (5.3 mmol/l)
1 hour	180 mg/dl (10.0 mmol/l)
2 hour	155 mg/dl (8.6 mmol/l)
3 hour	140 mg/dl (7.8 mmol/l)

Data from Carpenter and Coustan (1982), Sacks et al. (1989), Neiger and Coustan (1991a)

defined by WHO criteria as a 2-hour plasma glucose value above 140 mg/dl, plus at least 200 mg/dl at any other time point (30 min, 60 min, or 90 min). This opinion was echoed in the Third International Workshop-Conference on Gestational Diabetes (Metzger *et al.*, 1991).

An OGTT is administered after the patient has fasted for at least 10 hours prior to the test. The patient is instructed to consume at least 150 mg of carbohydrate each day for the 3 days preceding the OGTT, though one investigator has questioned the need for this recommendation (Harlass *et al.*, 1991b). During the test, the patient should not smoke, eat, or drink anything other than water.

Implications of testing

WHAT DOES AN ABNORMAL TEST RESULT MEAN?

An abnormal screen indicates the need for an OGTT unless serum glucose levels exceed 180 mg/dl (10.0 mmol/l) since this indicates overt diabetes. An abnormal OGTT is the diagnosis of gestational diabetes.

Women who are diagnosed with gestational diabetes are traditionally advised on appropriate dietary intake and instructed how to measure daily capillary blood glucose using either a chemical test strip or a home glucose reflectance monitor. Both the American College of Obstetricians and Gynecologists and the American Diabetes Association recommend that fasting and 2-hour postprandial blood glucose values be obtained. However, Lewis *et al.* (1976) found that the peak glucose response to a meal occurs 1 hour after eating. Moreover, Combs *et al.* (1992) and Jovanovic-Peterson *et al.* (1991) have observed that an elevated 1-hour postprandial blood glucose level is more strongly associated with birthweight and macrosomia in diabetic women than a fasting level. A 2-hour level was not evaluated. Currently there is no consensus as to whether 1-hour or 2-hour postprandial glucose determination is more appropriate. Many practitioners use both on alternating days. It is recommended that insulin therapy be initiated when the fasting plasma glucose concentration exceeds 105 mg/dl (5.8 mmol/l) /or the 2-hour postprandial plasma glucose concentration exceeds 120 mg/dl (6.7 mmol/l) on two or more occasions within a 2-week interval (American College of Obstetricians and Gynecologists, 1986; American Diabetes Association, 1986). In addition to blood glucose monitoring, a regular program of fetal surveillance should be added to the obstetric management of patients *who require insulin* (American College of Obstetricians and Gynecologists, 1986).

The effort to diagnose gestational diabetes makes several assumptions which may not be true in modern obstetric practice. It is assumed that if the goal of screening is to improve pregnancy outcome, women with gestational diabetes (i.e. excluding those whose prepregnancy disease was discovered during pregnancy) and their fetuses are at increased risk of an adverse outcome. Yet, as already noted, it is unclear whether this is true. Screening to improve pregnancy outcome also assumes that current therapy, diet modification (not restriction), improves outcome. The evidence for this too is scant. Santini and Ales (1990) observed that screening not only failed to decrease the rate of large infants, but also failed to improve any other outcome of pregnancy. If the goal is to identify women at risk later in life for the development of type 2 diabetes mellitus, screening assumes that postnatal intervention will either diminish that likelihood or decrease the associated morbidity. Unfortunately, no study – prospective or retrospective – has tested this assumption.

WHAT DOES A NORMAL TEST RESULT MEAN?

Women who have a normal 50 g 1-hour glucose challenge test at 28 weeks' gestation require no further testing. Watson (1989) studied 550 pregnant women serially at 20 weeks, 28 weeks, and 34 weeks of gestation and observed that 11% of gestational diabetes cases would have been undetected if a 34 week screen had not been performed. This raises again the issue of rescreening women who have a positive 50 g 1-hour glucose screen but only one abnormal value on the 100 g 3-hour OGTT as recommended by some investigators (Harlass *et al.*, 1991a; Neiger and Coustan, 1991b). Some (Langer *et al.*, 1987) but not all (Weiner, 1988) found that one abnormal value on an OGTT is strongly associated with adverse perinatal outcome if left untreated. It is unclear whether the improved outcome noted by Langer *et al.* (1987) is the result of specific therapy, or a general increase in the level of scrutiny that all patients might have benefited from.

What is the cost of testing?

The cost of screening for gestational diabetes depends on both the cut-off point and the methodology chosen. If the prevalence of gestational diabetes in the population is 2% and a glucose challenge cut-off of 130 mg/dl (7.2 mmol/l) is selected, then 230 (23%) of every 1000 pregnant womem screened will require an OGTT to diagnose the 20 cases of gestational diabetes expected. If we assume a cost of US $23.75 to screen and $57.50 for an OGTT, then screening would cost $1848.75 for every case of gestational diabetes diagnosed. If the cut-off is set instead at 140 mg/dl (7.8 mmol/l), then 140 OGTTs will be performed ($8050) for every 1000 women screened ($23 750) to identify the expected 18 cases of gestational diabetes at a cost of $1766.67 each. These costs can be greatly reduced using capillary samples and a reflectance meter (Weiner *et al.*, 1987).

In addition to the immediate cost of screening, Santini and Ales (1990) found that screening increases both the amount of intensive surveillance employed and the primary (or nonemergency) cesarean section rate. Much of this is attributed to either physician or patient anxiety resulting from the test rather than a perceived problem with the pregnancy. They concluded that to prevent one case of macrosomia (assuming current therapy could do so), 3716 women would need to be screened. As a result of this screening, 58 women would have 15 or more antenatal visits and 250 women would have supplemental fetal testing (ultrasonography, nonstress testing, etc.) as part of the follow-up. In addition, 134 more women would have had a primary cesarean section than in an unscreened population. All of this translates into increased medical cost without a demonstrable improvement in outcome.

CONCLUSIONS AND RECOMMENDATIONS

The health impact of gestational diabetes during pregnancy is unclear. Without this information, the cost-effectiveness of screening for gestational diabetes cannot be calculated. Current screening recommendations for gestational diabetes do not differentiate well between patients with diabetes that predates pregnancy and those who truly develop glucose intolerance during pregnancy. It seems likely that undiagnosed /or untreated diabetes which antedates pregnancy is a real health risk to the developing fetus. It may be sound policy to screen for diabetes during pregnancy if only to identify the patient who requires insulin therapy during pregnancy.

There is no consensus as to who should undergo screening and which cut-offs are most appropriate for the diagnosis of gestational diabetes. The Third International Workshop-Conference on Gestational Diabetes Mellitus (Metzger *et al.*, 1991) recommended universal 50 g, 1-hour glucose challenge testing at 24–28 weeks' gestation, with a full 100 g, 3-hour OGTT for screening values at or above 140 mg/dl (7.8 mmol/l). Recommended cut-off values for the OGTT are those given in the top half of Table 15.1. They acknowledge that the adjustments recommended by the NDDG for converting whole blood to plasma values may result in some overcorrection, but claim that it appears unlikely that this has a significant adverse clinical impact. They further state that 'because it is hoped that international agreement will soon be reached as to appropriate and globally acceptable diagnostic criteria, it seems inadvisable to introduce minor corrective modifications at present' (Metzger *et al.*, 1991).

Can screening for gestational diabetes be justified? Stephenson (1993) concluded after a critical review of the literature that there was insufficient evidence to justify routine universal screening. This conclusion was based on three facts: (a) there is uncertainty about the burden of illness of gestational diabetes; (b) major problems exist with the screening test and reference standard; and (c) there are no methodologically sound trials of therapy. Since these criteria were not satisfied, it was felt that there was no rationale for pursuing the remaining criteria important to justify screening: can the health system cope with the screening program? Does the program reach those who would benefit from it? Will patients with positive screens comply with subsequent advice and intervention? If untreated gestational diabetes presents a potential risk to the fetus, mother or neonate, then a screening regimen that would have a high positive predictive value would seem warranted. However, until such risks are well documented, a concerted effort to minimize the cost of performance and eliminate unnecessary follow-up is called for.

SUMMARY

1

WHAT IS THE PROBLEM THAT REQUIRES SCREENING?

GESTATIONAL DIABETES.

a What is the incidence/prevalence of the target condition?

About 2–15% depending upon the diagnostic criteria, geographic locale and patient demographic profile.

b What are the sequelae of the condition which are of interest in clinical medicine?

Sequelae may be long-term and short-term. There is a 6-fold to 18-fold increase in the likelihood of type 2 diabetes within 28 years. There is a higher prevalence of obesity, hyperlipidemia, atherosclerotic vascular disease, increased systolic blood pressure, and mortality in women who have had gestational diabetes. Whether the perinatal morbidity or mortality is altered by gestational diabetes in modern obstetrics is unclear.

2 THE TESTS

a What is the purpose of the tests?

The purpose of testing is to identify pregnant women with gestational diabetes, as assessed by oral glucose tolerance test. It is assumed but unproven that treatment and surveillance will reduce both short-term and longterm maternal and perinatal morbidity.

b The nature of the tests

Screening tests: neither history nor urine testing for glucose are effective. A 50 g glucose challenge with a blood sample obtained after 1 hour is common. There is controversy regarding the appropriate threshold value for diagnostic testing. Random blood testing is also effective.

Standard reference tests: it is unclear whether a 100 g 3-hour oral glucose tolerance test (OGTT) or a 75 g 2-hour OGTT is best. There is no consensus on the cut-offs.

c Implications of testing

1 *What does an abnormal test result mean?*

An abnormal screen indicates the woman should undergo diagnostic testing for gestational diabetes. The diagnosis of gestational diabetes is made when there are two abnormal values on the OGTT.

2 *What does a normal test result mean?*

A normal test means that no further testing is necessary. However, if the goal is to identify all cases of gestational diabetes, there is controversy as to whether women either negative at 28 weeks or screen positive but OGTT negative should be retested.

d What is the cost of testing?

The cost per case of gestational diabetes identified using a policy of universal screening with a glucose challenge test followed by an OGTT for screen positives ranges from US $1500 to $2000 US. This does not include repeat testing or the costs of additional tests that may be performed in response to the diagnosis.

3 CONCLUSIONS AND RECOMMENDATIONS

It is difficult to recommend universal screening since (a) there is uncertainty about the burden of illness of gestational diabetes, (b) major problems exist with cut-offs for the screening test and standard reference tests, and (c) there are no methodologically sound trials of therapy. It seems likely that undiagnosed or untreated diabetes which predates pregnancy is a potential health risk to the developing fetus. It may be sound policy to screen for diabetes during pregnancy, if only to identify the patient who requires insulin therapy during pregnancy. If untreated gestational diabetes presents a risk to the fetus, mother or neonate, then a screening regimen that would have a high positive predictive value would seem warranted. A concerted effort to minimize the cost of diagnosis and eliminate unnecessary follow-up is required.

REFERENCES

Amankwah KS, Prentice RL & Fleury FJ (1977) The incidence of gestational diabetes. *Obstet Gynecol* **49:** 497–498.

American College of Obstetricians and Gynecologists (1986) *Management of Diabetes Mellitus in Pregnancy.* ACOG Technical Bulletin. Washington, DC: ACOG.

American Diabetes Association (1986) Position statement on gestational diabetes mellitus. *Diabetes Care* **9:** 430–431.

Berkus MD, Stern MP, Mitchell BD, Newton ER & Langer O (1990) Does fasting interval affect the glucose challenge test? *Am J Obstet Gynecol* **163:** 1812–1817.

Carpenter MW & Coustan DR (1982) Criteria for screening tests for gestational diabetes. *Am J Obstet Gynecol* **144:** 768–773.

Combs CA, Gunderson E, Kitzmiller JL, Gavin LA & Main EK (1992) Relationship of fetal macrosomia to maternal postprandial glucose control during pregnancy. *Diabetes Care* **15:** 1251–1257.

Cousins L (1985) Pregnancy complications among diabetic women: review 1965–1985 (1987). *Obstet Gynecol Survey* **42:** 140–149.

Cousins L, Baxi L, Chez R *et al.* (1991) Screening recommendations for gestational diabetes mellitus. *Am J Obstet Gynecol* **165:** 493–496.

Coustan DR, Nelson C, Carpenter MW, Carr SR, Rotondo L & Widness JA (1989) Maternal age and screening for gestational diabetes: a population-based study. *Obstet Gynecol* **73:** 557–560.

Damm PD, Molsted-Pedersen LMP & Kuhl CK (1989) High incidence of diabetes mellitus and impaired glucose tolerance in women with previous gestational diabetes mellitus (abstract). *Diabetologia* **32:** 479A.

Davison JM & Hytten FE (1975) The effect of pregnancy on the renal handling of glucose. *Br J Obstet Gynaecol* **82:** 374–381.

Dong ZG, Beischer NA, Wein P & Sheedy MT (1993) Value of early glucose tolerance testing in women who had gestational diabetes in their previous pregnancy. *Aust NZ J Obstet Gynaecol* **33:** 350–375.

Dooley SL, Keller JD, Metzger BE, Ogata E & Freinkel N (1989) Screening for gestational diabetes mellitus (GDM): is the 140 mg/dl threshold appropriate? Abstract 52, *Society of Perinatal Obstetricians*, p. 66.

Dornhorst A, Paterson CM, Nicholls JSD *et al.* (1992) High prevalence of gestational diabetes in women from ethnic minority groups. *Diabet Med* **9:** 820–825.

Forsbach G, Contreras-Soto JJ, Fong G, Flores G & Moreno O (1988) Prevalence of gestational diabetes and macrosomic newborns in a Mexican population. *Diabetes Care* **11:** 235–238.

Freinkel N, Metzger RL, Phelps RL, *et al.* (1986) Gestational diabetes mellitus: a syndrome with phenotypic and genotypic heterogeneity. *Horm Metab Res* **18:** 427.

Freinkel N (1989) Fuel-mediated teratogenesis: an exercise in 'acquired' genetics. In Larkins RG, Zimmet PZ & Chisholm DJ (eds), *Diabetes 1988: Proceedings of the 13th Congress of the International Diabetes Federation*, p 831–840. Amsterdam: Excerpta Medica.

Friedman S, May JY, Hod M, Rusecki Y & Ovadia J (1985) Glucose tolerance test in Israeli pregnant women. *Isr J Med Sci* **21:** 639–643.

Green JR, Pawson IG, Schumacher LB, Perry J & Kretchmer N (1990) Glucose tolerance in pregnancy: ethnic variation and influence of body habits. *Am J Obstet Gynecol* **163:** 86–92.

Hadden DR (1985) Geographic, ethnic, and racial variations in the incidence of gestational diabetes mellitus. *Diabetes* **34:** 8–12.

Harlass FE, Brady K & Read JA (1991a) Reproducibility of the oral glucose tolerance test in pregnancy. *Am J Obstet Gynecol* **164:** 564–568.

Harlass FE, McClure GB, Read JA & Brady K (1991b) Use of a standard preparatory diet for the oral glucose tolerance test. *J Reprod Med* **36:** 147–150.

Jovanovic-Peterson L, Peterson CM, Reed GF *et al.* (1991) Maternal postprandial glucose levels and infant birth weight: The diabetes in early pregnancy study. *Am J Obstet Gynecol* **164:** 103–111.

Kirshon B, & Wait RB (1990) Incidence of gestational diabetes: effects of race. *J Texas Med* **86:** 88–90.

Landon MB & Gabbe SG (1985) Antepartum fetal surveillance in gestational diabetes mellitus. *Diabetes* **34:** 50–54.

Langer O, Brustman L, Anyaegbunam A & Mazze R (1987) The significance of one abnormal glucose tolerance test value on adverse outcome in pregnancy. *Am J Obstet Gynecol* **157:** 758–763.

Lewis SB, Wallin JD, Kuzuya H, *et al.* (1976) Circadian variation of serum glucose, C-peptide immunoreactivity and free insulin in normal and insulin-treated diabetic pregnant subjects. *Diabetologia* **12:** 343–350.

Lewis GF, McNally C, Blackman JD, Polonsky KS & Barron WM (1993) Prior feeding alters the response to the 50-g glucose challenge test in pregnancy. *Diabetes Care* **16**: 1551–1556.

Li DFH, Wong VCW, O'Hoy KMK, Yeung CY & Ma HK (1987) Is treatment needed for mild impairment of glucose tolerance in pregnancy? A randomized controlled trial. *Br J Obstet Gynaecol* **94**: 851–854.

Lind T (1985) Antenatal screening using random blood glucose values. *Diabetes* **34**: 17–20.

Lind T & Hytten FE (1972) The excretion of glucose during normal pregnancy. *J Obstet Gynaecol Br Commonw* **79**: 961–965.

Magee MS, Walden CE, Benedetti TJ & Knopp RH (1993) Influence of diagnostic criteria on the incidence of gestational diabetes and perinatal morbidity. *JAMA* **269**: 609–615.

Mello G, Macacci F, Meir YJ, *et al.* (1989) Nostra esperienza in terma di screening del Diabete Gestazionale. *Riv Ostet Ginecol* **II**: 90–95.

Metzger BE & the Organizing Committee (1991) Summary and recommendations of the Third International Workshop-Conference on Gestational Diabetes Mellitus. *Diabetes* **40**: 197–201.

Monteros A, Parra A, Carino N & Ramirez A (1993) The reproducibility of the 50-g, 1-hour glucose screen for diabetes in pregnancy. *Obstet Gynecol* **82**: 515–518.

Nahum GG & Huffaker BJ (1993) Racial differences in oral glucose screening test results: Establishing race-specific criteria for abnormality in pregnancy. *Obstet Gynecol* **81**: 517–522.

Neiger R & Coustan DR (1991a) Are the current ACOG glucose tolerance test criteria sensitive enough? *Obstet Gynecol* **78**: 1117–1120.

Neiger R & Coustan DR (1991b) The role of glucose tolerance tests in the diagnosis of gestational diabetes. *Am J Obstet Gynecol* **165**: 787–790.

O'Sullivan JB (1988) The interaction between pregnancy, diabetes and long-term maternal outcome. In Reece EA & Coustan DR (eds), *Diabetes Mellitus in Pregnancy*. New York: Churchill Livingstone.

O'Sullivan JB (1989) The Boston Gestational Diabetes Studies: review and perspectives. In Sutherland HW, Stowers JM & Pearson DWM (eds), *Carbohydrate Metabolism in Pregnancy and the Newborn*, Vol. 4. pp. 287–294. London: Springer-Verlag.

O'Sullivan JB (1991) Diabetes mellitus after GDM. *Diabetes* **29**: 131–135.

O'Sullivan JB & Mahan CM (1964) Criteria for the oral glucose tolerance test in pregnancy. *Diabetes* **13**: 278–285.

O'Sullivan JB, Charles D, Mahan CM & Dandrow RV (1973a) Gestational diabetes and perinatal mortality rate. *Am J Obstet Gynecol* **116**: 901–904.

O'Sullivan JB, Charles D, Mahan CM & Dandrow RV (1973b) Screening criteria for the high-risk gestational diabetic patient. *Am J Obstet Gynecol* **116**: 895–900.

Oh W (1988) Neonatal outcome and care. In Reece EA & Coustan DR, (eds), *Diabetes Mellitus in Pregnancy*. New York, Churchill Livingstone.

Pettit DJ, Knowler WC, Baird HR & Bennett PH (1980) Gestational diabetes: infant and maternal complications of pregnancy in relation to third trimester glucose tolerance in Pima Indians. *Diabetes Care* **3**: 458–464.

Pettit DJ, Bennett PH, Knowler WC, *et al.* (1985) Gestational diabetes mellitus and impaired glucose tolerance in the offspring. *Diabetes* **34**: 119.

Sacks DA, Abu-Fadil S, Greenspoon JS & Fotheringham N (1989) Do the current standards for glucose tolerance testing in pregnancy represent a valid conversion of O'Sullivan's original criteria? *Am J Obstet Gynecol* **161**: 638–641.

Santini DL & Ales KL (1990) The impact of universal screening for gestational glucose intolerance on outcome of pregnancy. *Surg Gynecol Obstet* **170**: 427–436.

Second International Workshop (1985) Summary and recommendations of the Second International Workshop Conference on Gestational Diabetes Mellitus. *Diabetes* **34** (Suppl. 2): 123–126.

Stangenberg M, Persson B & Nordlander E (1985) Random capillary blood glucose and conventional selection criteria for glucose tolerance testing during pregnancy. *Diabetes Res* **2**: 29–33.

Stephenson MJ (1993) Screening for gestational diabetes mellitus: A critical review. *J Fam Pract* **37**: 277–283.

Super DM, Edelberg SC, Philipson EH, Hertz RH & Kalhan SC (1991) Diagnosis of gestational diabetes in early pregnancy. *Diabetes Care* **14**: 288–294.

Watson WJ (1990) Screening for glycosuria during pregnancy. *South Med J* **83**: 156–158.

Watson WJ (1989) Serial changes in the 50-g oral glucose test in pregnancy: implications for screening. *Obstet Gynecol* **74**: 40–43.

Weiner CP, Fraser MM, Burns JM, Schnoor D, Herrig J & Whitaker LA (1986) Cost efficacy of routine screening for diabetes in pregnancy: 1-h versus 2-h specimen. *Diabetes Care* **9**: 255–259.

Weiner CP, Faustich MW, Burns J, Fraser M, Whitaker L & Klugman M (1987) Diagnosis of gestational diabetes using capillary blood samples and a portable reflectance meter: Derivation of threshold values and prospective validation. *Am J Obstet Gynecol* **156**: 1085–1089.

Weiner CP (1988) Effect of varying degrees of 'normal' carbohydrate metabolism upon maternal and perinatal outcome. *Am J Obstet Gynecol* **159**: 862–870, 1988.

WHO (1980) World Health Organization Expert Committee on Diabetes Mellitus. Technical Report Series 646. Geneva: WHO.

16

Antepartum & Postpartum Assessment of Hemoglobin, Hematocrit & Serum Ferritin

Christine Kirkpatrick & Sophie Alexander

ABNORMALITIES OF MATERNAL RED BLOOD CELL MASS – ANTEPARTUM.

What is the incidence/prevalence of the target condition?

About 8% to 40% of pregnant women are classified as having anemia (de Leeuw and Brunton, 1976). The wide range probably reflects differences in the definition of anemia. From 8% to 10% of women have an elevated red blood cell count.

Most healthy pregnant women experience a decrease in hemoglobin concentration and hematocrit during the second trimester due to a rapid increase in plasma volume. As red cell production catches up with intravascular volume, hemoglobin levels and hematocrit rise in the third trimester (Figure 16.1) (Scott and Pritchard, 1974; de Leeuw and Brunton, 1976). The initial decline in hemoglobin and hematocrit is often described as a physiologic or dilutional anemia. Iron deficiency is the most common cause of pathologic anemia during pregnancy. Unfortunately, there is no international agreement on the definition of pathologic anemia (i.e. anemia in excess of the normal dilution) during pregnancy. Between 10 g/dl (6.2 mmol/l) and 11 g/dl (6.8 mmol/l) is typically considered the arbitrary dividing line between dilutional and true anemia (Mahomed and Hytten, 1989). It is suggested that a more physiologic threshold would be the 5th percentile for gestational age (Yip, 1989). It is also possible that the distribution of hemoglobin values varies between populations (Blankson *et al.*, 1993). To what extent this reflects nutritional habits or other extrinsic factors has not been explored.

What are the sequelae of the condition which are of interest in clinical medicine?

A low hemoglobin/hematocrit value is generally secondary to iron deficiency anemia; a high hemoglobin/hematocrit value (polycythemia) is associated with preeclampsia, intrauterine growth restriction, and preterm delivery.

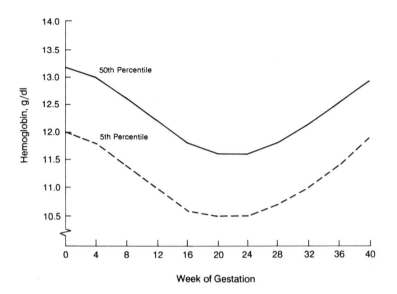

Figure 16.1 Normal hemoglobin values during pregnancy. Reprinted with permission from *Nutrition During Pregnancy*. Copyright 1990 by the National Academy of Sciences. Courtesy of the National Academy Press, Washington, DC.

Iron deficiency usually evolves slowly, progressing through several stages before presenting as frank anemia (Cook, 1982). The earliest stage is iron storage depletion, in which the iron reserves are low, but there is not yet a decrease in iron supply to the developing red cell. The second stage begins when the supply of iron available for erythropoiesis is diminished. The circulating hemoglobin content is not significantly decreased, but there is a decrease of the mean corpuscular volume (MCV). The final stage of iron deficiency is characterized by overt iron deficiency anemia.

The evidence that marked iron deficiency is associated with severe maternal and perinatal problems is compelling in nonindustrialized countries (Griswold and Cavanagh, 1966; de Leeuw and Brunton, 1976; Royston and Armstrong, 1989). The evidence is less convincing that iron deficiency is an important perinatal problem for women in industrialized countries. The underlying assumption pervading the literature is that a low hemoglobin content is associated with adverse perinatal outcome (Garn *et al.* 1981), and that the maintenance of an optimal hemoglobin and iron store is bound to be advantageous for mother and child (Murphy *et al*, 1986). However, few studies have actually addressed this issue. There are no maternal physical symptoms secondary to mild anemia (Elwood, 1973) and the evidence for adverse neonatal effects is conflicting. Rios and colleagues (Rios *et al.*, 1975) found no difference in the umbilical cord ferritin measurements of infants born to iron deficient and iron replete women. Thus, the fetus is quite efficient at extracting iron from its mother. In contrast, two other investigators observed either a limit to the iron extracting capacity of the placenta or a correlation between the maternal and neonatal ferritin levels (Colomer *et al.*, 1990; Puolakka *et al.*, 1980). Another study of children aged 10–12 years concluded that the child's mean systolic blood pressure adjusted for current weight rose by 2.6 mmHg for each 1 g/dl (0.6 mmol/l) fall in the mother's lowest hemoglobin level during pregnancy (Godfrey *et al.*, 1994). These results parallel animal experiments and suggest that impaired maternal nutrition may underlie the programming of adult hypertension during fetal life.

In contrast to low levels of hemoglobin/hematocrit, a high hemoglobin/hematocrit value (polycythemia) is a marker for an increased risk of preeclampsia, intrauterine growth restriction and preterm delivery (Mau, 1977; Koller *et al.*, 1979; Koller *et al.*, 1980; Koller, 1982; Garn *et al.*, 1981; Murphy *et al.*, 1986; Lieberman *et al.*, 1988; Klebanoff *et al.*, 1989). Duvekot *et al.* (1995) observed that the likelihood of poor intravascular volume expansion in early pregnancy is increased in pregnancies subsequently complicated by fetal growth restriction. Thus, the increase in hematocrit is not the result of excess RBC synthesis compared with normal pregnancy, but is due to decreased dilutional expansion.

THE TESTS

What is the purpose of the tests?

To identify women with either pathologic anemia or polycythemia for the purpose of initiating therapy to reduce their risk of an adverse pregnancy outcome.

The nature of the tests

The measurement of maternal red blood cell (RBC) mass and/or iron stores.

The assessment of hemoglobin, hematocrit, and MCV in industrialized countries is usually performed with automated equipment. In recent years, both the World Health Organization criteria – a hemoglobin level of less than 11 g/dl (6.8 mmol/l) – and a hematocrit of less than 33% (Yip, 1989) have become widely accepted definitions of pathologic anemia during pregnancy. The principal limitation of hemoglobin as an index of iron deficiency is the marked overlap in frequency distribution curves of anemic and nonanemic individuals. As a result, the use of this criterion is associated with a large number of false negative and false positive findings. The three erythrocyte indices, i.e. the mean corpuscular volume, the mean corpuscular hemoglobin concentration (MCHC), and the mean corpuscular hemoglobin (MCH), are commonly used to screen for the various types of anemia, including microcytic anemia due to iron deficiency, and macrocytic anemia due to either folate or B_{12} deficiency. These indices remain within the normal range during the dilutional anemia of pregnancy. The MCV is now regarded as the *most sensitive red cell index* for the identification of iron deficiency. Values below 70 fl occur only with iron deficiency anemia or thalassemia minor.

A hemoglobin level above 13 g/dl (8.1 mmol/l) has been associated with adverse pregnancy outcomes (Murphy *et al.*, 1986; Mitchell and Lerner, 1992). The RBC indices are not usually affected by polycythemia.

Serum ferritin is the most accurate indicator of available iron stores (Lipschitz *et al.*, 1974). However, the sensitivity of serum ferritin for true depletion of iron reserves is low. A concentration below 12 µg/l is diagnostic of depleted iron stores in white males (Cook, 1982). A low serum ferritin level (< 12 µg/l) in combination with a low hemoglobin level is strongly suggestive of iron deficiency anemia. However, ferritin behaves as an acute phase reactin. Several pathologic conditions, such as infection, chronic disease and active liver disease increase serum ferritin levels independent of the iron stores. Thus, a normal ferritin level does not exclude iron deficiency anemia. Methods for the measurement of serum ferritin include immunoradiometric assays (IRMA) using labelled antibody, radioimmune assays (RIA) using labelled antigen, and enzyme-linked immune assays (EIA) which eliminate the need for radioisotopes. Interlaboratory comparisons reveal that the differences between laboratories are not substantially greater then the intra-assay differences within the same laboratory (Cook, 1982). An important advantage of serum ferritin measurement is its reliability on serial study. In one study, day-to-day variability in serum ferritin in the same subject was 15%. This compares favorably with the 28% day-to-day variability in serum iron and transferrin levels (Pilon *et al.*, 1981).

Implications of testing

WHAT DOES AN ABNORMAL TEST RESULT MEAN?

Screening for anemia: A hemoglobin value below 11 g/dl (6.8 mmol/l) suggests the presence of a pathologic anemia. A normal MCV is more typical of dilution and argues against both iron deficiency anemia and thalassemia. Testing is typically done during the first antenatal visit and again sometime in the mid-second or third trimesters since an anemia may manifest over time. Some researchers have suggested that the serum ferritin also be routinely measured at the start of antenatal care, or by 20–24 weeks' gestation and at 6–8 week intervals thereafter (Romslo *et al.*, 1983). However, there is no evidence to support this recommendation. There are at least two routes to take once a pathologic anemia associated with a low MCV has been identified: either confirm the presence of iron deficiency anemia by measuring the serum ferritin, or proceed directly with iron replacement therapy. A reticulocytic response to iron replacement would confirm the diagnosis of iron deficiency anemia.

Iron supplementation does have a beneficial effect on maternal hematologic indices in women with iron deficiency anemia (Table 16.1). Observational studies and clinical trials of iron supplementation suggest a reduction in the risk of complications with therapy, especially in the nonindustrialized world (Table 16.2). The recommended daily dose of iron for the treatment of anemia during pregnancy is 60–180 mg elemental iron (300–600 mg ferrous sulfate). Neither blood transfusion nor parenteral iron administration is warranted for the treatment of iron deficiency anemia per se (Blankson, 1990; Morgan, 1961). Parenteral iron therapy is justified in women with malabsorption, women in the nonindustrialized world, women with intolerance to oral therapy, or when the iron loss exceeds the maximum oral replacement. One Kenyan study reported that women with moderate to severe anemia had a decreased risk of preterm birth and stillbirth when treated with iron (Macgregor, 1963). In another study, a beneficial effect on birthweight was noted (Harrison and Ibeziako, 1973). Since the true impact of anemia on pregnancy outcome in industrialized countries has never been established, it is impossible to evaluate the possible benefit of replacement therapy. It has been suggested that women begin iron supplementation if their hemoglobin level continues to fall in the third trimester, or if they have low serum ferritin values at the first antenatal visit (Bently, 1985).

Screening for preterm birth and low birthweight: A relationship between an elevated hemoglobin level or hematocrit and poor pregnancy outcome has been noted, though it is difficult to determine whether the relationship is direct or indirect (Table 16.3). Overall, the sensitivity of an elevated hemoglobin or hematocrit value for the prediction of an adverse pregnancy outcome varies between 5% and 36%, while specificity varies between 79% and 97%. Although there is no therapy for polycythemia known to reduce the risk of an adverse outcome, increased maternal and fetal surveillance seems warranted. Both high and low hematocrit levels are risk factors for intrauterine growth restriction and preterm birth (Murphy *et al.*, 1986). Many studies, however, have not considered the timing of the hematocrit measurements nor the physiologic U-shaped relationship between hematocrit and pregnancy duration (Figure 16.1) (Ogambode, 1980; Garn *et al.*, 1981; Lieberman *et al.*, 1988). Blankson *et al.* (1993) suggested that a mean

Table 16.1 Effect of iron supplementation on hemoglobin (g/dl).

AUTHOR AND YEAR	NO. OF WOMEN IRON/ CONTROLS	RANGE OF GESTATION (weeks)	PLACEBO OR NO TREATMENT	TYPE AND DOSE OF IRON/ DAY	IRON-TREATED (mean + SD)	PLACEBO OR NO TREATMENT (mean + SD)	SIGNIFICANCE
Paintin, 1966	55/54	36	placebo	105 mg iron aminoates	12.0 ± 1.04	10.7 ± 0.98	NS
Chanarin, 1971	49/46	37	placebo	120 mg elemental iron	12.2 ± 0.26	11.4 ± 0.14	NA
Svanberg, 1976	30/30	35	placebo	100 mg ferrous sulfate	12.4 ± 0.18	11.4 ± 0.17	NA
Puolakka, 1980	16/25	28	no treatment	200 mg ferrous sulfate	11.5 ± 8.00	9.9 ± 1.00	$P < 0.001$
Taylor, 1982	21/24	40	no treatment	325 mg ferrous sulfate	12.7 ± 0.7	11.2 ± 0.75	NA
Romslo, 1983	22/23	37–40	placebo	200 mg ferrous sulfate	12.6 ± 0.8	11.3 ± 1.0	$P < 0.001$

NA, not available; NS, not significant.

Table 16.2 Anemia and pregnancy outcome in developing countries.

AUTHOR AND YEAR	NO. OF WOMEN	Hct (%) OR Hb (g/dl)	BW (g) OR % OF LBW	GA (weeks) OR % PRETERM	PREECLAMPSIA (%)	NEONATAL BIRTHS (‰)	STILLBIRTH (‰)
Macgregor, 1963 (Kenya)	3 950	≥ 8.9 7.5–8.8 ≤ 7.4	13 32 42		14 22	22 29 50	51 150 147
Reinhardt, 1978 (Ivory Coast)	198	≥ 10.0 < 10.0	3 070 2 881**	38.60 38.37			
Lister, 1985 (Zaire)	20 025	≥ 30.0 < 30.0				29 60	55 190
Bhargava, 1989 (India)	225	< 6.0 > 10.0	2 183 2 599*	36.4 37.7			
Brabin, 1990 (New Guinea)	8 000	≥ 8.0 < 8.0	46 76	20 23			

* P < 0.05. ** P < 0.001. BW, birthweight; LBW, low birthweight.

Table 16.3 High hemoglobin/hematocrit and poor fetal outcome.

AUTHOR AND YEAR	TEST	RANGE OF GESTATION (weeks)	NO. OF WOMEN	OUTCOME	SENS.	SPEC.	PV+	PV−
Mau, 1977	Hb > 14.4 g/dl	≥ 28	4690	LBW Preterm	5 6	97 97	15 16	91 92
Sagen, 1984	Hb ≥ 13 g/dl	38–42	847	LBW	50	86	60	80
Knottnerus, 1986	Hb ≥ 13 g/dl	< 26	494	Preterm Preeclampsia	30 23	88 89	10 21	96 90
Lieberman, 1988	Hcte > 40%	38–40	8163	Preterm	6	86	2	95
Knottnerus, 1990	Hb ≥ 13 g/dl	31–32	796	Preterm Preeclampsia	26 15	88 87	9 24	96 80
Fukushima, 1991	Hb ≥ 13.5 g/dl	< 12	460	Preeclampsia Preterm	24 33	82 79	32 5	75 97
Hemminki, 1991	Hcte > 39%	28	2698	LBW	36	83	6	97
Heilman, 1993	Hb ≥ 13 g/dl	12–26	707	LBW Preterm	28 18	87 88	7 25	97 83

hematocrit above 40% is associated with an increased risk of intrauterine growth restriction and elective preterm deliveries, the latter mainly resulting from hypertension with or without fetal growth restriction. Studies that did not control for gestational age at sampling have tended to find a strong association between low hematocrit and preterm birth, especially among black women. However, a low hematocrit is not associated with adverse pregnancy outcome when adjusted for confounding factors.

WHAT DOES A NORMAL TEST RESULT MEAN?

Women with normal red blood cell mass and iron stores do not have anemia or polycythemia. A 3–5% decline is typical between the first measurement at booking and the second measurement later in pregnancy (Figure 16.1). Routine iron supplementation has been advocated because of the physiologic dilution and the 1 year necessary for the woman to recover from an uneventful pregnancy. Most randomized clinical trials conclude that supplemented women are less likely to develop anemia. However, this is the only difference in terms of outcome (Editorial, 1978; US Preventive Services Task Force, 1993; Mahomed, 1994). Iron supplementation has been associated with a lower cesarean section rate, and (not surprisingly) a reduction in need for blood transfusion (Mahomed, 1994). However, the reduction in the frequency of cesarean section was not predicted by prior hypotheses and may be a chance association. In addition, the sample sizes of these trials were small and their power to prove that routine iron supplementation is ineffective was low.

Routine iron supplementation has potential risks. Iron supplements may cause unpleasant gastrointestinal symptoms (e.g. nausea and constipation). These are dose-related and usually occur at doses higher than those recommended for iron supplementation. Iron supplements may exacerbate preexisting gastrointestinal disorders such as ulcerative colitis. Complications of excessive iron storage such as hemochromatosis and hemosiderosis are possible, but very uncommon in women taking oral supplements (US Preventive Services Task Forces, 1993). There is a documented risk of accidental iron overdosage in young children (Berkovitch et al., 1994).

Perhaps because of the lack of supporting evidence, patient and physician compliance is a potential problem with recommending routine iron supplementation. In Norway, where routine iron supplementation is officially recommended, only 11% of caregivers and 25% of pregnant women comply with the recommendation (Rytter et al., 1993). In fact, increased absorption of iron from food is a physiologic consequence of normal pregnancy. The increase is large enough to meet the requirements of pregnancy provided the dietary intake is adequate (Barrett et al., 1994). While the routine use of folate in multivitamins has virtually eliminated macrocytic anemia resulting from a folic acid deficiency, this category of anemia is still a problem in the nonindustrialized world and in populations not receiving antenatal care.

What is the cost of testing?

The cost of testing either red cell mass and/or iron stores in most industrialized countries is similar or higher than the cost of routine iron supplementation. The cheapest preparation of combined iron and folate supplementation for a whole pregnancy cost UK £3.57 (US $5.70, 1995) and a serum ferritin assay cost £2.50 (US $4.00, 1995) (Horn, 1988). However, the price of testing is considerably higher in the USA where a complete blood profile approximates US $17 and a serum ferritin measurement $36 (US, 1995). If routine screening of red cell mass is performed at booking and in the early third trimester, and 15% of the women have iron deficiency anemia on booking and 5% of the remaining women are anemic when tested later in pregnancy, the cost per case identified (per 1000 women, exclusive of treatment) is $164 if ferritin is not checked. In contrast to routine testing, the cost of iron and folate supplementation to the patient for 1 year approximates $17. Thus, in the US, the cost of routine supplementation to prevent one case of iron deficiency anemia is $89 without laboratory screening (US, 1995). Considering the lack of an identifiable improvement in outcome in industrialized nations, neither test seems necessary in women at low risk for iron deficiency anemia.

CONCLUSIONS AND RECOMMENDATIONS

In contrast to the nonindustrialized countries where the prevalence of iron deficiency anemia is high, there is no scientific justification for the age-old practice in industrialized countries of routine supplementation of iron in pregnancy (Blankson, 1990). The practice carries some theoretic risk and real costs. Routine iron supplementation or testing is advised only for pregnant women who are at increased risk of developing iron deficiency anemia (e.g. multiple fetus pregnancy, recurrent pregnancies within a 2-year interval, low socioeconomic status, or the mother is an adolescent) (Taylor *et al.*, 1982; Blankson, 1990). Any endorsement for routine testing or treatment in the future should be based on a randomized controlled trial conducted in an industrialized country. There does appear to be adequate data to conclude that either routine testing or supplementation is beneficial for pregnant women in the nonindustrialized world. On the other hand, what form of enhanced surveillance can be offered to women who have high hematocrits in pregnancy is not yet clear. We suggest that if Hb > 13 g/dl then a pregnancy should be considered at risk for an unfavorable outcome.

SUMMARY

1   WHAT IS THE PROBLEM THAT REQUIRES SCREENING?

ABNORMALITIES OF MATERNAL RED BLOOD CELL MASS – ANTEPARTUM.

a What is the incidence/prevalence of the target condition?

Eight per cent to 40% of pregnant women are classified as having anemia during pregnancy. The wide range probably reflects differences in the definition of anemia. 8–10% of women have an elevated red blood cell count.

b What are the sequelae of the condition which are of interest in clinical medicine?

In non-industrialized countries, marked iron deficiency is associated with severe maternal and perinatal problems. In industrialized countries, however, there is little evidence that iron deficiency is an important perinatal problem. Polycythemia is associated with preeclampsia, intrauterine growth restriction, and preterm delivery.

2 THE TESTS

a What is the purpose of the tests?

To identify women with either pathologic anemia or polycythemia for the purpose of initiating therapy to reduce their risk of an adverse pregnancy outcome.

b The nature of the tests

The measurement of maternal red blood cell mass and/or iron stores.

c Implications of testing

1 What does an abnormal test result mean?

A hemoglobin value below 11 g/dl (6.8 mmol/l) suggests the presence of a pathologic anemia, particularly when associated with an abnormal MCV value (1 < 70 fl). If anemia is associated with a low MCV, serum ferritin should be measured or iron replacement therapy instituted. A mean hematocrit above 40% is associated with an increased risk of interuterine growth restriction.

2 What does a normal test result mean?

Women with normal red blood cell mass and iron stores do not have anemia or polycythemia. A 3–5% decline is typical between the first measurement at booking and the second measurement later in pregnancy

d What is the cost of testing?

In the USA, a complete blood profile approximates US $17 and a serum ferritin measurement $36 (US, 1995). Routine testing of maternal red blood cell mass and/or iron stores is not cost-effective.

3 CONCLUSIONS AND RECOMMENDATIONS

There is no scientific justification for the age-old practice in industrialized countries of routine supplementation of iron in pregnancy, in contrast to the nonindustrialized countries where the prevalence of iron deficiency anemia is high. The practice carries some theoretic risk and real costs. Routine iron supplementation or testing is advised only for pregnant women who are at increased risk of developing iron deficiency anemia (e.g. multiple pregnancies, recurrent pregnancies within a 2-year interval, low socioeconomic status, and adolescent age). Any endorsement for routine testing or treatment in the future should be based on a randomized controlled trial. There does appear to be adequate data to conclude that either routine testing or supplementation is beneficial for pregnant women in the nonindustrialized world.

REFERENCES

Barrett JF, Whittaker PG, Williams JG & Lind T (1994) Absorption of non-haem iron from food during normal pregnancy. *Br Med J* **309**: 79–82.

Bentley DP (1985) Iron metabolism and anaemia in pregnancy. *Clin Haematol* **14** (3): 613–628.

Berkovitch M, Matsui D, Lamm SH, Rosa F & Koren G (1994) Recent increases in numbers and risk of fatalities in young children ingesting iron preparations. *Vet Hum Toxico* **36**: 53–55.

Bhargava M, Kumar R, Iyer PU et al. (1989) Effect of maternal anaemia and iron depletion on foetal iron stores, birthweight and gestation. *Acta Paed Scand* **78**: 321–322.

Blankson ML (1990) Maternal hematological status and pregnancy outcome. In Murkatz IR & Thompson JE (eds) *New Perspectives on Prenatal Care*, pp 409–418. New York: Elsevier.

Blankson ML, Goldenberg RL, Cutter G & Cliver SP (1993) The relationship between maternal haematocrit and pregnancy outcome: black-white differences. *J Nat Med Assoc* **85:** 130–134.

Brabin BJ, Ginny M, Sapau J, Galme K & Paino J (1990) Consequences of maternal anaemia on outcome of pregnancy in a malaria endemic area in Papua New Guinea. *Ann Trop Med Parasitol* **84:** 11–24.

Chanarin I & Rothman D (1971) Further Observations on the Relation between Iron and Folate Status in Pregnancy. *Br Med J* **2:** 81–84.

Colomer J, Colomer C, Gutierrez D et al. (1990) Anaemia during pregnancy as a risk factor for infant iron deficiency: report from the Valencia Infant Anaemia Cohort (VIAC) study. *Paed Perinat Epidemiol* **4:** 196–204.

Cook JD (1982) Clinical Evaluation of Iron Deficiency. *Semin Hematol* **19:** 6–18.

de Leeuw NKM & Brunton L (1976) Maternal hematologic changes, iron metabolism, and anaemias in pregnancy. In Goodwin JW, Godden JO and Chance GH (eds.) *Perinatal Medicine*. pp. 425–447, Baltimore: Williams & Williams.

Duvekot JJ, Cheriex EC, Pieters FAA et al. (1995) Maternal volume homeostasis in early pregnancy in relation to fetal growth restriction. *Obstet Gynecol* **85:** 361–367.

Editorial (1978) Do all pregnant women need iron? *Br Med J* **2:** 1317.

Elwood PC (1973) Evaluation of the clinical importance of anaemia. *Am J Clin Nutr* **26:** 958–964.

Fairbanks VF (1971) Is the peripheral blood film reliable for the diagnosis of iron deficiency anemia? *Am J Clin Pathol* **55:** 447–451.

Fleming AF, Martin JD, Hahnel R & Westlake AJ (1974) Effects of iron and folic acid antenatal supplements on maternal hematology and fetal wellbeing. *Med J Aust* **2:** 429–436.

Fukushima M & Watanabe H (1991) An observation on pregnancy outcomes in relation to haemoglobin levels. *Fukushima J Med Sci* **37** (1): 23–27.

Garby L, Irnell L & Werner I (1969) Iron deficiency in women of fertile age in a Swedish community. III. Estimation of prevalence based on response to iron supplementation. *Acta Med Scand* **185:** 113–117.

Garn SM, Keating MT & Falkner F (1981) Hematological status and pregnancy outcomes. *Am J Clin Nutr* **34:** 115–117.

Godfrey KM, Forrester T, Barker DJ et al. (1994) Maternal nutritional status in pregnancy and blood pressure in childhood. *Br J Obstet Gynaecol* **101:** 398–403.

Griswold DM & Cavanagh D (1966) Prematurity: the epidemiologic profile of the 'high risk' mother. *Am J Obstet Gynecol* **96:** 878–882.

Groner JA, Holtzman NA, Charney E & Mellits ED (1986) A randomized trial of oral iron on tests of short-term memory and attention span in young pregnant women. *J Adolesc Health Care* **7:** 44–48.

Harrison KA & Ibeziako PA (1973) Maternal anaemia and fetal birthweight. *J Obstet Gynaecol Br Commonw* **80:** 798–804.

Heilmann L, Hojnacki B, Herrle B, v. Tempelhoff G & Kriechbaum A (1993) Das Hämoglobin – ein geburtshilflicher Risikofaktor. *Geburtsh Frauenheilk* **53:** 235–239.

Hemminki E & Starfield B (1978) Routine administration of iron and vitamins during pregnancy: review of controlled clinical trials. *Br J Obstet Gynaecol* **85:** 404–410.

Hemminki E & Rimpela U (1991) Iron supplementation, maternal packed cell volume, and fetal growth. *Arch Dis Child* **66:** 422–425.

Horn E (1988) Iron and folate supplements during pregnancy: supplementing everyone treats those at risk and is cost effective. *Br Med J* **297:** 1325–1327.

Klebanoff MA, Shiono PH, Berendes HW & Rhoads GG (1989) Facts and artefacts about anaemia and preterm delivery. *JAMA* **262:** 511–515.

Knottnerus JA, Delgado LR, Knipschild PG, Essed GG & Smits F (1986) Maternal haemoglobin and pregnancy outcome. *Lancet* ii: 282.

Knottnerus JA, Delgado LR, Knipschild PG, Essed GG & Smits F (1990) Haematologic parameters and pregnancy outcome. A prospective cohort study in the third trimester. *J Clin Epidemiol* **43:** 461–466.

Koller O (1982) The clinical significance of hemodilution during pregnancy. *Obstet Gynecol Surv* **37:** 649–652.

Koller O, Sagen N, Ulstein M & Vaula D (1979) Fetal growth retardation associated with inadequate haemodilution in otherwise uncomplicated pregnancy. *Acta Obstet Gynecol Scand* **58:** 9–13.

Koller O, Sandvei R & Sagen N (1980) High haemoglobin levels during pregnancy and fetal risk. *Int J Gynecol Obstet* **18:** 53–56.

Lieberman E, Ryan KJ, Monson RR & Schoenbaum SC (1988) Association of maternal haematocrit with premature labor. *Am J Obstet Gynecol* **159:** 107–114.

Lipschitz DA, Cook JD & Finch CA (1974) A clinical evaluation of serum ferritin as an index of iron stores. *N Engl J Med* **290:** 1213–1216.

Lister UG, Rossiter CE & Chong H (1985) Perinatal mortality. *B J Obstet Gynaecol* Suppl. 5: 86–99.

Lu ZM, Goldenberg RL, Cliver SP, Cutter G & Blankson M (1991) The relationship between maternal hematocrit and pregnancy outcome. *Obstet Gynecol* **77:** 190–194.

Macgregor MW (1963) Maternal anemia as a factor in prematurity and perinatal mortality. *Scot Med J* 8: 134–140.

Mahomed K (1994) Routine iron supplementation in pregnancy. In Enkin MW, Keirse MJ, Renfrew MJ, Neilson JP (eds) *Pregnancy and Childbirth Module* Cochrane Database of Systematic Reviews: Review 03157. Oxford: Update Software, Disk Issue 1.

Mahomed K & Hytten F (1989) Iron and folate supplementation in pregnancy. In Chalmers I, Enkin M & Keirse M (eds). *Effective Care in Pregnancy and Childbirth*. pp. 301–17. Oxford University Press.

Mau A (1977) Hemoglobin changes during pregnancy and growth disturbances in the neonate. *J Perinat Med* 5: 172–177.

Mitchell MC & Lerner E (1992) Maternal hematologic measures and pregnancy outcome. *J Am Dietet Assoc* 92: 484–486.

Morgan EH (1961) Plasma-iron and haemoglobin levels in pregnancy. The effect of oral iron. *Lancet* i: 9–12.

Murphy JF, O'Riordan J, Newcombe RG, Coles EC & Pearson JF (1986) Relation of haemoglobin levels in first and second trimesters to outcome of pregnancy. *Lancet* i: 992–994.

Ogambode O (1980) The relationship between hematocrit levels in gravidae and their newborns. *Int J Gynaecol Obstet* 18: 57–60.

Paintin DB, Thomson AM & Hytten FE (1966) Iron and the haemoglobin level in pregnancy. *J Obstet Gynaecol Br Commonw* 73: 181–190.

Pilon VA, Howanitz PJ, Howanitz JH *et al.* (1981) Day-to-day variation in serum ferritin concentration in healthy subjects. *Clin Chem* 27: 78–82.

Prasad AN & Prasad C (1991) Iron deficiency; non-hematological manifestations. *Prog Food Nutr Sci* 15: 255–283.

Puolakka J, Jänne O & Vihko R (1980) Evaluation by serum ferritin assay of the influence of maternal iron stores on the iron status of newborns and infants. *Acta Obstet Gynaecol Scand* (suppl). 95: 53–56.

Ratten GJ & Beischer NA (1972) The significance of anaemia in an obstetric population in Australia. *J Obstet Gynaecol Br Commonw* 79: 228–237.

Reinhardt MC (1978) Maternal anaemia in Abidjan – its influence on placenta and newborns. *Helv Paed Acta* (suppl). 41: 43–63.

Rios E, Lipschitz DA, Cook JD & Smith NJ (1975) Relationship of maternal and iron stores as assessed by determination of plasma ferritin. *Pediatrics* 55: 694–699.

Romslo I, Haram K, Sagen N & Augensen K (1983) Iron requirement in normal pregnancy as assessed by serum ferritin, serum transferrin saturation and erythrocyte protoporphyrin determinations. *B J Obstet Gynaecol* 90: 101–107.

Royston E, Armstrong S (1989) *Preventing Maternal Deaths*. 233pp. Geneva: World Health Organization.

Rytter E, Forde R, Andrew M et al (1993) Graviditet og jerntilskudd-blir de offisielle retningslinjene fulgt? *Tidssk Norske Laegefor* 113: 2416–2419.

Sagen N, Tore Nilsen S, Chan Kim H, Bergsjø & Koller O (1984) Maternal hemoglobin concentration is closely related to birthweight in normal pregnancies. *Acta Obstet Gynecol Scand* 63: 245–248.

Scott DE & Pritchard JA (1974) Anaemia in pregnancy. *Clin Perinat* 1: 491–506.

Svanberg B, Arvidsson B, Norrby A, Rybo G & Sölvell L (1976) Absorption of supplemental iron during pregnancy – a longitudinal study with repeated bone-marrow studies and absorption measurements. *Acta Obstet Gynecol Scand* (Suppl.) 48: 87–108.

Taylor DJ, Mallen C, McDougall N & Lind T (1982) Effect of iron supplementation on serum ferritin levels during and after pregnancy. *Br J Obstet Gynaecol* 89: 1011–1017.

US Preventive Services Task Force (1993) Routine Iron Supplementation During Pregnancy. *JAMA* 270: 2846–2854.

Williams MD & Wheby MS (1992) Anemia in pregnancy. *Med Clin North Am* 76: 631–647.

Yip R (1989) Centers for Diseases Control criteria for anaemia in children and childbearing-aged women. *MMWR* 38: 400–404.

Willoughby MLN (1967) An investigation of folic acid requirements in pregnancy, II. *Br J Haematol* 13: 503–509.

WHAT IS THE PROBLEM THAT REQUIRES SCREENING?

ABNORMALITIES OF MATERNAL RED BLOOD CELL MASS – POSTPARTUM

What is the incidence/prevalence of the target condition?

The frequency of iron deficiency anemia in postpartum women who were not given supplementary iron is high. In one Danish study, 40% of women not supplemented with oral iron had a serum ferritin measurement below 20 µg/l and 4% had a hemoglobin level of less than 12.1 g/dl (7.5 mmol/l). The corresponding frequencies in women who received iron were 16% and 0% respectively (Milman *et al.*, 1991). These findings are in agreement with earlier observations (Taylor *et al.*, 1982).

What are the sequelae of the condition which are of interest in clinical medicine?

Delayed recovery from pregnancy and health sequelae secondary to severe, untreated anemia.

The estimated normal blood loss at delivery varies greatly. Mathie and Snodgrass (1967) reported a blood loss between 5 ml and 1600 ml, with a mean of 186 ml. Careful investigation using reliable laboratory techniques to actually measure blood loss reveals a mean blood loss at delivery of 339 ml (Newton *et al.*, 1961). Much of the loss represents excess RBC mass synthesized during pregnancy and need not be replaced. Nonetheless, the red blood cell loss constitutes a drain on iron stores which are typically low in menstruating women. Iron loss via lactation is insignificant (Underwood, 1977).

Massive postpartum hemorrhage is a serious problem in both the industrialized and non-industrialized worlds (Duthie *et al.*, 1990). One review of 2067 maternal deaths in the USA observed that hemorrhage was associated with over half the deaths, with one-third of these occurring postpartum (Kaunitz *et al.*, 1985). Another review of maternal deaths from 1987 to 1991 in the rural south of the USA revealed an alarming increase in the proportion of maternal deaths due to obstetric hemorrhage, with the majority occurring in the immediate postpartum period (Moore *et al.*, 1993).

Postpartum anemia secondary to iron deficiency and acute blood loss are intimately related. It is estimated that it takes the average woman approximately 1 year to recover her iron losses without supplementation. However, it remains unknown whether women who end their pregnancy with a serum ferritin level below normal, or who suffer a modest blood loss anemia, are in worse health during the first year postpartum than women with normal values. Such information is crucial for the formulation of informed public health policy.

THE TESTS

What is the purpose of the tests?

To identify women with postpartum anemia for the purpose of initiating therapy to reduce their risk of an adverse health outcome.

The nature of the tests

The tests are discussed in the previous section of this chapter on antepartum screening. Internationally accepted criteria for abnormal hemoglobin, hematocrit, and MCV levels in the puerperium have not been adopted. Nor is there any agreement on the optimal day for postpartum testing. This is important since there is an 400 ml increase in plasma volume within 48 hours after delivery, followed by a fall in plasma volume with hemoconcentration (Dewhurst, 1976). There is no practical way to assess and correct for plasma volume routinely. The measurement of serum ferritin to determine iron stores is not useful since ferritin rises during the first 2–4 days postpartum (Haram *et al.*, 1993). Moreover, serum ferritin levels may be normal in women who are mildly anemic, because of iron release precipitated by the acute decline in red cell mass (Puolakka *et al* 1980; Taylor *et al* 1982).

Implications of testing

WHAT DOES AN ABNORMAL TEST RESULT MEAN?

An abnormal test means that the woman has a pathologic anemia. Anemia following blood loss during delivery and following postpartum hemorrhage is usually assessed by estimation of hemoglobin and hematocrit levels. This approach was challenged by Goodlin (1990) who pointed out that the hematocrit is a poor index of blood loss, as women with hematocrit levels of less than 35% may actually have increased red cell masses. In addition, there are very little published data on criteria for iron supplementation of asymptomatic anemic women. As a result, there is no consensus on whom to treat.

There is also no consensus on when to transfuse the profoundly anemic woman postpartum. The literature is remarkable for the absence of carefully controlled trials that would permit definitive conclusions. A major factor associated with maternal death after obstetric hemorrhage is the underestimate of total blood loss, and subsequently inadequate volume replacement. An accurate assessment of blood loss is an important guide to management of postpartum hemorrhage. Certainly, massive hemorrhage associated with hypoperfusion requires immediate blood replacement with blood components, whole blood, or blood volume expanders, adequate to both restore and maintain adequate perfusion of vital organs. In healthy individuals, cardiac output does not increase dramatically until hemoglobin level decreases to less than 7.0 g/dl (4.3 mmol/l). The same conclusion probably applies to women with a hemorrhage large enough to produce postural hypotension. It is essential to recognize that the combination of hypovolemia and anemia may lead to mortality or severe maternal morbidity due to insufficient tissue oxygenation. Sheehan syndrome (hypopituitarism following ischemia and infarction of the pituitary gland) is a rare but well-known late complication of obstetric hemorrhage. The potential benefits of maternal transfusion should be balanced against the potential risks of adverse outcome, including red cell alloimmunization and chronic viral infection. Usually the amount of blood replaced does not completely restore the hemoglobin deficit following hemorrhage. However, once dangerous hypovolemia has been treated and hemostasis achieved, the residual anemia can be treated by oral iron supplementation. Transfusion is not normally indicated in hemodynamically stable postpartum women with moderate anemia (e.g. hemoglobin levels from 7 g/dl to 10 g/dl (4.3–6.2 mmol/l). Oral iron therapy for at least 3 months should restore the lost iron (Cunningham *et al.*, 1993; Inglis *et al.*, 1995).

WHAT DOES A NORMAL TEST RESULT MEAN?

Postpartum women with normal red cell mass need no further evaluation. Since most of the women who breastfeed do not menstruate, dietary iron is usually sufficient to meet daily iron requirements (de Leeuw and Brunton, 1976).

What is the cost of testing?

The costs of these tests are discussed in the previous section on antepartum screening. There is inadequate information to allow a cost-benefit analysis for the practice of routine postpartum screening. Since there are no known sequelae of asymptomatic post-partum anemia, it is not likely to be a necessary expenditure of funds.

CONCLUSIONS AND RECOMMENDATIONS

Blood loss at delivery can be considerable. Postpartum hemorrhage may lead to maternal death or severe maternal morbidity. No single laboratory test currently available can replace sound clinical judgment as the basis for the optimal management of excessive blood loss during the postpartum period.

There is no rationale in the industrialized world for the widespread practice of routinely prescribing iron postpartum. This is true for both lactating and nonlactating women. The estimated iron loss from lactation is about 1 mg per day (Fairbanks, 1971). On empirical grounds, iron supplementation is reasonable if the hemoglobin level is less than 10 g/dl (6.2 mmol/l) four days postpartum or the MCV is abnormal (< 70 fl), the diet is deficient of iron-containing foods, pregnancy within 1 year is likely, or the woman will breastfeed for more than 6 months.

SUMMARY

1 WHAT IS THE PROBLEM THAT REQUIRES SCREENING?

ABNORMALITIES OF MATERNAL RED BLOOD CELL MASS – POSTPARTUM.

a What is the incidence/prevalence of the target condition?

The frequency of iron deficiency anemia postpartum is high in women who were not given iron supplementation during pregnancy. In one study, 40% of women not supplemented had a serum ferritin level below 20 µg/l and 4% had a hemoglobin level of less than 12.1 g/dl (7.5 mmol/l). The corresponding frequencies in women who received iron were 16% and 0% respectively

b What are the sequelae of the condition which are of interest in clinical medicine?

Delayed recovery from pregnancy and health sequelae secondary to severe, untreated anemia or blood loss.

2 THE TESTS

a What is the purpose of the tests?

The purpose of the tests is to estimate the severity of anemia secondary to blood loss at delivery and to evaluate the woman's depletion of the iron stores.

b The nature of the tests

The measurement of maternal red blood cell mass and/or iron stores.

c Implications of testing

I What does an abnormal test result mean?

An abnormal test means that the woman has a pathologic anemia and therapy should be initiated.

2 What does a normal test result mean?
Postpartum women with normal red cell mass need no further evaluation, provided they are hemodynamically stable.

d What is the cost of testing?

There is inadequate information to allow a cost-benefit analysis for the practice of routine postpartum screening. Since there are no known sequelae of asymptomatic postpartum anemia, it is not likely to be a necessary expenditure of funds.

3 CONCLUSIONS AND RECOMMENDATIONS

There is no rationale in the industrialized world for the widespread practice of routinely prescribing iron postpartum. This is true for both lactating and nonlactating women.

REFERENCES

Bothwell TH & Charlton RW (1982) A general approach to the problems of iron deficiency and iron overload in the population at large. *Semin Hematol* **19**: 54–67.

Cunningham FG, MacDonald PC, Gant NF, Leveno KJ & Gilstrap LC (1993) Hematologic disorders. In *Williams Obstetrics*, 19th edn, pp. 1171–1199. Norwalk: Appleton & Lange.

de Leeuw NKM & Brunton L (1976) Maternal hematologic changes, iron metabolism, and anemias in pregnancy. In Goodwin JW, Godden JO & Chance GH (eds) *Perinatal Medicine*, pp 425–447. Baltimore: Williams & Williams.

Dewhurst CJ (1976) *Integrated Obstetrics and Gynaecology for Postgraduates*, 2nd edn, pp 316–339. Oxford: Blackwell.

Duthie SJ, Ven D, Yung GLK *et al.* (1990) Discrepancy between laboratory determination and visual estimation of blood loss during normal delivery. *Eur J Obstet Gynecol Reprod Biol* **38**: 119–124.

Fairbanks VF (1971) Is the peripheral blood film reliable for the diagnosis of iron deficiency anaemia? *Am J Clin Pathol* **55**: 447–451.

Goodlin RC (1990) Need for plasma volume estimation. *Am J Obstet Gynecol* **162**: 601.

Haram K, Sandberg S & Ulstein M (1993) High serum ferritin postpartum: an acute phase reaction. *Acta Obstet Gynecol Scand* **72**: 50–51.

Harrison KA (1982) Anaemia, malaria and sickle cell disease. *Clin Obstet Gynaecol* **9**: 445–477.

Kaunitz AM, Hughes JM, Grimes DA, *et al.* (1985) Causes of maternal mortality in the United States. *Obstet Gynecol* **65**: 605–612.

Inglis S, Stevens L, Udom-Rice I, Yun H & Chervenak FA (1995) Is observation of severe acute anemia in women safe? *Am J Obstet Gynecol* **172**: 290.

Liley AW (1970) Clinical and laboratory significance of maternal plasma volume in pregnancy. *Int J Gynecol Obstet* **8**: 358.

Mathie IK & Snodgrass CA (1967) The effect of prophylactic oxytocic drugs on blood loss after delivery. *J Obstet Gynaecol Br Commonw* **74**: 653–662.

Milman N, Agger AO & Nielsen OJ (1991) Iron supplementation during pregnancy. *Danish Med Bull* **38**: 471–476.

Moore JL, Chauman SP, Wiener WB, *et al.* (1993) Maternal mortality in Mississippi: 1987–1991. *J MS Med Assoc* **34**: 35–39.

Newton M, Mosey LM, Egli GE, Gifford WB & Hull CT (1961) Blood loss during and immediately after delivery. *Obstetr Gynecol* **17**: 9–18.

NIH Consensus Conference (1988) Perioperative red blood cell transfusion. *JAMA* **260**: 2700–2703.

Pritchard JA, Baldwin RM, Dickey JC *et al.* (1962) Blood volume changes in pregnancy and the puerperium. *Am J Obstet Gynecol* **84**: 1271–1282.

Puolakka J, Jänna O & Vihko J (1980) Evaluation by serum ferritin assay on the influence of maternal iron stores on the iron status of newborns and infants. *Acta Obstet Gynecol Scand* (suppl.) **95**: 53–56

Taylor DJ, Mallen C, McDougall N & Lind T (1982) Effect of iron supplementation on serum ferritin levels during and after pregnancy. *Br J Obstet Gynaecol* **89**: 1011–1017.

Ueland K (1976) Maternal cardiovascular dynamics VII. Intrapartum blood volume changes. *Am J Obstet Gynecol* **126**: 671–677.

Underwood EJ (1977) *Trace Elements in Human and Animal Nutrition*, 4th edn, p 23. New York: Academic Press.

17

Cervical Examination in Pregnancy

Lisan S. Schrevel, Hajo I. J. Wildschut & Sophie Alexander

PRETERM BIRTH.

Preterm birth (PTB) is defined as delivery before 37 completed weeks of gestation (Chiswick, 1986). Despite major improvements in socioeconomic conditions and in quality and accessibility of medical care since the 1960s, the rate of PTB in industrialized countries has remained essentially unchanged (Breart et al., 1995). Preterm birth is a heterogeneous condition which may occur spontaneously after the onset of labor or may result from an obstetric intervention, including induction and cesarian section. In spite of the many studies that have used PTB as the outcome of interest, its etiology remains obscure (Kramer, 1987; Bryce, 1991). Women with a history of PTB are at increased risk for PTB in a subsequent pregnancy (Bakketeig et al., 1979). However, this information is useful only to multiparous women. The vast majority (over 80%) of multiparous women who do experience a PTB have an uneventful reproductive history (Wildschut, 1994).

Strategies for the prevention of PTB are conflicting. In several European countries, serial vaginal examinations during pregnancy are regarded as standard practice, while in other countries vaginal examinations are generally avoided (Heringa and Huisjes, 1988). This chapter focuses on the value of routine cervical assessment by digital vaginal examination for the identification of women in unselected populations at risk for PTB.

What is the incidence/prevalence of the target condition?

Officially reported PTB rates in western Europe range from 4% to 8% (MacFarlane and Mugford, 1984; Mortensen et al., 1987; Masuy-Stroobant et al., 1992; Bréart et al., 1995). Crude PTB rates in the USA are higher, ranging from 8.5% in whites to 18% in blacks (Rowley et al., 1993).

What are the sequelae of the condition which are of interest in clinical medicine?

Preterm birth is the major determinant of fetal morbidity and mortality resulting primarily from the inability of the newborn to cope with extrauterine life. Longterm morbidity includes pulmonary disorders, retinopathy, and neuromotor disabilities. The relative frequency and severity of these adverse perinatal outcomes are inversely related to the duration of gestation. Escobar *et al.* (1991) concluded from a review of the literature that the median prevalence of cerebral palsy in newborns weighing less than 1500 g was 7.7% (95% confidence interval: 5.3, 9.0) and the median prevalence of disabilities was 25% (95% CI 20.9, 30.0). Hagberg *et al.* (1989a) reported that 45% of the infants with cerebral palsy were born prior to 37 weeks' gestation. Further, there is some concern that the severity of neuromotor disabilities among preterm children with cerebral palsy is increasing (Hagberg *et al.*, 1989b).

THE TEST

What is the purpose of the test?

The timely identification of a subgroup of women at increased risk for spontaneous PTB.

The nature of the test

Assessment of cervical maturation by digital vaginal examination.

The stage of cervical maturation is determined by its dilatation at the internal os, length, consistency, and position. Cervical dilatation is considered the most objective finding (Bergsjø and Koss, 1982; Blondel *et al.* 1990). Published policies concerning the frequency and timing of antenatal cervical assessment vary markedly (Table 17.1).

Implications of testing

WHAT DOES AN ABNORMAL TEST RESULT MEAN?

Criteria for an abnormal test result are given in Table 17.1. Women with an abnormal test result are often advised to restrict their daily physical activities. If it is deemed necessary by their health care provider, they may be admitted to hospital for strict bed-rest and frequent maternal and fetal surveillance. Tocolytic drugs in an attempt to inhibit preterm labor and corticosteroids to accelerate fetal surfactant production are often administered.

Table 17.2 summarizes the performance statistics of cervical examination for the identification of women who will experience PTB. Overall, cervical dilatation prior to 32 weeks is a poor predictor of PTB. In a large hospital-based prospective study, women were routinely examined after 32 weeks (Chalmers *et al.*, 1990). An open cervix, defined as a dilatation of the internal os of at least 1 cm prior to 37 weeks, was associated with a sensitivity of 41% and a specificity of 82% for PTB (positive predictive value 9%; negative predictive value 97%). These disappointing findings are in agreement with those of another study (Buekens *et al.*, 1994), whose authors conducted a multicenter randomized controlled trial comparing routine cervical examinations at each antenatal visit (study group) to a policy of avoiding cervical examination unless medically indicated. Preterm birth occurred in 5.7% (152 of 2669) of women assigned to routine cervical examination and 6.4% (172 of 2672) of women assigned to the control group. Based on these and other analyses, they concluded that routine cervical examination does not

Table 17.1   Criteria for abnormal cervical maturation.

REFERENCE	INTERNAL OS ASSESSMENT CRITERIA	TIMING AND FREQUENCY OF CERVICAL ASSESSMENT
Parikh et al. (1961)	accessible to one finger	2-week intervals from 21 weeks onward
Anderson et al. (1969)	accessible to one finger	repeated measurements at 28, 32, 34, and 36 weeks
Leveno et al. (1986)	dilatation greater than 1 cm	single measurement at 26–30 weeks
Papiernik et al. (1986)	dilatation of at least 1 cm	each antenatal visit
Stubbs et al. (1986)	dilatation of at least 1 cm	repeated measurements at 28, 32, and 34 weeks
Mortensen et al. (1987)	dilatation greater than 0.5 cm	repeated measurements at 24, 28, and 32 weeks
Chambers et al. (1990)	dilatation of at least 1 cm	each antenatal visit
Blondel et al. (1990)	dilatation of at least 1 cm	each antenatal visit
Buekens et al. (1994)	not mentioned	each antenatal visit
Copper et al. (1995)	dilatation of at least 1 cm	28 weeks

identify a subgroup of women at risk of PTB and that interventions prompted by an abnormal examination were ineffective in delaying delivery. Indeed, although bed rest and beta-mimetic drug treatment delay delivery by 24–48 hours, the actual incidence of PTB in treated patients remains unchanged from the period before their introduction (Keirse, 1994).

WHAT DOES A NORMAL TEST RESULT MEAN?

A normal cervical examination is fairly reassuring, as illustrated by the high specificities and negative predictive values (NPV) reported in most studies. However, serial vaginal examinations during pregnancy may cause pain, embarrassment or fear (Garcia, 1982; Kaufman, 1994). The claims that vaginal examination might induce prostaglandin release and thus preterm uterine contractions (Mitchell *et al.*, 1977) or be associated with preterm rupture of the membranes cannot be substantiated (Chalmers *et al.*, 1990; Buekens *et al.*, 1994; Kaufman, 1994).

Table 17.2 Prediction of preterm birth by cervical examination.

REFERENCE	PTB (%)	GA (weeks)	SENS. (%)	SPEC. (%)	PPV (%)	NPV (%)
Parikh et al. (1961)	8/37 (22)	24	25	93	50	82
	23/171 (13)	28	35	76	19	88
	20/161 (12)	32	65	47	15	90
Anderson et al. (1969)	4/77 (5)	32	100	73	17	100
Leveno et al. (1986)	7/185 (4)	30	57	94	27	98
Papiernik et al. (1986)	136/2387 (6)	28	18	95	17	95
Stubbs et al. (1986)	8/108 (7)	28	25	85	12	93
	10/136 (7)	32	40	78	13	94
Mortensen et al. (1987)	27/857 (3)	28	26	97	20	98
Blondel et al. (1990)	384/8050 (5)	28	17	97	20	96
	271/5768 (5)	31	21	94	15	96
Copper et al. (1995)	32/589 (5)	28	8	95	10	95

PTB, number of preterm births per number of subjects studied; GA, gestational age on which assessment was based; SENS., sensitivity; SPEC., specificity; PPV, positive predictive value; NPV, negative predictive value.

What is the cost of testing?

The initial costs of testing are extremely low for a cervical examination when performed as part of an antenatal visit (that is, little more than the cost of a pair of surgical gloves). Cervical examination is not associated with an increase in the total medical costs in one randomized controlled trial (Buekens et al., 1994).

CONCLUSIONS AND RECOMMENDATIONS

The effectiveness of routine digital cervical examination to identify women at risk for PTB is very limited. Second-trimester dilatation of the internal cervical os is a poor predictor of either preterm labor or PTB. The various management options currently available for the prolongation of pregnancy are effective for only 24–48 hours compared with controls (Keirse, 1994). There is no evidence that serial vaginal examinations are harmful to maternal or fetal health, but they may cause discomfort to the pregnant woman. In conclusion, routine digital cervical examination is not justified for the identification of women at risk of PTB, or for its prevention.

SUMMARY

1

WHAT IS THE PROBLEM THAT REQUIRES SCREENING?

PRETERM BIRTH (PTB).

a What is the incidence/prevalence of the target condition?

Officially reported PTB rates in western Europe range from 4% to 8%. Crude PTB rates in the USA are higher, ranging from 8.5% in whites to 18% in blacks.

b What are the sequelae of the condition which are of interest in clinical medicine?

Preterm birth is a major determinant of fetal morbidity and mortality resulting primarily from the inability of the newborn to cope with extrauterine life. Longterm morbidity includes pulmonary disorders, retinopathy, and neuromotor disabilities.

2

THE TEST

a What is the purpose of the test?

To identify a subgroup of women at risk of PTB.

b The nature of the test

Assessment of cervical maturation by digital vaginal examination.

c Implications of testing

1 What does an abnormal test result mean?

Women with an abnormal test result are frequently advised to restrict their daily physical activities. Overall, cervical dilatation prior to 32 weeks is a poor predictor of PTB.

2 What does a normal test result mean?

A normal cervical examination is fairly reassuring, as illustrated by the high specificities and NPVs.

d What is the cost of testing?

Cervical examination is not associated with an increase in total medical costs.

3

CONCLUSIONS AND RECOMMENDATIONS

Routine digital cervical examination is justified neither for the identification of women at risk of PTB, nor for its prevention.

REFERENCES

Anderson ABM & Turnbull AC (1969) Relationship between length of gestation and cervical dilatation, uterine contractility and other factors during pregnancy. *Am J Obstet Gynecol* **105**: 1207–1214.

Bakketeig LS, Hoffman HJ & Harley EE (1979) The tendency to repeat gestational age and birth weight in successive births. *Am J Obstet Gynecol* **135**: 1086–1103.

Bergsjø P & Koss KS (1982) Interindividual variation in vaginal examination findings during labor. *Acta Obstet Gynecol Scand* **61**: 509–510.

Blondel B, Le Coutour X, Kaminski M, Chavigny C, Bréart G & Sureau C (1990) Prediction of preterm delivery: is it substantially improved by routine vaginal examinations? *Am J Obstet Gynecol* **162**: 1042–1048.

Bréart G, Blondel B, Tuppin Ph, Grandjean H & Kaminski M (1995) Did preterm deliveries continue to decrease in France in the 1980s? *Paed Perinat Epidemiol* **9**: 296–306.

Bryce R (1991) The epidemiology of preterm birth. In Kiely M (ed.) *Reproductive and Perinatal Epidemiology*, pp 437–444 Boca Raton: CRC Press.

Buekens P, Alexander S, Boutsen M et al. (1994) Randomised controlled trial on routine cervical examinations in pregnancy. *Lancet* **344**: 841–844.

Chambers S, Pons JC, Richard A, Chiesa M, Bouyer J, & Papiernik E. (1990) Vaginal infections, cervical ripening and preterm delivery. *Eur J Obstet Gynecol* **38**: 103–108.

Chiswick ML (1986) Commentary on current World Health Organisation definitions used in perinatal statistics. *Br J Obstet Gynaecol* **93**: 1236–1238.

Copper RL, Goldenberg RL, Dubard MB, Hauth JC, & Cutter GR (1995) Cervical examination and tocodynamometry at 28 weeks' gestation: prediction of spontaneous preterm birth. *Am J Obstet Gynecol* **172**: 666–71.

Escobar GJ, Pittenberg B & Petitti DB (1991) Outcome among surviving very low birthweight infants: a meta-analysis. *Arch Dis Child* **66**: 204–211.

Garcia J (1982) Women's views of antenatal care. In Enkin M, Chalmers I (eds) *Effectiveness and Satisfaction in Antenatal Care* pp. 81–91. London, Spastics International Medical Publications.

Hagberg B, Hagberg G & Zetterstrom R (1989a) Decreasing perinatal mortality-increase in cerebral palsy morbidity? *Acta Paediatr Scand* **78**: 664–670.

Hagberg B, Hagberg G, Olow I & Van Wendt C (1989b) The changing panorama of cerebral palsy in Sweden. V. The birth year period 1979–82. *Acta Paediatr Scand* **78**: 283–290.

Heringa M & Huisjes HJ (1988) Prenatal screening: current policy in the EC countries. *Eur J Obstet Gynecol* **28** (suppl): 7–52.

Kaufman K (1994) Weekly vaginal examinations. In Enkin MW, Keirse MJNC, Renfrew MJ & Neilson JP (eds) *Pregnancy and Childbirth* module. Cochrane Database of Systematic Reviews. Review 06818. Oxford: Update Software.

Keirse MJNC (1994) Betamimetic tocolytics in preterm labour. In Enkin MW, Keirse MJNC, Renfrew MJ & Neilson JP (eds) *Pregnancy and Childbirth* module. Cochrane Database of Systematic Reviews. Review 03237. 1993. Oxford: Update Software.

Kramer MS (1987) Intrauterine growth and gestational duration determinants. *Pediatrics* **80**: 502–511.

Leveno KJ, Cox K & Roark ML (1986) Cervical dilatation and prematurity revisited. *Obstet Gynecol* **68**: 434–435.

MacFarlane A & Mugford M (1984) Variations in births and deaths. In A MacFarlane & M Mugford (eds) *Birth Count Statistics of Pregnancy and Childbirth*. London; HMSO.

Masuy-Stroobant G, Buekens P & Gourlin C (1992) Perinatal health in Belgium-1987. *Arch Publ Health* **50**: 217–39.

Mitchell MD, Flint APF, Bibby J, et al. (1977) Rapid increases in plasma prostaglandin concentration after vaginal examination and amniotomy. *Br Med J* **2**: 1183–1185.

Mortensen OA, Franklin J, Löfstrand T & Svanberg B (1987) Prediction of preterm birth. *Acta Obstet Gynecol Scand* **66**: 507–512.

Papiernik E, Bouyer J, Collin D, Winisdorffer G & Dreyfus J (1986) Precocious cervical ripening and preterm labour. *Obstet Gynecol* **67**: 238–242.

Parikh MN & Mehta AC (1961) Internal cervical os during the second half of pregnancy. *J Obstet Gynaecol Br Commonw* **68**: 818–821.

Rowley DL, Hogue CJR, Blackmore CA, Ferr CD, Hatfield-Timajchy K, Branch P & Atrash HK (1993) Preterm delivery among African-American women: a research strategy. *Am J Prev Med* **9** (suppl.): 1–6.

Stubbs TM, Van Dorsten JP & Miller MC (1986) The preterm cervix and preterm labor: relative risks, predictive values and change over time. *Am J Obstet Gynecol* **155**: 829–834.

Wildschut HIJ. (1994) *Risk assessment of preterm birth. Epidemiological considerations*. Thesis, University of Bristol.

18

Fetal Monitoring

George A. Macones & Richard Depp

Antepartum Fetal Monitoring

WHAT IS THE PROBLEM THAT REQUIRES SCREENING.

ANTEPARTUM UTEROPLACENTAL DYSFUNCTION SEVERE ENOUGH TO CAUSE FETAL METABOLIC ACIDOSIS OR ANTEPARTUM FETAL DEATH.

What is the incidence/prevalence of the target condition?

The overall rate of antepartum fetal death after 20 weeks' gestation is approximately 2–4 per 1000 normally formed singleton births (Grant *et al.*, 1989; Moore and Piacquadio, 1989). About 70% of these deaths are unexplained. The estimated birth prevalence of severe fetal metabolic acidemia is less than 0.5% (see next section for details).

What are the sequelae of the condition which are of interest in clinical medicine?

Transient episodes of hypoxemia (e.g. from cord compression) are common and generally well tolerated by the fetus. However, the fetus with metabolic acidemia from chronic hypoxemia secondary to uteroplacental dysfunction is likely to be growth restricted and is at increased risk of a progressive series of insults which include cesarean delivery for an inability to tolerate labor, ischemic multiorgan injury, neurodevelopmental abnormalities, and intrauterine death. There is an inverse relationship between the frequency of subsequent neurodevelopmental abnormalities and the umbilical cord pH and P_{O_2} (Goodwin *et al.*, 1992; Soothill *et al.*, 1992). Growth restricted fetuses may be less tolerant of intermittent exacerbations produced by transient cord occlusion. The linkage between hypoxemia as might be detected by current methods for antepartum surveillance and cerebral palsy is less clear.

THE TESTS

Tests currently used for routine antepartum fetal surveillance include formal fetal movement counting and the nonstress test.

What is the purpose of the tests?

The purpose of routine antepartum fetal surveillance is to detect fetal hypoxic compromise so that timely intervention occurs prior to the development of fetal acidemia and subsequent intrauterine death (Sadovsky and Yaffe, 1973; Sadovsky and Polishuk, 1977; Freeman et al., 1982a).

The nature of the test

Fetal movement counting.

Women are instructed to count fetal movements routinely every day. For this purpose the Cardiff 'count-to-ten' method is usually advocated. Women are trained to record methodically on a chart the time interval required to feel ten fetal movements (Grant et al., 1989; Moore and Piacquadio, 1989). In order to confirm the women's assessment, some investigators have advocated the use of a special device which records fetal movements (Sadovsky and Polishuk, 1977). According to Moore and Piacquadio (1989), the mean (± SD) time interval to perceive ten fetal movements is 20.9 (± 18.1) minutes, while after 1 hour 97% of women feel ten movements. The minimum number of fetal movements considered acceptable ranges from three in 1 hour to ten in 24 hours (Neldam, 1980; Grant et al., 1989). Various protocols have been proposed for the perceived decrease in fetal movements. These protocols either rely on a percentage change in the number of movements from the past baseline or on an absolute number of movements. In a randomized controlled trial involving 68 000 women, 'alarm' criteria included either no movements on a single day, or fewer than ten movements in 10 hours on two consecutive days (Grant et al., 1989). These definitions were chosen to limit the number of false positives to an acceptable level. Women are instructed to contact the hospital for further diagnostic work-up, such as cardiotocography (Sadovsky and Polishuk, 1976) or fetal biophysical profile, when they notice a reduction in fetal movements. Clinical action such as admission to hospital and early delivery is advocated where deemed necessary (Sadovsky and Polishuk, 1977).

Implications of testing

WHAT DOES AN ABNORMAL TEST RESULT MEAN?

Decreased maternal perception of fetal movement triggers the performance of a nonstress test (NST) with subsequent admission to hospital when indicated. However, given the low prevalence of fetal compromise and an estimated specificity of 90–95% (Nelson, 1980; Grant et al., 1989; Moore and Piacquadio, 1989), positive predictive values for fetal compromise are low, ranging from 2% to 7%. Hence, false alarms occur often in women who report infrequent fetal movements, creating undue anxiety. Based on the results of a randomized controlled trial, the policy of routine formal fetal movement counting cannot be recommended as its beneficial effect is very limited (Grant et al., 1989). According to Grant et al. (1989), the policy would have to be used by about 1250 women to prevent one unexplained death. Moreover, the policy of formal fetal movement counting has resource implications such as an increased rate of cardiotocography and hospital admissions compared with a policy of informal inquiry about fetal movements (Grant et al., 1989).

WHAT DOES A NORMAL TEST RESULT MEAN?

Given the low prevalence of fetal distress in low-risk pregnant women, normal findings are usually a sign of fetal wellbeing.

What is the cost of testing?

Any evaluation of the cost-effectiveness of formal fetal movement counting is hampered by the uncertainty of efficacy of this type of surveillance. Although multiple observational studies utilizing fetal movement counts suggest a decrease in perinatal mortality (Nelson, 1980; Moore and Piacquadio, 1989), the only randomized controlled trial of formal fetal movement counting failed to identify any decrease in perinatal mortality in the test group (Grant *et al.*, 1989). Fetal movement counting clearly generates additional costs from further diagnostic evaluation and admission to hospital. Such costs have not been objectively evaluated.

CONCLUSIONS AND RECOMMENDATIONS

The merits of antepartum surveillance by formal fetal movement counting have not been clearly demonstrated. Based on a randomized controlled trial involving 68 000 women, it must be concluded that the policy of formal fetal movement counting does not significantly decrease the risk of intrauterine death compared with a policy of informal inquiring about fetal movements at each antenatal visit (Grant et al., 1989). The absence of a beneficial effect of the policy of formal fetal movement counting could be partially explained by poor compliance with both recording and reporting 'alarmingly' reduced fetal movements.

The nature of the test

Nonstress test.

The antepartum nonstress cardiotocography or nonstress test (NST) is based on the observation of fetal heart rate (FHR) accelerations as a measure of fetal wellbeing. Fetal heart rate accelerations that occur independent of uterine contractions are nearly always associated with fetal movements and are not associated with acidemia. The FHR, uterine contractions, and fetal movements are continuously recorded with an electronic monitor while the woman is in a semirecumbent position for an NST. The interpretation of the NST is based on both the frequency and magnitude of FHR accelerations with a temporal reference to uterine activity. A *reactive* NST is variously defined as either two accelerations (i.e. a rise in FHR exceeding 15 beats/min in amplitude and lasting more than 15 seconds at any point during the test) in 20 minutes, or three accelerations in 15 minutes (Flynn and Kelly, 1977; Evertson, 1979; Keegan *et al.*, 1980; Phelan, 1981; Flynn *et al.*, 1982b; Freeman *et al.*, 1982a; Boehm *et al.*, 1986). However, the time required to achieve a *reactive* NST is normally distributed, and the number of falsely abnormal test results can be greatly reduced by extending the testing duration. There is no significant difference in the intra- and interobserver variability when the cardiotocogram is classified as either *reactive* or *nonreactive* (Flynn *et al.*, 1982b). A *nonreactive* NST usually triggers the performance of either a contraction stress test (CST) or a fetal biophysical profile (BPP) (Box

Box 18.1 The contraction stress test and biophysical profile.

Contraction stress test (CST)
The CST involves a study of the FHR in reaction to either spontaneous or induced uterine contractions. In fact the interpretation of a CST is based on the presence or absence of late decelerations in association with contractions. Uterine contractions could be induced by infusion or oxytocin or by nipple stimulation (Owen *et al.*, 1989). Possible CST interpretations include (Freeman *et al.*, 1982a, b):

positive	consistent and persistent late deceleration without excessive uterine activity (hyperstimulation)
negative	no late deceleration

Biophysical profile (BPP)
The BPP combines the NST with objective sonographic measurements of fetal movement, fetal tone, fetal breathing, and amniotic fluid (Manning *et al.*, 1980).

NST	2 points if reactive; 0 otherwise
tone and posture	2 points if there is a demonstration of active extension with rapid return of flexion of fetal limbs, or trunk rotation; 0 otherwise
gross body/limb movements	2 points if there are more than three discrete movements in a 30-minute period; 0 otherwise
breathing	2 points if there is more than one episode of 30 seconds duration, intermittent within a 30-minute period overall; 0 otherwise
amniotic fluid volume	2 points if there is one pocket > 3 cm without umbilical cord loops or more than 1 pocket of > 2 cm without cord loops; 0 otherwise

Thus, the BPP score can range from 0 to 10.

A positive CST or a BPP < 4 is often considered an indication for delivery. A BPP of 6 or more is reassuring and testing may continue semi weekly or weekly depending upon the indication.

18.1). The percentage of healthy fetuses with a *reactive* NST increases with advancing gestational age.

Implications of testing

WHAT DOES AN ABNORMAL TEST RESULT MEAN?

The response of the caregiver to a *nonreactive* NST depends on the underlying clinical condition, gestational age and the type of abnormality discovered. Clinical action prompted by abnormal test results shows marked variation between and within centers (Flynn *et al.*, 1982a). For instance, a *nonreactive* NST at a very early stage of gestation (i.e. up to 28 weeks) is typically followed by another – diagnostic – test of fetal wellbeing (e.g. a BPP), since a *nonreactive* NST may be normal and a reassuring secondary test result will provide justification to delay preterm delivery. The effectiveness of such a policy, however, has never been demonstrated by randomized controlled trials (Neilson, 1994). The response to an abnormal NST changes after 36 weeks. By that stage, active management such as induction of labor or cesarean section is often preferred to conservative management. Again, the effectiveness of such a policy in low-risk women remains to be established. There are only four published randomized controlled trials evaluating the effectiveness of antepartum nonstress cardiotocography in women at increased risk of fetal demise (Flynn *et al.*, 1982a; Brown *et al.*, 1982; Lumley *et al.*, 1983; Kidd *et al.*, 1985). From these trials, there is no evidence that the use of NST is beneficial (Neilson, 1994).

WHAT DOES A NORMAL TEST RESULT MEAN?

A *reactive* NST is generally considered to be indicative of fetal wellbeing, in particular in those at low risk of fetal demise. A *reactive* NST predicts that the fetus will be alive one week later (Lumley *et al.*, 1983). In women at risk of fetal compromise, testing is repeated either weekly, twice weekly or daily. Such a policy, however, has not yet been shown to be effective in reducing fetal demise (Neilson, 1994).

What is the cost of testing?

The NST has never been evaluated in the context of a randomized controlled trial in the general obstetric population. Large observational series with either historical or geographical controls suggest a decrease in perinatal mortality for women at risk using the NST for antepartum surveillance, with the CST and BPP as back-up tests. Although not tested prospectively, some estimates of the cost of routine antepartum surveillance can be made. Assuming the target population has a perinatal mortality rate of 15 per 1000 – approximately that of a postdates (i.e. 42 or more weeks) population – and that the NST at a total (physician plus hospital) cost of $150 (US, 1995) is used as primary test, a nonreactive NST is followed by either a CST or BPP (at a cost of US $250 each), and the protocol reduces perinatal mortality by 50%, then the average pregnant woman will undergo three NSTs and 0.3 CST or BPP. This results in a cost per pregnancy screened using NST/CST of $625 (US, 1995) and a cost per perinatal death averted of $83 000 (US, 1995). If the BPP were used as the back-up test, the cost per pregnancy screened would be $700 and the cost per perinatal death averted $92 000 (US, 1995).

CONCLUSIONS AND RECOMMENDATIONS

Antepartum nonstress cardiotocography is commonly employed for the assessment of fetal wellbeing but the effectiveness of this test has to date not been evaluated by randomized controlled trial in women at low risk of fetal demise. Using optimistic estimates for the NST, CST and BPP derived mostly from observational studies (Flynn and Kelly, 1977; Freeman *et al.*, 1981, 1982a; Manning *et al.*, 1981; Phelan, 1981; Johnson *et al.*, 1986), it is concluded that these tests employed for antepartum fetal surveillance are likely to be cost-effective for the prevention of perinatal mortality in at-risk pregnancies. Hence, in the absence of definitive findings, it is reasonable to confine nonstress cardiotocography to pregnancies deemed at increased risk for fetal demise (i.e. perinatal mortality rate over 15 per 1000 pregnancies).

SUMMARY

1 WHAT IS THE PROBLEM THAT REQUIRES SCREENING?

ANTEPARTUM UTEROPLACENTAL DYSFUNCTION SEVERE ENOUGH TO CAUSE FETAL METABOLIC ACIDEMIA OR INTRAUTERINE DEATH.

a What is the incidence/prevalence of the target condition?

The overall rate of antepartum fetal death is approximately 2–4 per 1000 normally formed singleton births. Approximately 70% of these deaths are unexplained.

b What are the sequelae of the condition which are of interest in clinical medicine?

The fetus with metabolic acidemia from chronic hypoxemia secondary to uteroplacental dysfunction is likely to be growth restricted and is at increased risk of a progressive series of insults including ischemic multiorgan injury, neurodevelopmental abnormalities, and intrauterine death.

2 THE TESTS

Tests currently used for routine and selective antepartum surveillance include fetal movement counting and the nonstress test.

a What is the purpose of the test?

To screen pregnancies deemed at risk of fetal compromise so that timely intervention occurs before the development of acidemia, thus preventing intrauterine death.

b The nature of the tests

Fetal movement counting: The minimum number of fetal movements considered acceptable ranges from three in 1 hour to ten in 24 hours.

Nonstress test: The interpretation is based on both the frequency and magnitude of fetal heart rate accelerations.

c Implications of testing

1 What does an abnormal test result mean?

Decreased maternal perception of fetal movement triggers the performance of an NST. However, given the low prevalence of fetal compromise and an estimated specificity of 90–95%, positive predictive values for fetal compromise are low, ranging from 2% to 7%. With regard to a *nonreactive* NST in early gestation is typically followed by another – diagnostic – test of fetal wellbeing. After 36 weeks' gestation, a *nonreactive* NST is usually followed by active management of labor, such as induction or cesarean section. However, the effectiveness of such a policy in low-risk women remains to be established.

2 What does a normal test result mean?

Both normal fetal movement counts and a *reactive* NST are considered to be indicative of fetal wellbeing, in particular in women deemed to be at low risk of fetal compromise. In women at risk, NST is repeated either weekly or twice weekly.

d **What is the cost of testing?**

Using optimistic estimates derived mostly from observational studies, it is concluded that the NST is likely to be cost-effective for the prevention of perinatal mortality in a selective group of women, i.e. those with a risk of perinatal death of at least 15 per 1000.

3 CONCLUSIONS AND RECOMMENDATIONS

The merits of antepartum surveillance by formal fetal movement counting have not been clearly demonstrated. Given the absence of a beneficial effect on fetal wellbeing, formal fetal movement counting cannot be recommended as an integral part of antenatal care.

Antepartum nonstress cardiotocography is commonly employed for the assessment of fetal wellbeing but the effectiveness of this test has not been evaluated to date by randomized controlled trials in women at low risk. Hence, in the absence of definitive findings, it is reasonable to confine nonstress cardiotocography to pregnancies deemed at increased risk of intrauterine demise.

REFERENCES

Boehm FH, Salyer S, Shah DM & Vaughn WK (1986) Improved outcome of twice weekly nonstress testing. *Obstet Gynecol* **67:** 566–568.
Brown VA, Sawers RS, Parsons RJ, Duncan SLB & Cooke ID (1982) The value of antenatal cardiotocography in the management of high-risk pregnancy – a randomized controlled trial. *Br J Obstet Gynaecol* **89:** 716–722.
Evertson LR, Gauthier RJ, Schifrin BS & Paul RH (1979) Antepartum fetal heart rate testing. I. Evolution of the nonstress test. *Am J Obstet Gynecol* **133:** 29–33.
Flynn AM & Kelly J (1977) Evaluation of fetal well-being by antepartum fetal heart monitoring. *Br Med J* **1:** 936–939.
Flynn AM, Kelly J, Mansfield H, Needham P, O'Connor M & Viegas O (1982a) A randomized controlled trial of non-stress antepartum cardiotocography. *Br J Obstet Gynaecol* **89:** 427–433.
Flynn AM, Kelly J, Matthews K, O'Conor M & Viegas O (1982b) Predictive value of, and observer variability in, several ways of reporting antepartum cardiotocograms. *Br J Obstet Gynaecol* **89:** 434–440.
Freeman RK, Garite TJ, Mondanlou H, Dorchester W, Rommal C & Devaney M (1981) Post-date pregnancy: Utilization of contraction stress testing for primary fetal surveillance. *Am J Obstet Gynecol* **140:** 128–35.
Freeman RK, Anderson G & Dorchester W (1982a) A prospective multi-institutional study of antepartum fetal heart rate monitoring. I. Risk of perinatal mortality according to antepartum fetal heart rate test results. *Am J Obstet Gynecol* **143:** 771–7.
Freeman RK, Anderson G & Dorchester W (1982b) A prospective multi-institutional study of antepartum fetal heart rate monitoring. II. Contraction stress test versus nonstress test from primary surveillance. *Am J Obstet Gynecol* **143:** 778–81.
Goodwin TM, Belai I, Hernandez P, Durand M & Paul RH (1992) Asphyxial complications in the term newborn with severe umbilical acidemia. *Am J Obstet Gynecol* **167:** 1506–12.
Grant AM, Elbourne DR, Valentin L & Alexander S (1989) Routine formal fetal movement counting and the risk of antepartum late death in normally formed singletons. *Lancet* **ii:** 345–49.
Johnson JM, Harman CR, Lange IR & Manning FA (1986) Biophysical profile scoring in the management of the postterm pregnancy: an analysis of 307 patients. *Am J Obstet Gynecol* **154:** 269–73.
Keegan KA, Paul RH, Broussard PM, McCart D & Smith MA (1980) Antepartum fetal heart rate testing. V. The non-stress test – an outpatient approach. *Am J Obstet Gynecol* **136:** 81–3.

Kidd LC, Patel NB & Smith R (1985) Non-stress antenatal cardiotocography – a prospective randomized clinical trial. *Br J Obstet Gynaecol* **92**: 1156–59.

Lumley J, Lester A, Anderson I, Renou P & Wood C (1983) A randomized trial of weekly cardiotocography in high risk obstetric patients. *Br J Obstet Gynaecol* **90**: 1018–26.

Manning FA, Platt LD & Sipos L (1980) Antepartum fetal evaluation: development of a fetal biophysical profile. *Am J Obstet Gynecol* 1980; **136**: 787–95.

Manning FA, Baskett TF, Morrison I & Lange I (1981) Fetal biophysical profile scoring: a prospective study in 1,184 high risk patients. *Am J Obstet Gynecol* **140**: 289–94.

Moore TR & Piacquadio K (1989) A prospective evaluation of fetal movement screening to reduce the incidence of antepartum fetal death. *Am J Obstet Gynecol* **160**: 1075–80.

Neilson JP (1994) Cardiotocography for antepartum fetal assessment. In Enkin MW, Keirse MJNC, Renfrew MJ & Neilson JP (eds) *Pregnancy and Childbirth Module* Cochrane Database of Systematic Reviews 03881 (Disk Issue 1). Oxford: Update Software.

Neldam S (1980) Fetal movements as an indicator of fetal well-being. *Lancet* **ii**: 1222–4.

Owen J, Hauth JC, Williams G, Davies RO, Goldenberg RL & Brumfield CG (1989) A comparison of perinatal outcome in patients undergoing contraction stress testing by nipple stimulation versus spontaneously occurring contractions. *Am J Obstet Gynecol* **160**: 1081–5.

Phelan JP (1981) The nonstress test: a review of 3,000 cases. *Am J Obstet Gynecol* **139**: 7–10.

Sadovsky E & Polishuk WZ (1976) Fetal heart rate monitoring in cases of decreased fetal movements. *Int J Gynecol Obstet* 285–8.

Sadovsky E & Polishuk WZ (1977) Fetal movements in utero. Nature, assessment, prognostic value, timing of delivery. *Obstet Gynecol* **50**: 49–55.

Sadovsky E & Yaffe H (1973) Daily fetal movement recording and fetal prognosis. *Obstet Gynecol* **31**: 845–50.

Soothill PW, Ajuyi RA, Campbell S, Ross EM, Candy DCA, Snijders RM & Nicolaides KH (1992) Relationship between fetal acidemia at cordocentesis and subsequent neurodevelopment. *Ultrasound Obstet Gynecol* **2**: 80–83.

Intrapartum Fetal Monitoring

WHAT IS THE PROBLEM THAT REQUIRES SCREENING?

INTRAPARTUM FETAL HYPOXIC INJURY.

The current goal of fetal heart rate (FHR) monitoring is the detection of fetal hypoxia-acidemia which can cause multiorgan complications in the newborn. This is a change from the mid-1970s when the goal of FHR monitoring was to decrease the occurrence of intrapartum fetal death with an implied reduction in cerebral palsy. As medicine evolved, it has become clear that intrapartum death is unusual and that cerebral palsy is usually the result of events occurring prior to the onset of labor. Hence, the morbidity associated with metabolic acidemia is more relevant from the standpoint of prevention.

What is the incidence/prevalence of the target condition?

Neither the incidence nor the prevalence of clinically 'significant' metabolic acidemia can be stated with certainty since a critical threshold which reliably predicts morbidity has not been established. It appears to be in the proximity of an umbilical artery pH below 7.00 or a base deficit of at least 16 mmol/l (Low *et al.*, 1994). Applying this definition, less than 0.5% of all newborns have severe metabolic acidosis (Low *et al.*, 1994).

Table 18.1 Newborn complications in term acidotic and control infants.

REPORTED CLINICAL COMPLICATION	METABOLIC ACIDOSIS[a] (n = 59)	MATCHED CONTROLS[b] (n = 59)	P VALUE
meconium staining of amniotic fluid	33%	19%	< 0.02
Apgar score < 7 at 1 min	64%	20%	< 0.01
Apgar score < 8 at 5 min	41%	13%	< 0.01
mean birthweight (g)	3257	3273	NS
newborns with one or more complications[c]	78%	27%	< 0.01
CNS	61%	15%	—
cardiovascular	59%	19%	—
respiratory	47%	14%	—
kidneys	14 (24%)	2 (3%)	—

[a] The criterion of severe metabolic acidosis used in this study was an umbilical artery buffer base < 30 mmol/l (equivalent to a base deficit greater than 16 mmol/l); [b] No metabolic or respiratory acidosis at delivery. Matching was on the basis of gestational age, birthweight, and date of delivery (within 12 months); [c] Newborn complications – minor, moderate, or severe; From: Low et al. (1994)

What are the sequelae of the condition which are of interest in clinical medicine?

The fetus or newborn with metabolic acidemia secondary to a sustained and progressive hypoxia is at risk for multiorgan injury including the brain, kidneys, heart, lung, bowel and the hemopoietic system (Table 18.1). Central nervous system injury *cannot* be attributed to intrapartum ischemia in the absence of coexisting acute injury to the respiratory, renal or gastrointestinal systems (ACOG, 1989). It may have been nonphysiologic to consider cerebral palsy a target of fetal monitoring since the prevalence of cerebral palsy has not diminished in the last 20 years despite a reduction in the frequency of hypoxic newborns (Rosen and Dickenson, 1994). This strongly suggests that cerebral palsy has its origins in events that occur remote from labor and delivery. There have been reports of an increase in the prevalence of cerebral palsy (Hagberg *et al.*, 1993), particularly among preterm infants. These reports may reflect improved survival of low birthweight infants, since the birthweight specific prevalence rates of cerebral palsy among infants weighing more than 2500 grams has remained largely stable (Mutch *et al.*, 1992). In addition, the effect of hypoxemia/acidemia on any organ system is likely to be dependent on gestational age. Low *et al.* (1995) found fetal metabolic acidemia had little or no impact on the baseline morbidity rates of newborns delivered prior to 32 weeks. Although not often used prospectively to guide newborn management, scoring systems which include the umbilical cord blood gases, buffer base and Apgar scores are predictive of subsequent newborn multi-organ injury in newborns above 32 weeks and could serve as a basis for an informed plan of neonatal management (Low *et al.*, 1994).

THE TEST

What is the purpose of the test?

To detect fetal hypoxemia during labor.

Intrapartum fetal heart rate monitoring, whether by intermittent auscultation or continuous FHR monitoring permits the detection and quantification of FHR alterations indicative of fetal hypoxemia. If not corrected, hypoxemia could lead to a clinically relevant metabolic acidemia which is generally regarded as an indirect measure of fetal compromise.

The nature of the test

Fetal heart rate monitoring.

Intrapartum cardiotocography consists of an evaluation of both the FHR (baseline heart rate and periodic changes) and uterine activity. The FHR is monitored either intermittently, using an obstetric stethoscope or Doppler ultrasonography, or continuously, externally by Doppler ultrasound or internally by an electrode applied to fetal scalp or fetal buttocks after the membranes have ruptured. The method chosen reflects the availability of trained personnel, the presence of risk factors for hypoxia/acidosis, as well as pragmatic and medicolegal considerations.

The widespread implementation of electronic fetal monitoring (EFM) during labor was based on its promotion as a diagnostic tool that provided more reliable and accurate information than intermittent auscultation. For example, Kelly (1973) concluded that intermittent auscultation samples only 1–2% of the available FHR and uterine activity data. Further, an earlier report from a national collaborative project concluded that FHR alterations detected by intermittent auscultation were those of serious fetal problems at the extremes (Benson *et al.*, 1968). Good agreement between auscultation and EFM exists only for severe variable decelerations (Applegate *et al.*, 1979). The relationship is reduced for less serious patterns and beat-to-beat variability and mild to moderate late decelerations cannot be determined by intermittent auscultation.

There are no data from low-risk women that permit identification of the optimal time interval for auscultation. It is traditionally recommended that the FHR be evaluated at least every 30 minutes during and immediately after a contraction in the active phase of labor, and at least every 15 minutes in the second stage of labor. Should risk factors for hypoxia/acidemia be present during labor, the FHR should be assessed by one of the following methods (American Academy of Pediatrics, American College of Obstetricians and Gynecologists, 1988).

Intermittent auscultation at 15-minute intervals after a uterine contraction during the first stage of labor, and at 5-minute intervals (at least) after a uterine contraction during the second stage of labor, which is equivalent to EFM as a means to assess fetal condition (ACOG, 1995). Intermittent auscultation typically requires a one-to-one nurse–patient ratio.

Continuous monitoring of FHR and uterine activity. The FHR is obtained either with an external Doppler ultrasound or an internal electrode to fetal scalp or buttocks. The identification of uterine activity provides a temporal reference for FHR alterations. It is determined either with an external tocodynamometer or an internal intrauterine pressure system. Fetal heart rate data are categorized by the baseline rate (the modal heart rate between contractions and/or periodic change) and the presence of periodic changes. Included in the assessment of baseline FHR are fluctuations about the baseline, i.e. long-term and short-term variability. Variability is generally considered a more reliable predictor of fetal cardiovascular status than the baseline rate itself. Periodic (i.e. less than 10 minutes' duration) FHR alterations include accelerations as well as decelerations. Decelerations, which are defined as a decline in the heart rate below the baseline FHR, are either uniform in configuration with regard to shape, magnitude, time of onset and offset, and symmetry, or nonuniform. Early and late decelerations are uniform decelerations. Any deceleration that is not uniform is by definition nonuniform, or variable. Variable and late decelerations may combine to form mixed decelerations. Late decelerations result from hypoxemia and variable decelerations from umbilical cord compression. Early decelerations are thought to be secondary to fetal head compression.

Full documentation of neonatal outcome measures is important for the neonatologist and the obstetrician. Umbilical arterial and/or venous blood gas measurements allow the objective categorization of the type (metabolic, mixed, respiratory), degree, and indirectly the duration of fetal acidemia. Such information enhances the interpretation of newborn findings. The umbilical cord is doubly clamped prior to the first newborn breath. The blood gases are reasonably stable within the cord for at least 90 minutes. Umbilical arterial and/or venous blood samples are aspirated into heparinized syringes. Blood gas parameters commonly measured include pH, calculated base deficit, P_{CO_2}, P_{O_2} and bicarbonate. While the Apgar score reflects the newborn's immediate adaptation to life ex utero, it is not a reliable means for the evaluation of the acid-base status.

Implications of testing

WHAT DOES AN ABNORMAL TEST RESULT MEAN?

The fetus is at risk for intrapartum hypoxemia. An abnormal test may result from either FHR or uterine activity. It is important that periodic FHR changes be appropriately designated to avoid unnecessary interventions (Box 18.2). Interventions to reduce the frequency and severity of these changes include fluid administration (intravenous or intrauterine), oxygen administration by mask (8–10 l/min) and position change (ACOG,

Box 18.2   Abnormal patterns of the cardiotocogram

(a) *Uterine contractions*: Tachysystole (an aaverage of fove or more contractions per 10-minute window), prolonged contractions (lasting more than 90 seconds) and tetanic contractions each increase the risk of fetal hypoxemia by decreasing recovery time.

(b) *Fetal Heart Rate*: The phrase 'non-reassuring' is preferred to 'abnormal' since positive findings are not highly predictive of a specific adverse end-point. A nonreassuring FHR on auscultation is indicated by either a baseline rate between uterine contractions of less than 100 beats/min; a rate less than 100 beats/min 30 seconds after a contraction; unexplained baseline tachycardia of more than 160 beats/min, especially in an at-risk patient in whom the tachycardia persists through three or more contractions (10–15 minutes) despite corrective measures (ACOG, 1989). Either continuous EFM or another ancillary test (fetal capillary blood gas sampling or vibroacoustic stimulation) may provide supplemental information to aid management decisions should abnormal auscultatory findings be encountered.

A nonreassuring FHR or EFM can result from either a change in the baseline or the presence of repetitive periodic changes (variable or late decelerations); the latter generally have greater clinical significance. Nonreassuring findings include significant variable decelerations to less than 70 bpm, lasting more than 60 seconds, and persistent late decelerations (i.e. present with most contractions) (ACOG, 1995).

Late decelerations may be a response to uteroplacental dysfunction (e.g. that associated with severe fetal growth restriction and fetal hypoxia).

Fetal tachycardia may result from a fetal tachyarrhythmia, maternal fever, chorioamnionitis or a compensatory response to hypoxemia. Persistent fetal tachycardia in most instances is not associated with adverse outcome unless associated with either a decrease in variability or periodic changes. Absent or minimal baseline variability or progressive loss of variability in association with repetitive periodic decelerations is also considered nonreassuring, as in a sinusoidal heart rate pattern.

1995). Where there is uncertainty regarding the fetal status, ancillary testing such as fetal scalp blood sampling or fetal vibroacoustic stimulation may be helpful (Smith *et al.*, 1986; Newham *et al.*, 1990). The reduction/discontinuation of oxytocin or, in some cases, the administration of a tocolytic agent may be useful to decrease contraction frequency. Cesarean delivery may be indicated if the severe decelerations are nonremediable and vaginal delivery is not imminent (typically considered to be < 1 hour).

Electronic fetal monitoring is a poor predictor of the neonatal Apgar score, having a reasonable association only with scores of 0 or 1. In early series, positive predictive values for a 1-minute Apgar score of 6 or less ranged from 43% to 66%, while negative predictive values varied from 91% to 93% (Schifrin *et al.*, 1972; Gabert and Stenchever, 1973). On the basis of these results, clinicians tend to place greater reliance on normal and reassuring findings than on abnormal and nonreassuring findings. This conclusion is likely to be a reflection of the low prevalence of low Apgar scores and not just the predictive ability of EFM. In addition, the poor predictive value of EFM for a low Apgar score may have more to do with the poor association between Apgar scores and newborn metabolic status (Sykes *et al.*, 1982; Steer *et al.*, 1989).

The available literature indicates little benefit from continuous compared with intermittent FHR monitoring (Neilson, 1994) (Tables 18.2 and 18.3). The only consistent exception has been an apparent reduction in the number of newborns who develop seizures. Electronic fetal monitoring may be beneficial in the low birthweight fetus (Neutra et al, 1978) but no randomized controlled trial has been conducted to substantiate this observation. Continuous EFM results in a significantly increased rate of cesarean delivery (Tables 18.2, 18.3). Inaccurate reading or overinterpretation of the cardiotocograph (CTG) is likely to be the cause of much of the increased rate. The chance of performing an unnecessary cesarean section can be minimized by utilizing fetal scalp blood sampling whenever the caregiver is unsure of a fetal heart rate tracing's interpretation.

The impact of EFM on perinatal outcome measures such as the frequency of hypoxic fetal-neonatal organ injury is not well documented. However, the finding that neonatal seizures are reduced, especially when interpretation of the CTG is underpinned by the availability of fetal scalp blood sampling (Table 18.2), strongly suggests that there is benefit in identifying the hypoxic fetus during labor. Our inability to document clearly an altered perinatal outcome may indicate that the underlying pathophysiology is modified only marginally by our interventions, or that these events are so rare they almost prohibit study. For example, it is thought that the fetus is at increased risk of organ

Table 18.2 Results from a systematic review of randomized controlled trials of EFM **without** resort to fetal scalp blood sampling compared to intermittent auscultation.

OUTCOME	TYPICAL ODDS RATIO	95% CONFIDENCE INTERVAL
all perinatal deaths	1.94	0.20 to 18.62
all cesarean sections	2.70	1.92 to 3.81
Apgar score < 7 at 1 min	1.13	0.83 to 1.54
admission to special care unit	1.03	0.76 to 1.38
neonatal seizures	0.80	0.21 to 2.90

From: Neilson (1994)

Table 18.3 Results from a systematic review of randomized controlled trials of EFM **with** the option to assess fetal acid–base status versus intermittent auscultation.

OUTCOME	TYPICAL ODDS RATIO	95% CONFIDENCE INTERVAL
all perinatal deaths	0.98	0.58 to 1.64
all cesarean sections	1.29	1.08 to 1.54
Apgar score < 7 at 1 min	0.98	0.84 to 1.14
admission to special care unit	1.00	0.90 to 1.12
neonatal seizures	0.49	0.29 to 0.82
cerebral palsy	1.79	0.98 to 1.64

From: Neilson (1994)

injury when the arterial pH is below 7.00 as a result of metabolic or mixed-metabolic acidosis. In one study of 14 453 newborns delivered between 1984 and 1992, only 59 (0.4%) had severe metabolic acidemia and 51 (0.75%) severe respiratory acidemia (Low et al., 1994).

WHAT DOES A NORMAL TEST RESULT MEAN?

Fetal hypoxemia is unlikely. Accelerations 15 beats/min above baseline are generally considered reassuring and inconsistent with significant acidemia. Fetal acidemia is not generally seen in the absence of periodic changes. Reassuring FHR findings do not require additional testing. However, reassuring FHR data do not guarantee the absence of later central nervous system dysfunction/cerebral palsy arising from insults prior to the onset of FHR evaluation. Normal umbilical blood gas measurements in the absence of acute cessation of fetal cardiac output exclude a causal role of intrapartum metabolic acidemia in the development of cerebral palsy and suggest that the labor was appropriately managed.

What is the cost of testing?

Medical care costs include those of delivering continuous FHR monitoring services, but it should be remembered that there are also subsequent costs such as those associated with complications affecting either mother or newborn above baseline rates as well as the additional medical costs of cesarean delivery and maternal infectious morbidity. An early report by Quilligan (1975) estimated the costs of delivering continuous FHR monitoring to be $33.50 (US, 1974) per patient. Banta and Thacker (1979) subsequently estimated that EFM added $50 (US, 1979) in the medical care costs of each delivery. Based on the available randomized controlled trials, they estimated that 25% of cesarean deliveries in 1979 could be attributed to EFM. Although this is probably an overestimate, the impact of EFM is nonetheless likely to be important. Based on the linkage of EFM to an increased risk of neonatal scalp abscesses, cesarean delivery and its suspected linkage to newborn RDS, Banta and Thacker estimated that EFM would add $411 million to the annual cost of childbirth if 50% of deliveries were monitored electronically. Though continuous EFM is associated with an increased rate of obstetric intervention, the true impact of EFM on the cesarean delivery rate independent of other trends in perinatal care is extremely difficult to evaluate. The complexity of determining the exact cause for the rise in cesarean deliveries with EFM was in one report attributed to such factors as liberalization of the diagnoses of cephalopelvic disproportion, 'fetal distress', a decrease in vaginal breech delivery, routine repeat cesarean delivery, alterations in residency training programs, a more interventionistic attitude on the part of the obstetric community, as well as possible financial incentives favoring cesarean delivery (Marieskind, 1978). The increased use of epidural anesthesia during labor and the relative increase in the frequency of nulliparous women may also contribute fractionally to the rise in the cesarean delivery rate.

The absence of demonstrated therapeutic efficacy for continuous EFM imposes limitations on any attempt to evaluate its cost-effectiveness from the health standpoint. However, assuming continuous EFM is equal to intermittent auscultation and the latter requires one-to-one nursing, EFM will be cost-effective in many countries where labor is the primary expense. However, the CTG must be observed constantly, interpreted carefully and appropriate action taken when indicated.

Though umbilical cord blood gas analysis has not been demonstrated to improve neonatal outcome, this may reflect its lack of integration into newborn care since it can be used for the triage of newborns. Further, improved neonatal outcome is a surrogate measure. Umbilical blood gas measurements provide important validation of the intrapartum management in the face of unexpectedly poor Apgar scores. Although the patient charge for umbilical cord gas analysis may exceed $80 (US, 1995), this is not necessarily reflective of the actual costs, much of which may be borne by Hospital Risk Management programs. If one assumes that the expense of necessary equipment, personnel and space is already covered and that there is excess capacity, only marginal costs (heparinized syringes and laboratory supplies) are relevant. At Thomas Jefferson University Hospital the marginal cost of umbilical blood gas measurement is only $3.50 (US, 1995) per specimen.

Care must be exercised in arguing that umbilical cord blood gas analyses are cost-effective because of their potential to decrease the number or magnitude of malpractice awards. If society at large is the payer, the portion of money in a malpractice award which goes toward care can be viewed as a 'transfer payment' between parties, i.e. whoever pays for longterm care. Money saved by reducing expenses such as those arising from court costs, loss of defendant productivity, payments to lawyers and experts, would be the only moneys considered under such an analysis as legitimate cost savings.

CONCLUSIONS AND RECOMMENDATIONS

The current rate of cerebral palsy (2–3 per 1000 live births) has not changed since the 1970s despite dramatic advances in prenatal, intrapartum and neonatal care. While FHR monitoring has not noticeably decreased the prevalence of cerebral palsy, it has decreased the rate of intrapartum fetal death. Although the number of newborns hypoxic from labor has declined, intrapartum fetal 'asphyxia' accounts for only 8–15% of cerebral palsy (Nelson and Ellenberg, 1986; Gaffney *et al.*, 1994; Richmond *et al.* 1994). Despite this small contribution, the American College of Obstetricians and Gynecologists estimates that 70% of claims alleging a causal role for intrapartum asphyxia end out of court with a payment.

Though there is no proven clinical benefit to the measurement of the umbilical blood gases, there is no other method which provides the caregiver information on the degree and type of fetal acidemia present at the moment of birth. The Apgar score is not reliable as a means to make such an assessment. Thus, an umbilical cord segment be doubly clamped at each delivery and the gases measured in the event of perceived need.

Electronic fetus monitoring has dramatically changed the management of high-risk pregnancies. For example, reassuring intrapartum EFM findings in diabetic and preeclamptic patients provide the necessary level of reassurance to justify a trial of labor. Prior to the late 1970s such patients were commonly subjected to elective cesarean delivery.

While intermittent auscultation is apparently equal to continuous FHR monitoring for the reduction of perinatal mortality and adverse longterm neurologic outcomes in low-risk women, it will be difficult for health care providers to discontinue its use. However, EFM provides documentation that can be viewed retrospectively should the nurse leave the room; it requires only modest additional training of nurses and has a low maintenance cost. As health care systems continue to reduce costs, they will reduce nursing staff. It will become increasingly difficult to provide the one-to-one nursing care which is a requirement for acceptable intermittent auscultation, the alternative to continuous EFM. Further research to address the comparative effectiveness of continuous EFM versus intermittent auscultation, particularly with regard to the detection of fetal acidemia and the prevention of newborn multiorgan system injury is highly desirable and justifiable.

SUMMARY

1 WHAT IS THE PROBLEM THAT REQUIRES SCREENING?

INTRAPARTUM FETAL HYPOXIC INJURY.

a What is the incidence/prevalence of the target condition?

Less than 0.5% of all newborns have a significant metabolic or mixed acidemia.

b What are the sequelae of the condition which are of interest in clinical medicine?

The fetus/newborn with metabolic acidemia secondary to a sustained and progressive hypoxemia is at risk for multiorgan system injury.

2 THE TEST

a What is the purpose of the test?

To detect fetal hypoxemia during labor.

b The nature of the test

Fetal heart rate monitoring.

c Implications of testing

1 What does an abnormal test result mean?

The fetus is at risk for intrapartum hypoxemia. An abnormal test may result from either uterine activity or FHR. Abnormal cardiotocographic findings frequently lead to a modification of labor management (maternal position change, supplemental oxygen, intravenous and intrauterine fluids). Where there is uncertainty about the fetal status, ancillary testing such as fetal scalp blood sampling or vibroacoustic stimulation may be helpful. Cesarean section is indicated if there are severe nonremedial decelerations and prompt vaginal delivery is unlikely. The available literature indicates little increased benefit from continuous EFM when compared with intermittent auscultation. The likelihood of cesarean section is increased by continuous EFM during labor.

2 What does a normal test result mean?

Fetal hypoxemia is unlikely. Accelerations 15 beats/min above baseline are generally considered reassuring and inconsistent with significant acidemia. Fetal acidemia is not generally seen in the absence of periodic changes.

d What is the cost of testing?

The absence of demonstrated therapeutic efficacy imposes limitations on any attempt to evaluate its cost-effectiveness from the health standpoint. However, assuming continuous FHR monitoring is equal to intermittent auscultation and the latter requires one-to-one nursing, continuous FHR monitoring will be cost-effective in many countries where labor is the primary expense.

3 CONCLUSIONS AND RECOMMENDATIONS

Intrapartum FHR monitoring has reduced the rate of intrapartum fetal death but has had no effect on the rate of cerebral palsy. While intermittent auscultation is apparently equal to continuous EFM for the reduction of perinatal mortality and adverse longterm neurologic outcomes in low-risk women, it will be difficult for health care providers to discontinue its use. Continuous EFM provides documentation that can be viewed retrospectively should the nurse leave the room; it does not require a large amount of nursing training and has a low maintenance cost. As health care systems continue to reduce costs, they will reduce nursing staff. Though there is no proven clinical benefit to the measurement of umbilical blood gases, there is no other method that provides the caregiver information on the degree and type of fetal acidemia present at the moment of birth.

REFERENCES

American Academy of Pediatrics, American College of Obstetricians and Gynecologists (1988) *Guideline for Perinatal Care*, 2nd edn, p. 67. Washington DC: AAP, ACOG.

ACOG (1977) *Intrapartum Fetal Heart Rate Monitoring*. Technical Bulletin 44, January.

ACOG (1989) *Intrapartum Fetal Heart Rate Monitoring*. Technical Bulletin 132, September.

ACOG (1995) *Fetal Heart Rate Patterns: Monitoring, Interpretation, and Management*. Technical Bulletin 207, July.

Applegate J, Haverkamp AD, Orleans M & Taylor C (1979) Electronic fetal monitoring: Implications for obstetrical nursing. *Nursing Res* **6**: 369–371.

Banta HD & Thacker SB (1979) *Costs and Benefits of EFM: a Review of the Literature*. US Dept HEW PHEW Publication 79–3245.

Benson RC, Schubec F, Deutchberger J *et al.* (1968) Fetal heart rate as a predictor of fetal distress. A report from a collaborative project. *Obstet Gynecol* 32: 259–266.

Cunningham FG, MacDonald PC & Gant NF (1989) *Williams Obstetrics*, 18th edn, pp. 298–300. Englewood Cliffs: Prentice-Hall Int.

Gabert HA & Stenchever MA (1973) Continuous electronic monitoring of fetal heart rate during labor. *Am J Obstet Gynecol* 115: 919–923.

Gaffney G, Flavell V, Johnson A, Squier M & Sellers S (1994) Cerebral palsy and neonatal encephalopathy. *Arch Dis Child* 70: F195–F200.

Gilstrap LC, Levano KJ, Burris J, Williams Ml & Little BB (1989) Diagnosis of birth asphyxia on the basis of fetal pH, Apgar score, and newborn cerebral dysfunction. *Am J Obstet Gynecol* 161: 825–30.

Goldaber KG, Gilstrap LC, Levano KJ, Dax JS & McIntyre DD (1991) Pathologic fetal acidemia. *Obstet Gynecol* 78: 1103–7.

Goodwin TM, Belai I, Hernandez P, Durand M & Paul RH (1992) Asphyxial complications in the term newborn with severe umbilical acidemia. *Am J Obstet Gynecol* 162: 1506–12.

Hagberg B, Hagberg G & Olow I (1993) The changing panorama of cerebral palsy in Sweden. VI. Prevalence and origin during the birth year period 1983–1986. *Acta Paediatr* 387–93.

Kelly VC & Kulkarni D (1973) Experiences with fetal monitoring in a community hospital. *Obstet Gynecol* 41: 818–824.

Low JA, Panagiotopoulos C & Derrick EJ (1994) Newborn complications after intrapartum asphyxia with metabolic acidosis in the term fetus. *Am J Obstet Gynecol* 170: 1081–7.

Low JA, Panagiotopoulos C & Derrick EJ (1995) Newborn complications after intrapartum asphyxia with metabolic acidosis in the preterm fetus. *Am J Obstet Gynecol* 172: 805–10.

Marieskind H (1978) *An Evaluation of Cesarean Section in the USA*. A report submitted to the Department of Health, Education and Welfare.

Mutch L, Alberman E, Hagberg B, Kodama K & Perat MV (1992) Cerebral palsy epidemiology: where are we now and where are we going? *Dev Med Child Neurol* 34: 547–51.

Neilson JP (1994) EFM alone versus intermittent auscultation in labour. In: Enkin MW, Keirse MJNC, Renfrew MJ, & Neilson JP (eds) *Pregnancy and Childbirth Module* Cochrane Database of Systematic Reviews 03298 (Disk Issue 1).

Nelson KB & Ellenberg JH (1986) Antecedents of cerebral palsy. Multivariate analysis of risk. *N Engl J Med* 315: 81–6.

Neutra RR, Fienberg SE, Greenland S *et al.* (1978) The effect of fetal monitoring on neonatal death rates. *N Engl J Med* 299: 324–6.

Newham JP, Burns SE & Roberman BD (1990) Effect of vibratory acoustic stimulation on the duration of fetal heart rate monitoring tests. *Am J Perinatol* 7: 232–4.

Quilligan EJ & Hall RH (1975) Fetal monitoring: Is it worth it? *Obstet Gynecol* 45: 96–100

Richmond S, Niswander K, Snodgrass CA & Wagstaff I (1994) The obstetric management of fetal distress and its association with cerebral palsy. *Obstet Gynecol* 83: 643–6.

Rosen MG & Dickenson JC (1992) The incidence of cerebral palsy. *Am J Obstet Gynecol* 167: 417–23.

Schifrin BS & Dame L (1972) Fetal heart rate patterns prediction of Apgar score. *JAMA* 219: 1322–5.

Smith CV, Phelan JP, Platt LD, Broussard P & Paul RH (1986) Fetal acoustic stimulation testing. II. A randomized clinical comparison with the nonstress test. *Am J Obstet Gynecol* 155: 131–4.

Steer PJ, Eigbe F, Lisauer TJ & Beard RW (1989) Interrelationships among abnormal cardiotocograms in labor, meconium staining of the amniotic fluid, arterial cord blood pH, and Apgar score. *Obstet Gynecol* 74: 715–21.

Sykes GS, Molloy PM, Johnson P *et al.* (1982) Do Apgar scores indicate asphyxia? *Lancet* 1982; i: 494–6.

Winkler CL, Hauth JC, Tucker MJ, Owen J & Brumfield CG (1991) Neonatal complications at term as related to the degree of umbilical artery acidemia. *Am J Obstet Gynecol* 164: 637–41.

19

Intrapartum Coagulation Studies

Jami Star & Jeffrey F. Peipert

WHAT IS THE PROBLEM THAT REQUIRES SCREENING?

BLEEDING ABNORMALITIES DURING LABOR.

Several obstetric conditions that predispose the patient to hemorrhage. These include preeclampsia, placental abruption, intrauterine fetal demise (IUFD), amniotic fluid embolus and thrombocytopenia.

What is the incidence/prevalence of the target condition?

Preeclampsia complicates approximately 3–7% of pregnancies (Roberts, 1994) (see also Chapter 13). It is most common in nulliparous women and women with underlying vascular disease (e.g. chronic hypertension, renal disease, and connective tissue disease).

Placental abruption complicates approximately 1% of pregnancies (Green, 1994).

Disseminated intravascular coagulation (DIC) in the setting of IUFD occurs in 25% of patients by 4 weeks after fetal death has occurred (Dixon, 1973). Generally, the coagulopathy is not acute; rather, it is a chronic DIC defined by abnormalities of the primary coagulation tests, the magnitude of which depend on the length of time that the fetus is retained.

Amniotic fluid embolism occurs in 1 per 8 000 to 1 per 80 000 deliveries. It is fatal in more than 80% of cases (Killam, 1985).

Maternal thrombocytopenia ($< 150\ 000/\mu l^3$) of any cause complicates 6–7% of pregnancies (Burrows and Kelton, 1993a). One cause of thrombocytopenia, immune thrombocytopenia (ITP), has a 3:1 female preponderance. It is probably the most common autoimmune disorder of pregnancy, occurring in approximately 2–3 per 1000 pregnancies (Burrows and Kelton, 1993b).

What are the sequelae of the condition which are of interest in clinical medicine?

While hemorrhage is a major cause of maternal morbidity and mortality in the industrialized world, most events occur secondary to postpartum uterine atony. Antepartum-hemorrhage is most often associated with placental abruption or previa. Intrapartum coagulopathy is an uncommon event.

Preeclampsia is a leading cause of maternal and perinatal morbidity and mortality as a result of significant multisystemic manifestations.

Placental abruption releases tissue thromboplastin into the maternal circulation triggering the coagulation cascade (Sher and Statland, 1985). About 10% of patients with placental abruption will manifest clotting abnormalities (Sher, 1977). Hypofibrinogenemia, thrombocytopenia and increased fibrin degradation products (FDPs) are uncommon with minimal placental separation. A separation of more than 50% of the placental surface area is associated with fetal distress and fetal loss, and the risk of a clotting abnormality approximates 25–30% (Pritchard, 1973).

Between 0.5% and 2% of women with a retained IUFD *and* abnormal primary coagulation tests develop a hemorrhagic complication if untreated.

Amniotic fluid embolus is a rare event characterized by two clinical phases. In the first, cardiopulmonary collapse occurs. Approximately 40% of women who survive the initial cardiopulmonary insult develop clotting abnormalities that often present as hemorrhage (uterine atony, bleeding from wounds) (Taenaka *et al.*, 1981). The exact pathophysiology of DIC in the setting of amniotic fluid embolus is unknown, although amniotic fluid has procoagulant activity (Courtney and Allington, 1972; Phillips and Davidson, 1972; Salem *et al*, 1982).

Spontaneous bleeding secondary to thrombocytopenia is uncommon provided platelet function is normal and the platelet count is greater than 20 000/μl^3. Excessive surgical bleeding secondary to thrombocytopenia is rare when the count is greater than 50 000/μl^3 (Fellin and Murphy 1987). Bleeding in the adult with ITP is usually mild to moderate consisting of ecchymoses, gingival bleeding, epistaxis, menorrhagia, and hematuria. The most serious complication of ITP in nonsurgical patients is intracranial hemorrhage which occurs in less than 1% of untreated patients. It is often stated that the fetus of the woman with ITP is at risk for intracranial hemorrhage during labor and delivery. This has not been substantiated. The risk of a fetal hemorrhage intrapartum is so low that there is not a single well-documented case in the English language literature (Burrows and Kelton, 1993b). This is not to say it has not happened, or cannot do so, but even a most liberal estimate of the risk is below 0.5%.

THE TESTS

What is the purpose of the tests?

To detect coagulation abnormalities that would place the laboring woman at increased risk of hemorrhage; to identify women likely to develop acute, decompensated DIC during the intrapartum period; to ensure the safety of conduction anesthesia.

The nature of the tests

The laboratory assessment of clotting is approached in stages. In the clinical environment, a series of primary tests are most commonly employed. A platelet count is the key test in the pregnant woman since thrombocytopenia frequently accompanies the disorders of interest and is typically due to increased consumption rather than decreased synthesis. The bleeding time, defined as the time required for bleeding to stop after a standardized puncture of the forearm (Giddings and Peake, 1985) is not a reliable indi-

Table 19.1   Cost of common coagulation tests.

	COST (US$)[a]
complete blood count (with platelets)	25.35
WBC differential	18.00
manual platelet count	14.00
prothrombin time	26.50
activated partial thromboplastin time	29.45
fibrinogen	35.70
fibrin degradation products	30.00
Ivy bleeding time	13.30

[a] These 1995 costs are typical of the authors' hospital, but may vary by laboratory

cator of in vivo platelet function. Rodgers and Levin (1990) concluded after an extensive review of the literature that there is no consistent relationship between the platelet count and the bleeding time, nor was there evidence that the bleeding time accurately predicted hemorrhagic risk.

The prothrombin time (PT) evaluates the extrinsic (vitamin K-dependent) and common clotting pathways (Suchman and Griner, 1986). A normal PT requires a minimum of 100 mg/dl of fibrinogen to be present (Bick, 1978). The activated partial thromboplastin time (APTT) evaluates the intrinsic and common pathways and is most sensitive to a deficiency of factors early in the cascade sequence, such as factors XII, XI, IX and VIII (Naumann and Weinstein, 1985). Both the PT and APTT can be prolonged if a factor level falls below 25% of normal (Burns *et al.*, 1993) or by a high concentration of FDPs when the fibrinogen level is also decreased (Ockelford and Carter, 1982). When used as a screening test for DIC, the sensitivity of the APTT is about 57%, with a false positive rate of 33%. A normal PT and APTT virtually rule out clinically significant soluble clotting cascade coagulopathies (Suchman and Griner, 1986).

A fibrinogen content less than 100 mg/dl intrapartum indicates either consumptive coagulopathy (Suchman and Griner, 1986) or extrinsic loss. Elevated FDP levels (greater than 40 µg/ml) indicate a stimulated fibrinolytic system but not necessarily an ongoing activation owing to their long half-life (Dixon, 1973). Additional tests can be performed depending on the results of these primary tests. The costs of standard coagulation tests are described in Table 19.1.

ACUTE DISSEMINATED INTRAVASCULAR COAGULOPATHY

Disseminated intravascular coagulopathy is not a disease, but rather a symptom of underlying pathology. It is defined as abnormal activation of the coagulation system with enhanced consumption of platelets and coagulation proteins (Ockelford and Carter, 1982). Fibrinolysis creates FDPs which impair fibrin monomer polymerization and platelet function. The DIC may be chronic or acute, compensated, decompensated, or hypercompensated. Acute DIC is usually associated with hemorrhage and rarely requires laboratory testing for diagnosis. The more common low-grade DIC typical of pregnancy complications is often detected only through laboratory abnormalities (Weiner, 1986).

Implications of testing

WHAT DOES AN ABNORMAL TEST RESULT MEAN?

The diagnosis of acute DIC is supported by findings of increased serum FDPs and/or schistocytes on a peripheral blood smear. The sensitivity, specificity, and predictive values of these tests cannot be determined owing to difficulties in the precise diagnosis of DIC (Ockelford and Carter, 1982). The approximate percentage of time these tests are abnormal in patients with acute DIC (sensitivity) is shown in Table 19.2.

Table 19.2 Sensitivity of laboratory abnormalities associated with DIC.

LABORATORY FINDING	SENSITIVITY (%)	REFERENCE
thrombocytopenia	> 90	Viner (1982)
increased PT	90	Viner (1982)
increased PTT	20–50	Bick (1978), Viner (1982)
decreased fibrinogen	70	Viner (1982)
increased FDPs (>5 µg/ml)	95	Viner (1982)
schistocytes	40	Jacobson and Jackson (1974)
decreased AT-III	97	Naumann and Weinstein (1985)

Laboratory testing is indicated should the diagnosis of acute DIC require confirmation, or if pharmacologic therapy is planned. These tests should include a complete blood count (with platelets and a peripheral smear), PT/APTT, fibrinogen and FDPs. A bedside clotting assessment ('hanging clot') can be easily performed by obtaining 5 ml of blood in a tube free of preservative or anticoagulant. The lack of a clot within 10 minutes indicates a fibrinogen level below 50 mg/dl; rapid clot breakdown indicates the presence of FDPs (Weiner, 1993). Where available, a measurement of either antithrombin III or thrombin-antithrombin complexes is the most sensitive indicator of DIC (Weiner, 1986)

PREECLAMPSIA

Early studies demonstrating fibrin deposition and microvascular thrombosis in the organs of preeclamptic women established the presence of accelerated coagulation (Pritchard *et al.*, 1976). Subsequent laboratory studies have shown that preeclampsia is associated with a chronic compensated DIC characterized by enhanced activation of the intrinsic pathway causing increased levels of fibrinopeptide A, decreased antithrombin III, increased D-dimer, increased FDPs and increased platelet activation (Bonnar *et al.*, 1971; Douglas *et al.*, 1982; Weiner and Brandt, 1982; Borok *et al.*, 1984; Vaziri *et al.*, 1986; Trofatter *et al.*, 1989). Antithrombin III consumption is similar to that seen in septic shock (Weiner *et al.* 1990).

Implications of testing

WHAT DOES AN ABNORMAL TEST RESULT MEAN?

Thrombocytopenia is usually the only primary clotting test abnormality in women with preeclampsia, occurring in 15–50% of patients. In the absence of thrombocytopenia, disturbances of other clotting tests are rare (Leduc *et al.*, 1992) and additional testing is not indicated. Fibrinogen levels are generally unchanged. In several small studies, FDPs have been shown to be increased (Gibson *et al.*, 1982). Less than 20% of women with severe disease have a prolonged PT/APTT. When prolonged, it is usually in the setting of a decompensated DIC (Perry and Martin, 1992). Laboratory or clinical evidence of DIC has been reported in 38–100% of patients with HELLP syndrome (Van Dam *et al.*, 1989). However, this additional testing does not change clinical management.

Some anesthesiologists require a bleeding time and/or a PT/APTT in women with preeclampsia before placing a conduction anesthetic. However, it has been observed that coagulation abnormalities occur only in patients with 'severe' preeclampsia and thrombocytopenia (Barker, 1991). Coagulation studies are not necessary if the platelet count is normal. Though the data is limited with respect to risk of hemorrhage in women with counts below 100 000/µl, many authors advise against regional anesthesia unless the presence of a coagulopathy is ruled out (Rolbin *et al.*, 1988).

PLACENTAL ABRUPTION

Implications of testing

WHAT DOES AN ABNORMAL TEST RESULT MEAN?

Abnormalities of coagulation in women with placental abruption are usually associated with more than a 50% separation. Fetal distress is the rule in this situation. The treatment of clinically significant placental abruption is usually delivery and a full coagulation work-up is indicated. In cases of mild abruption unassociated with either fetal distress or death, the only additional testing required is either a hanging clot or measurement of serum fibrinogen.

INTRAUTERINE FETAL DEMISE

The nature of the tests

Hypofibrinogenemia is the most consistent laboratory abnormality; thrombocytopenia is uncommon (Pritchard, 1973).

Implications of testing

WHAT DOES A NORMAL TEST RESULT MEAN?

Normal fibrinogen levels indicate that the woman is not currently at risk of hemorrhage from DIC.

WHAT DOES AN ABNORMAL TEST RESULT MEAN?

Hypofibrinogenemia may indicate the need for delivery in either singleton or advanced age multiple gestations. In the setting of a multiple gestation, low dose heparin therapy may be indicated if there has been a demise of a co-twin and the surviving twin is extremely premature. In this instance, hypofibrinogenemia may be reversed allowing the pregnancy to continue (Romero *et al.*, 1985).

AMNIOTIC FLUID EMBOLUS

Acute DIC can occur up to 12 hours after the initial symptoms of an amniotic fluid embolus (Killam, 1985). Laboratory abnormalities such as decreased platelet counts, decreased fibrinogen, increased FDPs and increased PT/APTT develop before there is clinical evidence of DIC (for example uterine atony, bleeding from wounds).

Implications of testing

WHAT DOES A NORMAL TEST RESULT MEAN?

Normal results for PT/APTT, platelet count and FDPs are reassuring. These laboratory tests should be followed serially when the diagnosis is suspected.

WHAT DOES AN ABNORMAL TEST RESULT MEAN?

Abnormal primary coagulation tests indicate the need for blood product replacement and pharmacologic therapy.

IMMUNE THROMBOCYTOPENIA

Implications of testing

WHAT DOES AN ABNORMAL TEST RESULT MEAN?

It has been suggested that maternal ITP indicates the need for a fetal platelet count because of the risk of intrapartum intracranial hemorrhage. Fortunately, there is little evidence that the thrombocytopenic fetus of the woman with ITP is at increased risk or that cesarian section alters the risk to the fetus. While the intrapartum diagnosis of fetal thrombocytopenia secondary to ITP by a scalp platelet count poses little risk to the fetus in the setting of maternal ITP, the risk to the fetus from antepartum diagnosis by in the setting of maternal ITP fetal blood sampling is death. Even in the most skilled hands, the risk of fetal death as a complication of cordocentesis is greater than the risk of fetal hemorrhage due to thrombocytopenia. Cordocentesis is therefore not indicated for the diagnosis of fetal thrombocytopenia secondary to ITP. The risk of antepartum diagnosis to the thrombocytopenic woman is intraoperative hemorrhage, possibly culminating in cesarean hysterectomy.

CONCLUSIONS AND RECOMMENDATIONS

There is no indication for routine evaluation of the coagulation system of the normal laboring woman. Pregnancies complicated by a disorder potentially associated with the development of a clinically significant DIC should be screened with either a platelet count or fibrinogen measurement as appropriate for clinical care. While clinical information is often sufficient for diagnostic purposes, a laboratory evaluation consisting of a complete blood count, platelet count, fibrinogen, FDPs, PT/APTT and bedside hanging clot studies can aid patient assessment and guide replacement therapy when needed.

A platelet count is the primary screening test for the detection of coagulation abnormalities in the laboring preeclamptic patient. If normal, no further testing is indicated. Other coagulation studies may be appropriate when there is thrombocytopenia (below 100 000/μl³). A full coagulation profile may also be useful in patients with predisposing conditions such as placental abruption or fetal death in addition to preeclampsia.

Since clinical signs may be limited and the disorder is treatable (subcutaneous heparin; Romero *et al.*, 1985), all women presenting with intrauterine fetal demise should be assessed for the development of a clotting abnormality by the measurement of serum fibrinogen on a weekly basis until delivery. When DIC accompanies the demise of a single fetus in a multiple gestation, subcutaneous heparin is an option.

In women with ITP, spontaneous vaginal delivery without antepartum or intrapartum diagnosis of fetal thrombocytopenia is the most prudent approach for mother and child. Because the thrombocytopenic fetus may be at increased risk of a bleeding complication during an instrumented vaginal delivery, a scalp platelet count may be considered before a nonemergent, operative vaginal delivery.

SUMMARY

1

WHAT IS THE PROBLEM THAT REQUIRES SCREENING?

BLEEDING ABNORMALITIES DURING LABOUR.

a What is the incidence/prevalence of the target condition?

Preeclampsia complicates approximately 3–7% of pregnancies. Placental abruption complicates approximately 1% of pregnancies. The coagulopathy of an intrauterine fetal demise rises to 25% by 4 weeks after death. Amniotic fluid embolism occurs in 1 per 8000 to 1 per 80 000 deliveries. Maternal thrombocytopenia (less than 150 000/μl) of any cause complicates 6–7% of pregnancies. One cause of thrombocytopenia, immune thrombocytopenia (ITP), has a 3 to 1 female preponderance. It is likely the most common autoimmune disorder of pregnancy occurring in approximately 2–3 per 1000 pregnancies.

b What are the sequelae of the condition which are of interest in clinical medicine?

Maternal hemorrhage causing maternal morbidity and mortality.

2 THE TESTS

a What is the purpose of the tests?

To detect women at risk during labor of a symptomatic disseminated intravascular coagulopathy.

b The nature of the tests

Platelet count, measurement of the fibrinogen level, PT, and PTT.

c Implications of testing

1 What does an abnormal test result mean?

The woman is at risk of developing a clinically important coagulopathy. Regional anesthesia may be contraindicated.

2 What does a normal test result mean?

The woman is likely to be at low risk of developing a clinically important coagulopathy.

d What is the cost of testing?

See Table 19.1.

3 CONCLUSIONS AND RECOMMENDATIONS

There is no indication to evaluate the coagulation system of the normal laboring woman. Pregnancies complicated by a disorder potentially associated with the development of a clinically significant DIC should be screened with either a platelet count or fibrinogen measurement as appropriate for clinical care.

REFERENCES

Barker P (1991) Coagulation screening before epidural analgesia in pre-eclampsia. *Anaesthesia* **46**: 64–67.

Bick RL (1978) Disseminated intravascular coagulation and related syndromes: etiology, pathophysiology, diagnosis and management. *Am J Hematol* **5**: 265–282.

Bonnar J, McNicol GP & Douglas AS (1971) Coagulation and fibrinolytic systems in preeclampsia and eclampsia. *Br Med J* **2**: 12–16.

Borok Z, Weitz J, Owen J, Auerbach M & Nossel HL (1984) Fibrinogen proteolysis and platelet alpha-granule release in preeclampsia/eclampsia. *Blood* **63**: 525–531.

Burns ER, Goldberg SN & Wenz B (1993) Paradoxic effect of multiple mild coagulation factor deficiencies on the prothrombin time and activated partial thromboplastin time. *Am J Clin Pathol* **100**: 94–98.

Burrows RF & Kelton JG (1993a) Fetal thrombocytopenia and its relation to material thrombocytopenia. *N Engl J Med* **329**: 1463–1466.

Burrows RF & Kelton JG (1993b) Pregnancy in patients with idiopathic thrombocytopenic purpura: assessing the risks for the infant at delivery. *Obstet Gynecol Surv* **48**: 781–788.

Courtney LD & Allington M (1972) Effect of amniotic fluid on blood coagulation. *Br J Haematol* **22**: 353–355.

Dixon RE (1973) Disseminated intravascular coagulation: a paradox of thrombosis and hemorrhage. *Obstet Gynecol Surv* **28**: 385–95.

Douglas JT, Shah M, Lowe, GDO *et al.* (1982) Plasma fibrinopeptide A and beta-thromboglobulin in pre-eclampsia and pregnancy hypertension. *Thromb Haemost* **47**: 54–55.

Fellin F & Murphy S (1987) Hematologic problems in the preoperative patient. *Med Clin North Am* **71:** 477–87.

Gibson B, Hunter D, Neame PB & Kelton JG (1982) Thrombocytopenia in preeclampsia and eclampsia. *Sem Thromb Hemost* **8:** 234–47.

Giddings JC & Peake IR (1985) Laboratory support in the diagnosis of coagulation disorders. *Clin Haematol* **14:** 571–95.

Green JR (1994) Placenta previa and abruptio placentae. In Creasy RK & Resnik R (eds) *Maternal–Fetal Medicine, Principles and Practice,* p. 610. Philadelphia: WB Saunders.

Jacobson RJ & Jackson DP (1974) Erythrocyte fragmentation in defibrination syndromes. *Ann Intern Med* **81:** 207–09.

Killam A (1985) Amniotic fluid embolism. *Clin Obstet Gynecol* **28:** 32–36.

Leduc L, Wheeler JM, Kirshon B, Mitchell P & Cotton DB (1992) Coagulation profile in severe preeclampsia. *Obstet Gynecol* **79:** 14–18.

Naumann RO & Weinstein L (1985) Disseminated intravascular coagulation – the clinician's dilemma. *Obstet Gynecol Surv* **40:** 487–92.

Ockelford PA & Carter CJ (1982) Disseminated intravascular coagulation: the application and utility of diagnostic tests. *Sem Thromb Hemost* **8:** 198–216.

Perry KG Jr & Martin JN (1992) Abnormal hemostasis and coagulopathy in preeclampsia and eclampsia. *Clin Obstet Gynecol* **35:** 338–50.

Phillips LL & Davidson EC (1972) Procoagulant properties of amniotic fluid. *Am J Obstet Gynecol* **113:** 911–19.

Pritchard JA (1973) Haematological problems associated with delivery, placental abruption, retained dead fetus and amniotic fluid embolism. *Clin Haematol* **2:** 563–86.

Pritchard JA, Cunningham FG, & Mason RA (1976) Coagulation changes in eclampsia: their frequency and pathogenesis. *Am J Obstet Gynecol* **124:** 855–64.

Roberts JM (1994) Pregnancy-related hypertension. In Creasy RK & Resnik R (eds) *Maternal–Fetal Medicine, Principles and Practice,* p. 807. Philadelphia: WB Saunders.

Rodgers RPC & Levin J (1990) A critical reappraisal of the bleeding time. *Semi Thromb Hemost* **16:** 1–20.

Rolbin SH, Abbott D, Musclow E et al (1988) Epidural anesthesia in pregnant patients with low platelet counts. *Obstet Gynecol* **71:** 918–20.

Romero R, Copel JA & Hobbins JC (1985) Intrauterine fetal demise and hemostatic failure: the fetal death syndrome. *Clin Obstet Gynecol* **28:** 24–31.

Salem HH, Walters WA, Perkin JL, Handley CJ & Firkin BG (1982) Aggregation of human platelets by amniotic fluid. *Br J Obstet Gynaecol* **89:** 733–37.

Sher G (1977) Pathogenesis and management of uterine inertia complicating abruptio placentae with consumption coagulopathy. *Am J Obstet Gynecol* **129:** 164–70.

Sher G & Statland BE (1985) Abruptio placentae with coagulopathy: a rational basis for management. *Clin Obstet Gynecol* **28:** 15–23.

Suchman AL & Griner PF (1986) Diagnostic uses of the activated partial thromboplastin time and prothrombin time. *Ann Intern Med* **104:** 810–16.

Taenaka N, Shimada Y, Kawai M, Yoshiya I & Kosaki G (1981) Survival from DIC following amniotic fluid embolism. *Anaesthesia* **36:** 389–93.

Trofatter KF, Howell ML, Greenberg CS & Hage ML (1989) Use of the fibrin D-dimer in screening for coagulation abnormalities in preeclampsia. *Obstet Gynecol* **73:** 435–39.

Van Dam PA, Renier M, Baekelandt M, Buytaert P & Uyttenbroeck F (1989) Disseminated intravascular coagulation and the syndrome of hemolysis, elevated liver enzymes, and low platelets in severe preeclampsia. *Obstet Gynecol* **73:** 97–102.

Vaziri ND, Toohey J, Powers D et al (1986) Activation of the intrinsic coagulation pathway in preeclampsia. *Am J Med* **80:** 103–7.

Viner ED (1982) Disseminated intravascular coagulation and other bleeding disorders in the critically ill patient: differential diagnosis and therapy. *Surg Ann* **14:** 1–23.

Weiner AE, Reid DE, Roby CC & Diamond LK (1950) Coagulation defects with intrauterine death from Rh isosensitization. *Am J Obstet Gynecol* **60:** 1015.

Weiner CP (1986) The obstetric patient and disseminated intravascular coagulation. *Clin Perinatol* **13:** 705–17.

Weiner CP (1993) Evaluation of clotting disorders during pregnancy. In Depp R, Eschenbach DA & Sciarra JJ (eds) *Gynecology and Obstetrics,* Vol.3 pp.1–14. Philadelphia: JB Lippincott.

Weiner CP & Brandt J (1982) Plasma antithrombin III activity: an aid in the diagnosis of preeclampsia-eclampsia. *Am J Obstet Gynecol* **142:** 275–81.

Weiner CP, Herrig J, Pelzer G & Heilskov J (1990) Elimination antithrombin III in healthy pregnant and preeclamptic women with an acquired antithrombin III deficiency. *Thromb Res* **58:** 395–406.

Postpartum Cord Blood Testing

Delores G. Cordle & Ronald G. Strauss

NEWBORN RH STATUS, HEMOLYTIC ANEMIA OF THE NEWBORN.

What is the incidence/prevalence of the target condition?

From 3% to 5% of pregnant women exhibit red blood cell (RBC) alloimmunization (isoimmunization) (Weinstein, 1982); a small fraction of their infants develop clinically significant hemolytic disease of the newborn. The incidence of clinically apparent hemolytic disease of the newborn for Rh antibodies is about 1 per 1000. Antibodies for other RBC antigens occur in 3 per 1000 births, of which approximately 10% (3 per 10 000) exhibit significant hemolytic disease of the newborn (Moise, 1994).

What are the sequelae of the condition which are of interest in clinical medicine?

Women who are Rh negative and deliver an Rh positive child are at risk for alloimmunization to D. Alloimmunization to Rh(D) can be prevented by the administration of anti-D immunoglobulin. Severe RBC alloimmunization, whether secondary to Rh(D) or another alloantibody may cause profound hemolytic anemia ending in intrauterine fetal death, preterm delivery and, after delivery, hyperbilirubinemia and kernicterus. Though fetal blood obtained from the umbilical cord at the time of birth can be tested for RBC incompatibilities, the results are poorly predictive of the clinical severity in the neonate.

What is the purpose of the tests?

To determine the newborn blood type to identify Rh(D) negative women at risk of developing alloimmunization. Such women should be given anti-D immunoglobulin prophylaxis to prevent the subsequent development of alloimmunization.

The nature of the tests

When indicated by clinical history, the blood obtained from the umbilical cord at delivery may be tested for ABO grouping and Rh type, as well as a direct antiglobulin test (DAT) and RBC antibody screen. Obtaining blood from the umbilical vessels avoids direct sampling of the neonate. While any blood test might be performed (e.g. serum chemistry analyses), the blood banking tests of interest are ABO group, Rh(D) type, direct antiglobulin test (also called a direct Coombs test) and RBC antibody screen. The results of these tests can help determine whether hemolytic disease of the newborn is a threat – particularly when viewed within the context of the maternal blood group and RBC antibody screen, the clinical setting, the serum bilirubin concentration, the blood hematocrit and the stained blood smear. Another purpose for cord blood testing is to determine the Rh(D) type of the neonate so that anti-D immunoglobulin can be given to unimmunized, Rh negative women during the immediate postpartum period.

The ABO grouping of neonates relies entirely on RBC antigen grouping, eliminating serum grouping for confirmation, because alloantibodies present in cord blood serum are of maternal, not infant, origin. Rh typing, including testing for weak D (formerly called D^u) is indicated for infants born to Rh negative mothers who are not already immunized to the Rh(D) antigen. Accurate Rh testing can be difficult if RBCs are heavily coated with immunoglobulin G (IgG) antibodies (positive direct antiglobulin test) or if samples are contaminated with Wharton's jelly (Walker, 1993).

The RBC antibody screen is intended to detect and identify maternal antibodies that have been transported across the placenta and are free in neonatal plasma. The DAT detects in vivo coating of cord blood RBCs by maternal IgG antibody. A negative direct antiglobulin test, however, does not guarantee absence of coating antibody, since antiglobulin reagents require approximately 200 molecules of IgG per RBC to give a positive reaction (Petz and Garratty, 1980) (see also Chapter 4).

Implications of testing

WHAT DOES AN ABNORMAL TEST RESULT MEAN?

A positive direct antiglobulin test usually indicates the presence of a red blood cell alloantibody. The antibody can be identified by *eluting* it from the RBCs and testing the *eluate* for specificity using a RBC panel. It is usually unnecessary to *elute* if the maternal serum contains clinically significant unexpected antibodies. However, this additional information occasionally can be of value in determining the type of antibodies responsible for hemolytic disease of the newborn (e.g. multiple maternal alloantibodies and unusually difficult instances of ABO hemolytic disease). A positive direct antiglobulin test on RBCs from infants of mothers with negative antibody screening tests – using standard group O screening RBCs – suggests the presence of ABO hemolytic disease of the newborn or a hemolytic disease of the newborn due to a low-incidence antigen not expressed on the screening cells. An *eluate* from the cord blood RBCs is required to confirm the diagnosis. The RBC antibody screen using cord blood plasma or serum serves the same purpose, particularly when reacted with group A_1 or B RBCs to establish the diagnosis of ABO hemolytic disease of the newborn. Because these tests are poorly predictive of hemolytic disease of the newborn, it is preferable to study only those infants who exhibit features of hemolytic disease of the newborn, such as anemia and/or indirect hyperbilirubinemia.

WHAT DOES A NORMAL TEST RESULT MEAN?

Women who are Rh negative and deliver an Rh positive child with a negative DAT should receive anti-D immunoglobulin (125–375 µg), depending upon local practices. These women should receive additional testing to detect the occurrence of a fetal to maternal hemorrhage greater than 30 ml, such as a peripheral blood smear stained with a Kleihauer-Betke stain to detect fetal RBCs. If a hemorrhage of this magnitude has occurred, additional anti-D immunoglobulin should be given to the mother (Judd et al., 1990; Crowther et al., 1993).

No testing is necessary on the cord blood from babies born to Rh positive mothers who have negative antibody screening tests in the absence of clinical signs and symptoms of hemolytic disease of the newborn.

What is the cost of testing?

Actual reagent and supply costs for cord blood ABO group, Rh(D) type and DAT screen are approximately US $1.25. Labor costs are $2, based on 10 minutes per test at $12 per hour. Thus, the total laboratory costs are about US $3.25. Patient charges include reagent costs, labor, and an overhead cost (e.g. space, utilities, insurance, etc.), and they often exceed laboratory costs several-fold. At the University of Iowa, the current charge is $63. When making economic decisions, it is perhaps better to focus on laboratory costs, not patient charges. The latter vary greatly among hospitals and do not reflect a true picture because of incomplete reimbursement.

It is possible to reduce health care costs by limiting cord blood testing to women with clinically significant maternal RBC antibodies or who are Rh negative. In the latter, the cord blood Rh type is used to determine need for anti-D immunoglobulin administration. But is this cost-effective? Assume 100 Rh(D) negative women who are not immunized to the Rh(D) antigen deliver infants of unknown Rh(D) type. Statistically, 60 newborns will be Rh positive and 40 Rh negative. The pharmacy cost at the University of Iowa for one 300 µg vial of anti-D immunoglobulin is approximately $50; the cost of administering it (nursing and materials) is another $25. Thus, the total cost of testing the 100 umbilical cord blood samples for their red blood cell ABO group, Rh(D) type, and DAT ($63 each), and of treating ($75 each) the 60 women with Rh positive children is $10 800. In comparison, the cost of simply treating the 100 women with anti-D immunoglobulin is $7500. Unfortunately, the second approach will miss the 1 in 200 to 1 in 400 women who experience a fetal to maternal transfusion greater than 30 ml whole blood.

CONCLUSIONS AND RECOMMENDATIONS

It is prudent to collect and accurately label an umbilical cord blood sample from all neonates at delivery. This sample can be used to determine the Rh(D) type from all neonates delivered of Rh negative women who have not been immunized to the Rh(D) antigen. This eliminates the need to sample neonates directly. It is neither wise nor cost-effective to test all cord blood samples routinely for ABO group, Rh(D) type, and DAT or anti-RBC antibody screen. It is better to study blood samples of only those infants who exhibit features of hemolytic disease of the newborn.

Although it is recommended that blood samples be collected from the umbilical cords of all neonates, it is not necessary to test cord blood samples routinely, except when the maternal serum contains clinically significant RBC antibodies or the mother is Rh negative (Judd *et al.*, 1990).

SUMMARY

1 WHAT IS THE PROBLEM THAT REQUIRES SCREENING?

NEWBORN RH STATUS, NEONATAL HEMOLYTIC ANEMIA.

a What is the incidence/prevalence of the target condition?

About 3–5% of pregnant women exhibit red blood cell (RBC) alloimmunization. The incidence of clinically apparent hemolytic disease of the newborn for Rh antibodies is about 1 per 1000. Antibodies for other RBC antigens occur in 3 per 1000 births, of whom approximately 10% (3 per 10 000) exhibit significant hemolytic disease of the newborn.

b What are the sequelae of the condition which are of interest in clinical medicine?

Women who are Rh negative and deliver an Rh positive child are at risk for alloimmunization to D. Severe RBC alloimmunization, whether secondary to Rh(D) or another alloantibody may cause profound hemolytic anemia ending in intrauterine fetal death, preterm delivery, and after delivery, hyperbilirubinemia and kernicterus.

2 THE TESTS

a What is the purpose of the tests?

To determine the newborn blood type to identify Rh(D) negative women at risk of developing alloimmunization. Such women should be given anti-D immunoglobulin prophylaxis to prevent the subsequent development of alloimmunization.

b The nature of the tests

Tests may include ABO grouping, Rh type, direct antiglobulin test, and RBC antibody screen.

c Implications of testing

1 What does an abnormal test result mean?

Rh(D) negative women who deliver an Rh(D) positive child with a negative direct antiglobulin test should receive anti-D immunoglobulin. Direct antiglobulin tests are unnecessary if the mother is Rh positive and the newborn is asymptomatic.

2 What does a normal test result mean?

No testing is necessary on the cord sample from newborns of Rh positive mothers who have negative antibody screening tests in the absence of clinical signs and symptoms of hemolytic disease of the newborn.

d What is the cost of testing?

It is possible to reduce costs by limiting cord blood testing to women with significant maternal RBC antibodies or who are Rh negative. In the latter, the cord blood Rh type is used to determine need for anti-D immunoglobulin administration.

3 CONCLUSIONS AND RECOMMENDATIONS

It is prudent to collect and accurately label an umbilical cord blood sample from all neonates at delivery. It is neither wise nor cost-effective to test all cord blood samples routinely for ABO group, Rh(D) type, direct antiglobulin test or anti-RBC antibody screen. It is better to study blood samples of only those infants who exhibit features of hemolytic disease of the newborn.

REFERENCES

Crowther CA & Keirse MJNC (1994) Anti-Rh-D prophylaxis postpartum. In Enkin MW, Keirse MJNC, Renfrew MJ & Neilson JP (eds) *Pregnancy and Childbirth Module.* Cochrane Database of Systematic Reviews. 03314 (Disk Issue 1). Oxford: Update Software.

Judd WJ, Luban NLC, Ness PM *et al.* (1990) Prenatal and perinatal immunohematology: recommendations for serologic management of the fetus, newborn infant, and obstetric patient. *Transfusion* 30: 175–183.

Moise KJ Jr (1994) Changing trends in the management of red blood cell alloimmunization in pregnancy. *Arch Path Lab Med* 118: 421–428.

Petz LD & Garratty G (1980) *Acquired Immune Hemolytic Anemias.* New York: Churchill Livingstone.

Walker RH, ed. (1993) *Technical Manual,* 11th edn, p. 445. Bethesda, M: American Association of Blood Banks.

Weinstein L (1982) Irregular antibodies causing hemolytic disease of the newborn: a continuing problem. *Clin Obstet Gynecol* 25: 321–322.

21

Antepartum & Postpartum Pap Smear

Clare Wilkinson & Alison Bigrigg

WHAT IS THE PROBLEM THAT REQUIRES SCREENING?

CARCINOMA OF THE CERVIX.

What is the incidence/prevalence of the target condition?

Carcinoma of the cervix is the second most common cancer of women worldwide. In developing countries, it is the most common female cancer (Austoker, 1994). Invasive cervical carcinoma is preceded by characteristic premalignant lesions whose treatment is almost always curative. Thus, screening programs must also consider the incidence of these premalignant lesions. It is difficult to determine accurately the incidence and prevalence of the premalignant lesion – carcinoma in situ – because of the effects of established screening programs, treatment, and the long latent period of transition between the premalignant and malignant states on the incidence and prevalence. While the overall mortality from cervical cancer declined during the 1980s in most parts of the world, several countries reported an increased rate in younger women. The incidence rate of cervical cancer in the UK during 1988 was 169 new cases per million population. Although only 15.5% of affected women were under 35 years old, it was the most common cancer in this age group (Austoker, 1994, 1995). The incidence rate of carcinoma in situ of the uterine cervix appears to have tripled in British women between 1971 and 1983 (Office of Population Censors and Surveys 1971–1984). These trends require careful interpretation, as the only method of calculating true incidence rates for carcinoma in situ is by the collection of data expressed per 1000 women screened and by age group, and such data are not readily available.

What are the sequelae of the condition which are of interest in clinical medicine?

Carcinoma of the cervix can be prevented by the identification and treatment of the precurser lesion – cervical intraepithelial neoplasia (CIN). A very high cure rate for CIN is possible using outpatient methods that preserve fertility. Survival of invasive cervical cancer is greatly improved by diagnosis and treatment at an early stage. There is a marked difference in survival between stages. A large percentage of women in the industrialized world who currently develop cervical cancer have never had a cervical smear.

THE TEST

What is the purpose of the test?

To obtain a sample of cells from the cervical squamocolumnar junction which is then examined cytologically for evidence of dyskaryotic changes (the Papanicolaou or 'Pap' smear).

The nature of the test

A doctor or a suitably trained nurse inserts an appropriate speculum into the vagina to visualize the cervix. A wooden spatula is inserted into the cervical os and rotated 360° to obtain a sample of cells from the cervical transformation zone. In addition, either a cotton swab or a purpose-designed brush is inserted into the os and rotated to obtain cells from the endocervical canal. The cells are spread evenly onto a glass slide, a fixative applied, and the sample allowed to air-dry.

Implications of testing

WHAT DOES AN ABNORMAL TEST RESULT MEAN?

A woman whose smear shows evidence of either a premalignant lesion is advised to undergo additional tests and, when indicated, treatment. These additional tests include colposcopically directed cervical biopsy, possibly followed by treatment at a second visit, or one-stage diagnosis and treatment by the performance of a large loop excision biopsy. A woman with a clearly malignant lesion is referred urgently for staging and subsequent treatment. Other treatments for CIN include carbon dioxide laser ablation, cold coagulation and cold-knife cone biopsy.

The risk of physical harm from cervical cancer screening is minimal. The treatments used for precancerous conditions of the cervix have a low associated morbidity. There is also some evidence that while the program may cause psychological morbidity this can be minimized by good communication (Wilkinson *et al.*, 1990).

The specificity of the cervical smear is between 90% and 99% (US Preventive Services Task Force, 1989). Any degree of cytological abnormality is a good predictor that there is some degree of cervical intraepithelial neoplasia present. However, the degree of dyskaryosis visualized on the smear does not necessarily reflect the severity of the CIN. Up to one-third of women with mild dyskaryosis cytologically have CIN-3 found in their cervical biopsy specimen. A lesion characterized by borderline changes or mild dyskaryosis is likely to regress if untreated. A woman with moderate or severe dyskaryosis should be offered colposcopy. Pregnant women can safely undergo this procedure, but generally feel more anxious about such an investigation than nonpregnant women. In addition, the vaginal walls become lax and the endocervical mucous becomes tenacious, obscuring vision as gestation advances. Many of the colposcopic features suggestive of disease in the nonpregnant woman occur during pregnancy as physiologic variants. If necessary, colposcopically directed punch biopsy can be carried out with relative safety (Economos *et al.*, 1993). Mild cytological abnormalities of the cervix may be particularly difficult to interpret during the postnatal period because of atrophic changes and the presence of large glycogen-packed parabasal cells. Colposcopy is safe postpartum but the histologic interpretation may be compromised by the reparative changes. In summary, extreme conscientiousness is required to exclude invasive disease by careful colposcopic, histological and cytological review in both nonpregnant and pregnant women (Campion and Sedlacek, 1993).

WHAT DOES A NORMAL TEST RESULT MEAN?

The recommended interval between normal tests varies across different countries. In practice, a normal test means that the woman should be recalled at an appropriate interval for future screening. However, the sensitivity of the smear test is a concern, with false negative rates ranging from about 20% to 45% for the various grades of cervical intraepithelial neoplasia. This explains in part why the screening intervals are set 2, 3 or 5 years in various programs, even though the natural evolution from CIN to invasive cancer is closer to a decade. Most programs offer cervical screening to all sexually active women between the ages of 20 years and 65 years (Eddy, 1990), though the precise upper age limit varies.

What is the cost of testing?

Cost of further investigation and treatment of screened positives: In the Netherlands, the costs of diagnosis and treatment of abnormal smears are relatively small compared with the costs of the cervical smear program itself (Koopmanschap *et al.*, 1990; van Ballegooijen 1992).

Total cost in the target population: The total cost of a cervical screening program is typically unknown at either the national or local level. For example, an activity-based approach to costing the cervical screening program carried out in the Oxford region of the UK summarized the complexity of the program and the elements that need to be included to establish the costs associated with a well-organized screening program (Havelock, 1994). These include the supra- and administrative structure of the screening program itself, the cost of screening and the cost of treatment. It is difficult to identify the total cost of a cervical screening program in most countries without an extensive economic evaluation. Nevertheless, the following data illustrate some of the detailed costs of the cervical screening program in the USA. It has been estimated that the average cost of the smear test itself is US $76, the cost of investigating a false positive smear (assuming colposcopy is performed) is $150, and the cost of treating a preinvasive lesion is $5641 (Eddy, 1990). A broader view of costs, however, suggests the true cost of the program – Eddy (1990) estimated that the marginal cost per year of life expectancy achieved by three annual smear tests prior to 3-yearly testing was about $721 310.

CONCLUSIONS AND RECOMMENDATIONS

The cervical smear test fits the criteria for a fairly good screening tool in terms of acceptability and performance statistics. It is relatively simple and the results are generally valid, reliable and reproducible (IARC, 1986).

Cervical screening programs with well-organized call and recall systems have been in operation in parts of Europe and North America since the early 1970s. Although no randomized controlled trials were initially carried out, there is increasing indirect evidence that cervical screening is effective. For instance, the incidence of invasive cancer has fallen, despite a concomitant rise in the incidence of preinvasive disease in British

Columbia and northern Scotland, where excellent coverage has been achieved over several decades (Anderson *et al.*, 1988; McGregor *et al.* 1994). The optimal screening schedule over a woman's lifetime is debated, but intervals of less than 3 years offer little return in terms of decline in mortality (Koopmanschap *et al.* 1990). It is well established that poorly coordinated screening efforts are ineffective, often costly, and fail to reduce the incidence of invasive cervical cancer (Miller, 1995). Innovative methods of targeting women at highest risk from the disease may prove beneficial (Wilkinson, 1992), and new methods of identifying oncogenic strains of human papillomavirus may be useful in the future.

A majority of the target population for screening are seen during the course of antenatal care. Women who are defaulters or have never had a first test can be opportunistically screened. The postnatal period is also a worthwhile time to offer a smear test as part of a woman's proposed lifetime schedule, if this has been omitted during the antenatal period. Antenatal cervical screening may be particularly useful in developing countries as an opportunistic way to include women in the cervical screening program. Antenatal testing may also be useful in the developed countries which have a poor coverage of some groups within the population who could be targeted for any type of opportunistic screening. However, if resources are limited, a concentration on antenatal screening should not replace concentration on the older, unscreened population. In countries where cervical screening is carried out without attention to resource allocation, many recommend a cervical smear as part of the first antenatal visit, but the rationale for this is hard to defend if there is already good population coverage. If a woman has never had a cervical smear, the antenatal period is a worthwhile time to offer a smear test. It is not, however, an ideal time for a smear test to be carried out for a number of reasons. The interpretation of smears and colposcopy findings is more difficult and the discovery of a mild abnormality will lead to a delay in investigation and treatment and therefore increased anxiety.

In summary, in countries with organized programs, antenatal or postnatal testing is only appropriate as part of a woman's lifetime schedule. Based on current knowledge and trends, such women should not be offered additional tests during pregnancy or the postnatal period.

SUMMARY

1
WHAT IS THE PROBLEM THAT REQUIRES SCREENING?

CARCINOMA OF THE CERVIX.

a What is the incidence/prevalence of the target condition?

Carcinoma of the cervix is the second most common cancer of women worldwide. The incidence and prevalence of premalignant lesions are very difficult to ascertain as a result of established screening programs and treatment, and long latent periods.

b What are the sequelae of the condition which are of interest in clinical medicine?

Survival of invasive cervical cancer is greatly improved by early detection and treatment.

2 **THE TEST**

a **What is the purpose of the test?**

The Pap smear obtains a sample of cells from the cervical squamocolumnar junction, which is then examined cytologically for dyskaryosis.

b **The nature of the test**

An appropriate speculum is inserted into the vagina, and the sample obtained by a wooden spatula and swab or brush inserted into the cervical os and rotated.

c **Implications of testing**

1 What does an abnormal test result mean?

There is evidence of dyskaryosis and the woman is advised to undergo additional tests and, possibly, treatment.

2 What does a normal test result mean?

The woman should attend for future screening after an appropriate interval. False negative rates vary from about 20% to 45%.

d **What is the cost of testing?**

Given the complexity of many programs, costs are difficult to gauge definitively. Nevertheless, though the smear test itself costs US $76, investigation of false positives $150 and treatment $5641, the costs per year of life expectancy gained has been estimated at $721 310 for three annual smears followed by a 3-year recall interval.

3 **CONCLUSIONS AND RECOMMENDATIONS**

Women who are defaulters from a screening program could be screened opportunistically during the course of antenatal care, particularly in developing countries or where coverage is poor. Pregnancy is not, however, an ideal time for a smear test to be performed. If antenatal testing is omitted then the postnatal period offers an opportunity to return to a lifetime schedule. In summary, in the context of a well-organized program women should not be offered additional tests during pregnancy or the postnatal period.

REFERENCES

Anderson GH, Boyes DA & Benedet JL (1988) Organisation and results of the cervical cytology screening programme in British Columbia, 1955–1985. *Br Med J* **296**: 975–978.
Austoker J (1994) *Cancer of the Cervix Uteri*. Cancer Research Campaign Factsheets 12.1–12.3.
Austoker J (1995) *Cancer Prevention in Primary Care*. London: BMJ Publishing Group.
Brown J & Sculpher MJ (1993) Economics of screening programmes to prevent cervical cancer. *Cont Rev Obstet Gynaecol* **5**: 221–229.
Campion MJ & Sedlacek TV (1993) Colposcopy in pregnancy. *Obstet Gynecol Clin North Am* **20**: 153–163.
Economos K, Veridiano NP, Delke I, Collado ML & Tancer ML (1993) Abnormal cervical cytology in pregnancy: a 17 year experience. *Obstet Gynecol* **81**: 915–918.
Eddy DM (1990) Screening for cervical cancer. *Ann Intern Med* **113**: 214–226.

Havelock C (1994) *NHS Cervical Screening Programme. The Cost of the Cervical Screening Programme – an Activity Based Approach*. Oxford: Hall.

IARC (1986) Working Group on Evaluation of Cervical Cancer Screening Programmes. Screening for squamous cervical cancer: duration of low risk after negative results of cervical cytology and its implications for screening policies. *Br Med J* **293:** 659–664.

Koopmanschap MA, Lubbe KTN, van Oortmarssen GJ, Agt HMA, van Ballegooijen M & Habbema JDF (1990) Economic aspects of cervical cancer screening. *Soc Sci Med* **30:** 1081–87.

McGregor JE, Cambell MK, Mann EMF & Swanson KY (1994) Screening for cervical intraepithelial neoplasia in north east Scotland shows fall in incidence and mortality from invasive cancer with concomitant rise in pre-invasive disease. *Br Med J* **308:** 1407–1411.

Miller AB (1995) Failures of cervical screening (editorial). *Am J Publ Health* **85:** 761.

US Preventive Services Task Force (1989) *Guide to Clinical Preventive Services. An Assessment of the Effectiveness of 169 Interventions*. New York: Williams & Wilkins.

van Ballegooijen M, Habbema JDF, Oortmarssen GJ, Koopmanschap MA, Lubbe JTN & van Agt HME (1992) Preventive pap-smears: balancing costs, risks and benefits. *Br J Cancer* **65:** 930–933.

Wilkinson C, Jones JM & McBride J (1990) Anxiety caused by abnormal result of cervical smear test: a controlled trial. *Br Med J* **300:** 440.

Wilkinson CE, Peters TJ, Harvey IM & Stott NCH (1992) Risk targeting in cervical screening: a new look at an old problem. *Br J Gen Pract* **42:** 435–438.

22

The Annual Bimanual Examination

Susan R. Johnson & Ann Laros

WHAT IS THE PROBLEM THAT REQUIRES SCREENING?

GYNECOLOGIC MALIGNANCIES.

The bimanual examination is widely recommended as a routine component of a complete gynecological screening examination to assess the pelvic structures. The bimanual examination is of clear clinical value in the evaluation of symptomatic women who have benign anatomic abnormalities such as uterine leiomyoma, endometriosis or adnexal masses. However, these diagnoses are of little consequence in the asymptomatic woman. They usually require no treatment and their identification with a screening test would not be cost-effective.

The identification of malignant masses which are often asymptomatic, particularly cancer of the ovary, is potentially of more use. This chapter reviews the evidence regarding the effectiveness of the annual bimanual examination to screen for ovarian cancer. We recognize that on rare occasions other, asymptomatic gynecologic malignancies will also be detected.

What is the incidence/prevalence of the target condition?

The incidence of ovarian cancer varies from 12–15 per 100 000 per year in industrialized nations to 3–8 per 100 000 per year in the developing world. Japan is a notable exception, with an incidence of between 4 and 6 per 100 000 women per year (Muir, 1987). The incidence of ovarian cancer rises with age, reaching a peak of 54 per 100 000 per year in the seventh decade. Eighty per cent of ovarian malignancies occur in women over 50 years old (DiSaia, 1993; Frame and Carlson, 1975; Goldstein *et al.*, 1989).

Another group of women at high risk are those in families with a genetically transmitted cancer syndrome. Women with two or more first-degree relatives with ovarian cancer have a lifetime risk as high as 50%, and women with a single first-degree relative with ovarian cancer may have a 5% risk. In contrast to these high-risk groups, the average lifetime risk in the USA is 1 in 70, about 1.4% (Steele *et al.*, 1994). Screening strategies usually focus on women over 50 years old, and on women with a high genetic risk.

What are the sequelae of the condition which are of interest in clinical medicine?

Ovarian cancer is the seventh leading cause of cancer deaths among women worldwide and accounts for almost 50% of gynecological cancer-related deaths in the developed countries (Tortolero-Luna *et al.*, 1994; Parkin, 1993). The mortality rate for ovarian cancer has changed little over the past 30 years. The overall 5-year survival rate continues to be only 40%. Survival is associated with the stage of the disease at diagnosis. Unfortunately, most cases are diagnosed at an advanced stage where the 5-year survival is only 5–20%. Indicating the potential importance of early detection, localized disease has a reported 5-year survival rate approximating 90% (Young, 1990).

THE TEST

What is the purpose of the test?

The purpose of an annual bimanual examination as a screening test is to identify women with early stage ovarian cancer by the detection of a pelvic mass.

The nature of the test

The bimanual examination is part of the physical examination. The examiner places one or two fingers in the vagina and the opposite hand on the abdomen, allowing palpation of the uterine cervix and corpus, and the adnexal structures. The examiner can then assess the location, size, consistency, and mobility of an abnormal mass.

The size of the normal ovary in a premenopausal woman approximates 3.5 cm × 2 cm × 1.5 cm; in the postmenopausal woman it is 2.0 cm × 0.5 cm or less. In the premenopausal woman, asymptomatic masses of 5 cm or larger are considered abnormal, and require follow-up. The finding of a palpable ovary or any other pelvic mass in a postmenopausal woman mandates further evaluation, since the normal postmenopausal ovary is not palpable and there are few benign causes of enlargement (Barber and Graber, 1971).

The bimanual examination is difficult to standardize, and many factors affect accuracy and reproducibility. These include the experience of the examiner, and the habitus and cooperation of the patient. Jacobs *et al.* (1988) suggested that a positive predictive value of at least 10% is required for either a single test or combination of tests to be cost-effective in screening for ovarian cancer. Assuming 40 women per 100 000 screened have ovarian cancer, it would require a sensitivity of 60% and a specificity of 99.6% for screening to be cost-effective. Test performance characteristics have not been well studied for the bimanual examination, but the data available suggest that while the sensitivity is sufficient, the specificity is not.

Ferris and Schapira (1991) found that internal medicine residents could detect adnexal masses of 3 cm and 6 cm in diameter in a synthetic model of the pelvis with a sensitivity and specificity of 67% and 100% respectively. Frederick *et al.* (1991) studied the agreement between the preoperative bimanual examination and the actual findings at surgery in 133 women. The study group had a mean age of 38 years, and there were a wide variety of pelvic findings, including a majority with uterine leiomyomas. The results are shown in Table 22.1. Unfortunately, the high positive predictive value is due in part to the high prevalence of pelvic abnormalities, which would not be expected in a screening setting. Further, the group with adnexal masses was not separately analyzed. Thus, these figures may not be generally applicable to the detection of ovarian cancer.

Masses smaller than 5 cm are frequently missed on the bimanual examination, and even larger masses can go undetected. Rulin and Preston (1987) compared the accuracy of a

Table 22.1 Percentage of pelvic masses identified by bimanual examination in 133 women.

	IDENTIFICATION OF PELVIC MASS (%)
sensitivity	65.7
specificity	92.5
positive predictive value	77.5

preoperative bimanual examination with surgical findings in 150 women. Examiners (either staff or resident physicians) failed to identify 10% of the masses that were 10 cm or less in size. The accuracy in assessing the size of those masses palpated was approximately 70%. Popp *et al.* (1993) found that almost half of the masses less than 5 cm were not detected.

Only one study has directly investigated the usefulness of the bimanual examination ovarian cancer screening. Jacobs *et al.* (1988) screened 1010 postmenopausal women using bimanual examination, pelvic ultrasonography, and CA-125 testing (see Chapter 24). Bimanual examination alone had a specificity of 97.3%. Its combination with either ultrasonography, CA-125 testing, or both, increased specificity to between 99% and 100%. Only one cancer was detected in this study, so the sensitivity could not be adequately assessed. Piver *et al.* (1976) found that only 15% of 100 consecutive patients with ovarian cancer were initially identified by a routine pelvic examination.

Implications of testing

WHAT DOES AN ABNORMAL TEST RESULT MEAN?

The differential diagnosis of an adnexal mass varies with the age and menopausal status of the patient. Many benign conditions cause enlargement of the ovaries in premenopausal women and the risk of ovarian cancer is low. However, a cystic mass greater than 5 cm that persists after one or two menstrual cycles, or any mass that has worrisome characteristics (i.e. solid, bilateral, nodular, or very large) should be investigated immediately (Spanos, 1973).

It has been recommended that any palpable mass in a postmenopausal woman be surgically explored (Barber and Graber 1971). However, a more conservative approach is now suggested for cystic masses less than 5 cm in diameter since these are unlikely to be malignant (Creasman and Soper, 1986; Rulin and Preston, 1987). Using this approach, a postmenopausal woman with a small mass is first evaluated with an ultrasound examination, preferably using the transvaginal approach (see Chapter 23). If the mass proves to be a unilocular cyst, periodic ultrasound examinations are performed to monitor its size. Levels of CA-125 can be measured simultaneously. Observation can continue as long as there is no significant enlargement or ominous changes in the consistency of the cyst.

WHAT DOES A NORMAL TEST RESULT MEAN?

While a normal examination does not exclude the presence of disease, the pelvic examination does have a reasonable level of specificity. Women who have a normal examination and remain asymptomatic should simply be reexamined at the time of their next scheduled pelvic examination.

What is the cost of testing?

The bimanual examination adds little direct cost to the health care system when performed at the time of a recommended Pap smear. The examination typically takes less than a minute of provider time, and the provider fee is generally included as part of the consultation fee. The cost of evaluating abnormal findings, however, can be high. In the USA, a pelvic ultrasound examination typically costs between US $250 and $350, and a serum CA-125 measurement costs approximately $50. The total cost will be much higher if the tests must be repeated two or three times yearly. Although such outpatient tests are costly, they are much less expensive than routine surgical exploration of every postmenopausal woman with a pelvic mass, which in the USA would cost at least $4000.

CONCLUSIONS AND RECOMMENDATIONS

An annual bimanual examination is not sufficient as a screening test for ovarian cancer. However, because it is inexpensive, minimally invasive, and a small percentage of asymptomatic ovarian cancers will be identified, a bimanual examination should be performed if a pelvic examination is being done for other reasons.

SUMMARY

1 WHAT IS THE PROBLEM THAT REQUIRES SCREENING?

THE IDENTIFICATION OF MALIGNANT MASSES, PARTICULARLY CANCER OF THE OVARY.

a What is the incidence/prevalence of the target condition?

The incidence of ovarian cancer varies from 12–15 per 100 000 per year in industrialized nations to 3–8 per 100 000 per year in the developing world. The incidence rises with age: 80% of ovarian malignancies occur in women over 50 years old. Women with two or more first-degree relatives with ovarian cancer have a lifetime risk as high as 50%, and women with a single first-degree relative with ovarian cancer may have a 5% risk. In contrast to these high-risk groups, the average lifetime risk in the USA is 1 in 70, about 1.4%.

b What are the sequelae of the condition which are of interest in clinical medicine?

Ovarian cancer is the seventh leading cause of cancer deaths among women worldwide, and accounts for almost 50% of gynecological cancer-related deaths in the developed countries.

2 THE TEST

a What is the purpose of the test?

To identify women with early stage ovarian cancer by the detection of a pelvic mass.

b The nature of the test

The bimanual examination is part of the physical examination.

c Implications of testing

I What does an abnormal test result mean?

The differential diagnosis of an adnexal mass varies with the age and menopausal status of the patient. A cystic mass of greater than 5 cm that persists after one or two menstrual cycles, or any mass that has worrisome characteristics (i.e. solid, bilateral, nodular, or very large) should be investigated immediately. Cystic masses smaller than 5 cm in diameter are unlikely to be malignant and should first be evaluated by ultrasonography. If the mass proves to be a unilocular cyst, periodic ultrasound examinations are performed to monitor its size. Levels of CA-125 can be measured simultaneously. Observation can continue as long as there is no significant enlargement or ominous changes in the consistency of the cyst.

2 What does a normal test result mean?

Women who have a normal examination and remain asymptomatic should simply be reexamined at the time of their next scheduled pelvic examination.

d What is the cost of testing?

The bimanual examination represents little direct cost to the health care system when performed during recommended Pap smear screening.

3 CONCLUSIONS AND RECOMMENDATIONS

An annual bimanual examination is not sufficient as a screening test for ovarian cancer. However, because it is inexpensive and minimally invasive, and a small percentage of asymptomatic ovarian cancers will be identified, a bimanual examination should be performed if a pelvic examination is being performed for other reasons.

REFERENCES

Barber HR & Graber EA (1971) The postmenopausal palpable ovary syndrome. *Obstet Gynecol* **38**: 921–923.
Creasman WT & Disaia PJ (1991) Screening in ovarian cancer. *Am J Obstet Gynecol* **165**: 7–10.
Creasman WT & Soper JT (1986) The undiagnosed adnexal mass after menopause. *Clin Obstet Gynecol* **29**: 446–448.
DiSaia PJ (1993) *Clinical Gynecologic Oncology*, 4th edn, St Louis: Mosby Yearbook, p 336.
Ferris AK & Schapira MM (1991) Accuracy of pelvic examination (letter). *Ann Intern Med* **114**: 522.
Frederick JL, Paulson RJ & Sauer MV (1991) Routine use of vaginal ultrasonography in the preoperative evaluation of gynecologic patients: an adjunct to resident education. *J Reprod Med* **36**: 779–782.
Frame PS & Carlson SJ (1975) A critical review of periodic health screening using specific screening criteria, part 3: selected diseases of the genitourinary system. *J Fam Pract* **2**: 189–194.
Goldstein SR, Subramanyam B, Snyder JR, Bellwe U, Raghavendra BN & Beckman EM (1989) The postmenopausal cycstic adnexal mass: the potential role of ultrasound in conservative management. *Obstet Gynecol* **73**: 8–10.
Jacobs I, Bridges J, Reynolds C *et al.* (1988) Multimodal approach to screening for ovarian cancer. *Lancet* **i**: 268–271.
Muir C (1989) *Cancer Incidence in Five Continents*, IARC Sci. P. 88. pp. 8/92–8/93. Lyon: IARC.

Parkin, DM (1993) Estimates of the worldwide incidence of eighteen major cancers in 1985. *Int J Cancer* **54:** 594–606.

Piver MS & Barlow JJ (1976) Preoperative and intraoperative evaluation in ovarian malignancy. *Obstet Gynecol* **48** (3): 312–315.

Popp, LW, Gaetje R & Stoyanov M (1993) Accuracy of bimanual palpation vs. vaginosonography in determination of the measurements of pelvic tumors. *Arch Gynecol Obstet* **252:** 197–202.

Rulin MC & Preston AL (1987) Adnexal masses in postmenopausal women. *Obstet Gynecol* **70:** 578–581

Spanos, WJ (1973) Preoperative hormone therapy of cystic adnexal masses. *Am J Obstet Gynecol* **116:** 551–556.

Steele KD, Osteen RT, Winchester DP, Murphy GP & Menck HR (1994) Clinical highlights from the National Cancer Data Base. *Cancer*, **44** (2): 71–80.

Tortolero-Luna G, Mitchell MF & Rhodes-Morris HE (1994) Epidemiology in screening of ovarian cancer. *Obstet Gynecol Clin North Am*, **21** (1): 1–23.

Young, RC (1990) Adjuvant therapy in stage I and stage II epithelial ovarian cancer: results of 2 prospective randomized trials. *N Engl J Med* **322:** 1021.

23

Transvaginal Ultrasonography as a Screening Method for Ovarian Cancer

P. D. DePriest, H. H. Gallion & J. R. van Nagell Jr

OVARIAN CANCER.

Most women present with advanced disease at the time they first consult a physician because early ovarian cancer produces no symptoms.

What is the incidence/prevalence of the target condition?

It is estimated that over 140 000 women worldwide will develop ovarian cancer in 1996. In the USA there will be 24 000 new cases diagnosed and 13 600 women will die of their disease (Boring *et al.*, 1994). The annual incidence of ovarian cancer in the general population increases with age to approximately 1 per 2000 women over 50 years old (Surveillance Program, 1988).

Other factors that increase the risk of ovarian cancer include family history, nulliparity, early menarche, and delayed childbearing (Greene *et al.*, 1984; Koch *et al.*, 1988). Ovarian cancer rates are highest in the industrialized countries of Europe and North America, and lowest in the developing countries of Asia and Africa. As many as 10% of ovarian cancer cases may be due to predisposing genes which have a small but definite effect on risk (Ponder *et al.*, 1989). As a result, the risk of ovarian cancer is higher in women with a family history of the disease. For example, the incidence of ovarian cancer in English women who have at least one close relative with the disease is 390 per 100 000 per year, or approximately ten times the risk of ovarian cancer in the general population (Bourne *et al.*, 1991). In contrast, oral contraceptive pills and breastfeeding each have a protective effect on the development of ovarian cancer. It is unclear whether the use of fertility drugs alters the risk of ovarian cancer (Shoham, 1994).

What are the sequelae of the condition which are of interest in clinical medicine?

Despite effective tumor debulking and appropriate chemotherapy, the prognosis is poor. Five-year survival rates are typically 5–20% in women with stage III and IV disease. In contrast, cancer confined to the ovary itself (stage I disease) is highly curable, with 5-year survival rates approaching 90% (Young et al., 1990). Any such comparison should acknowledge lead time bias (see Chapter 1).

THE TEST

What is the purpose of the test?

To identify patients with ovarian cancer at an early stage.

The nature of the test

Transvaginal ultrasonography of the ovaries.

Transvaginal sonography (TVS) is performed using a standard ultrasound unit with a high-resolution (5.0 MHz or higher) vaginal transducer. Color Doppler capability may be a useful adjunct. The test is essentially painless, takes approximately 5 minutes to perform, and is well accepted by women (van Nagell et al., 1990). Each ovary is measured in three dimensions, and the ovarian volume calculated using the prolate ellipsoid formula (length × height × width × 0.523). An ovarian volume of at least 20 cm³ in premenopausal women and at least 10 cm³ in postmenopausal women is considered abnormal. These results are based on volume measurements in excess of 2 standard deviations above published normal ovarian volumes for premenopausal and postmenopausal women (Goswamy et al., 1983, 1988). In addition, any papillary projection from the tumor wall is classified as abnormal.

Who are the potential candidates for screening for ovarian cancer? General screening of the premenopausal population is not advocated. Most screening protocols are open to postmenopausal women over 50 years old, since ovarian volume varies cyclically during the menstrual cycle (van Nagell et al., 1991) and the prevalence of ovarian cancer is highest in women over the age of 50 years. Screening may also be indicated in women over 30 years old when there is a documented family history of ovarian cancer.

At least three distinct cancer syndromes have been identified in which susceptibility appears to be inherited. The most common is the breast–ovarian cancer syndrome, in which multiple cases of breast cancer and ovarian cancer are observed in the same family (Lynch et al., 1978; Schildkraut et al., 1989). The next most frequent familial ovarian cancer syndrome is Lynch type II (Lynch and Lynch, 1987). In these families, there are multiple cases of proximal colon cancer associated with both endometrial and ovarian cancers. The least common is the site-specific ovarian cancer syndrome, in which excessive cancer risk appears to be restricted to the ovary (Lurain and Piver, 1979). In each of these syndromes, susceptibility to cancer is inherited as an autosomal dominant trait. Therefore, the siblings and children of an affected individual from an ovarian cancer family each have a 50% chance of inheriting the disease trait themselves. Epidemiologic studies suggest that in such families, gene carriers have at least an 80% lifetime chance of becoming affected (Easton et al., 1993). The age of onset of familial ovarian cancer is significantly earlier than that of ovarian cancer that is not genetically associated, and some women have contracted the disease as early as the third decade of life.

Implications of testing

WHAT DOES AN ABNORMAL TEST RESULT MEAN?

In most screening protocols, women with an abnormal sonogram have a repeat TVS in 4–6 weeks. If the repeat sonogram is abnormal, the patient undergoes morphologic indexing of the tumor, and may have additional adjuvant tests such as Doppler flow assessment of tumor blood flow or a serum CA-125 determination. The patient then undergoes operative removal of the persisting ovarian tumor. This may be accomplished through the laparoscope or by open laparotomy.

WHAT DOES A NORMAL TEST RESULT MEAN?

A normal test indicates that there is no sonographic evidence of an abnormality in ovarian size or morphology. Women with a normal test are screened annually because of the potential for a fast-growing tumor.

What is the cost of testing?

There are no published data concerning the cost of TVS screening. Cost estimates based on data from the University of Kentucky ovarian cancer screening project are shown in Table 23.1. Subsequent costs are based on the following published assumptions concerning TVS screening for ovarian cancer (DePriest and van Nagell, 1992):

  sensitivity 100%
  specificity 98.1%
  positive predictive value (PPV) 7%
  negative predictive value (NPV) 100%

These figures assume 143 of 100 000 screened women have ovarian cancer. Though a sensitivity of 100% may be too high with widespread application, slightly lower sensitivities should not lower the PPV dramatically. Assuming a PPV of TVS screening of 7%, for each case of ovarian cancer detected 13 women will undergo surgery. The cost per hospitalization for removal of a benign ovarian tumor is $3000 for a laparoscopic procedure and $6000 for laparotomy. If it is assumed that the majority of ovarian tumors

Table 23.1 Cost estimates for transvaginal ultrasonographic screening.

	US$
equipment: ultrasound unit and vaginal transducer	30 000
technician salary (year)	30 000
coordinator salary (year)	25 000
sonogram review by doctor ($50 per hour, 5 hours a week for 50 weeks)	12 500
space rental for screening	5 000
miscellaneous costs: postage, telephone, ultrasound supplies	7 500
Total	**$110 000**
number of screens per technician per year (20 a day for 5 days a week, for 50 weeks)	5 000
Cost per screening test (110 000/5000)	**$22**

would be removed laparoscopically, the mean cost of tumor removal would approach $5000 per case. Thus, the total cost of benign ovarian tumor removal per case of ovarian cancer detected is 13 × $5000, i.e. $65 000.

If a morphology index score of 5 or more is used as a prerequisite for surgery, the PPV increases to 47% since the false positive rate decreases (DePriest *et al.*, 1994), so two patients with benign ovarian tumors would undergo surgery per case of ovarian cancer detected. Therefore, the total cost of benign ovarian tumor removal per case of ovarian cancer detected would be 2 × $5000, i.e. $10 000.

Although the prevalence of ovarian cancer in women 50 years old or more is estimated to be 50 per 100 000 screened, the authors have detected approximately 1 new case of ovarian cancer per 1000 women screened (van Nagell *et al.*, 1991; DePriest *et al.*, 1993). Using the above assumptions, the total cost of detecting one case of ovarian cancer can be calculated as follows:

(a) $22 per test × 1000 .... $22 000
13 benign ovarian tumors removed (PPV = 7%) at $5000 per case.......... $65 000
cost of surgical removal of 1 ovarian cancer (stage 1) $10 000

total cost per case of ovarian cancer.. $97 000

(b) Alternatively, if a morphology index of at least 5 is used as a prerequisite for surgery:
$22 per test × 1000 .... $22 000
2 benign ovarian tumors removed (PPV = 47%) at $5000 per case.......... $10 000
cost of surgical removal of 1 ovarian cancer (stage 1) =............................ $10 000

total cost per case of ovarian cancer.. $42 000

These screening costs should be examined in the context of the medical costs required for a patient with stage III or IV ovarian cancer (over $200 000 per case) versus the costs for a patient with stage I ovarian cancer ($10 000 per case). Therefore, ovarian cancer produces not only tremendous loss of life and productivity, but is also associated with significant financial costs to society. To date, 13 of 14 of patients whose ovarian cancers have been detected by TVS screening have had stage I disease. In contrast, three-fourths of patients presenting with ovarian cancer in the absence of screening have had stage III or IV disease.

CONCLUSIONS AND RECOMMENDATIONS

Since ovarian cancer produces no symptoms until it is advanced, most women are virtually incurable at the time they present to a physician. Despite advances in surgery and chemotherapy, there has been no significant change in the 5-year survival rate of ovarian cancer since the 1970s (Boring *et al.*, 1994). Ovarian cancer now ranks as the fourth leading cause of female cancer mortality in the USA, and more women are dying each year of this disease. Clearly, methods for the early detection of ovarian cancer are highly desirable.

Data from existing ovarian cancer screening studies indicate that sonographic screening can reduce the stage at detection, and has the potential to reduce ovarian cancer mortality (van Nagell *et al.*, 1991; DePriest *et al.*, 1992). In the University of Kentucky ovarian cancer screening project, over 5000 postmenopausal women have been screened. Five ovarian cancers have been detected, four of which are stage 1, and all patients are presently alive and well with no evidence of disease. Similarly, there have been no deaths from ovarian cancer in the screened population. Not all centers have met with the same success. A properly designed, national, randomized controlled trial is needed to determine the effect of ovarian cancer screening on site-specific ovarian cancer mortality. Such a trial would also provide valuable data concerning the cost of screening, as well as the optimal population to be screened. Until such a screening trial is completed, it is premature to proceed with routine ovarian cancer screening.

SUMMARY

1 WHAT IS THE PROBLEM THAT REQUIRES SCREENING?

OVARIAN CANCER.

a What is the incidence/prevalence of the target condition?

It is estimated that over 140 000 women worldwide will develop ovarian cancer in 1996. The annual incidence of ovarian cancer in the general population increases with age to approximately 1 per 2000 women over 50 years old.

b What are the sequelae of the condition which are of interest in clinical medicine?

Death. Five-year survival rates are typically 5–20% in women with stage III and IV disease.

2 THE TEST

a What is the purpose of the test?

To detect ovarian cancer in a high-risk population at an early stage.

b The nature of the test

Transvaginal ultrasonography of the ovaries.

c Implications of testing

1 What does an abnormal test result mean?

In most protocols, women with an abnormal sonogram have a repeat TVS in 4–6 weeks. If it is still abnormal, the patient undergoes morphologic indexing of the tumor, and may have additional adjuvant tests such as Doppler assessment of tumor blood flow or a serum CA-125 determination. The patient undergoes operative removal of a persisting abnormality either through the laparoscope or by open laparotomy.

2 What does a normal test result mean?

A normal test indicates there is no sonographic evidence of an ovarian abnormality. Patients are screened annually.

d What is the cost of testing?

The cost depends upon the acceptable level of surgery for benign ovarian disorders. The cost ranges between US $40 000 and $100 000 per case of ovarian cancer identified, including the cost of surgery for benign lesions. These costs should be examined in the context of the medical costs required for a patient with stage III or IV ovarian cancer (over $200 000 per case) versus the costs for a patient with stage I ovarian cancer ($10 000 per case).

3 CONCLUSIONS AND RECOMMENDATIONS

A properly designed, national, randomized controlled trial is needed to determine the effect of ovarian cancer screening on site-specific ovarian cancer mortality. Such a trial would also provide valuable data concerning the cost of screening, as well as the optimal population to be screened.

REFERENCES

Boring CC, Squires TS, Tong T & Montgomery S (1994) Cancer statistics, 1994, *Cancer Clin* **44:** 7–26.

Bourne TH, Whitehead M, Campbell S, Royston P, Bhan V & Collins WP (1991) Ultrasound screening for familial ovarian cancer. *Gynecol Oncol* **43:** 92–97.

DePriest PD & van Nagell JR (1992) Transvaginal ultrasound screening for ovarian cancer. *Clin Obstet Gynecol* **35:** 40–44.

DePriest PD, Varner E, Powell J *et al.* (1994) The efficacy of a sonographic morphology index in identifying ovarian cancer: A multi-institutional investigation. *Gynecol Oncol* **55:** 174–178.

Easton DF, Bishop DT, Ford D, Crockford GP & the Breast Cancer Linkage Consortium (1993) Genetic linkage analysis in familial breast and ovarian cancer: Results from 214 families. *Am J Hum Genet* **52:** 678–701.

Goswamy RK, Campbell S & Whitehead MI (1983) Screening for ovarian cancer. *Clin Obstet Gynecol* **10:** 621–643.

Goswamy RK, Campbell S, Royston JP, Bhan V, Battersby RH, Hall VJ, Whitehead Ml & Collins WP (1988) Ovarian size in postmenopausal women. *Br J Obstet Gynaecol* **95:** 795–801.

Greene M, Clark J & Blayney D (1984) The epidemiology of ovarian cancer. Semin Oncol 1984; 11: 209–226.

Koch M, Jenkins H & Gaedke H (1988) Risk factors of ovarian carcinoma of epithelial origin: A case control study. Cancer Detect Prevent **13:** 131–136.

Lurain JR & Piver MS: Familial ovarian cancer. Gynecol Oncol 1979; 8: 185–192.

Lynch HT & Lynch J (1987) Genetic predictability and minimal cancer clues in Lynch Syndrome II. Dis Colon Rectum **30:** 243–246.

Lynch HT, Harris RE, Guirgis HA, Maloney K, Carmody LL & Lynch JF (1978) Familial association of breast/ovarian cancer. *Cancer* **41:** 1543–1548.

Ponder BAJ, Easton DF & Peto J (1989) Risk of ovarian cancer associated with a family history. In Sharp F, Mason WP, Leake RE (eds) (1994) *Ovarian Cancer*, pp 3–6. London: Chapman & Hall.

Shoham Z. Epidemiology, etiology, and fertility drugs in ovarian epithelial carcinoma: where are we today. Fertil Steril **62:** 433–48.

Schildkraut JM, Risch N & Thompson WD (1989) Evaluating genetic association among ovarian, breast and endometrial cancer. Evidence for a breast/ovarian relationship. *Am J Hum Genet* **45:** 521–529.

Surveillance Program (1988) Division of Cancer Prevention and Control. *Cancer Statistics Review 1973–1987.* Pub. 90–2789. Washington, DC: National Cancer Institute.

van Nagell JR, Higgins RV, Donaldson ES *et al.* (1990) Transvaginal sonography as a screening method for ovarian cancer: A report of the first 1000 cases screened. *Cancer* **65:** 573–577.

van Nagell JR, DePriest PD, Puls LE, *et al.* (1991) Ovarian cancer screening in asymptomatic postmenopausal women by transvaginal sonography. *Cancer* **68:** 458–462.

Young RC, Walton LA, Ellenberg SS, *et al.* (1990) Adjuvant therapy in stage I and stage II epithelial ovarian cancer: Results of two prospective randomized trials. *N Engl J Med* **322:** 1021–1027.

24

Serum CA-125 Screening for Ovarian Cancer

Kees A. Yedema & Peter Kenemans

OVARIAN CARCINOMA.

The potential roles for the measurement of CA-125 antigen in the diagnosis and management of ovarian carcinoma include: (1) the early identification of ovarian epithelial cancer in asymptomatic women, (2) the distinction between benign and malignant ovarian tumors in women with a pelvic mass, (3) the monitoring of therapy following surgical debulking and adjuvant chemotherapy in women with ovarian cancer, and (4) the detection of recurrent disease following treatment for ovarian cancer (see for review Yedema et al., 1994). This chapter focuses on the first two issues: the value of CA-125 as a tumor marker for ovarian cancer in asymptomatic women and the role of CA-125 in the evaluation of women presenting with a pelvic mass.

What is the incidence/prevalence of the target condition?

Approximately 1 out of 80 female newborns in the USA will develop ovarian cancer during their lifetime (DiSaia et al, 1989). Ovarian cancer may occur at any age. The median age is 53 years at detection (Katsube et al., 1982). The incidence of ovarian cancer increases with age, i.e. from 15.7 per 100 000 women per year in the 40–44 year age group, to an estimated 50 per 100 000 women per year in the higher age groups. Fewer than 25% of affected women have ovarian tumors confined to one ovary at diagnosis (Petterson et al., 1988). Familial cases of ovarian cancer account for 3% to 5% of all women with the disease (Oram and Jeyarajah, 1994). Pedigrees exhibit an autosomal dominant mode of inheritance with variable penetrance. Overall, these women have at least a three-fold risk of developing ovarian cancer (Schiltkraut and Thompson, 1988; Houlston et al., 1992).

What are the sequelae of the condition which are of interest in clinical medicine?

In Europe and North America, ovarian cancer is the most common cause of death in women with genital tract malignancies (Parkin et al., 1988; Henderson et al., 1991). Since women with early stage disease (stage I or stage II) usually do not have any clinical signs or symptoms, the majority of women with ovarian cancer are detected after their disease has progressed to stage III or IV. Despite appropriate therapy, 5-year survival rates (relative to diagnosis) in women with stage III and IV disease are poor, ranging from 5% to 20% (Friedlander and Dembo, 1991; Neijt et al., 1991). While complete clinical response following cytoreductive surgery and adjuvant chemotherapy is achieved in about 50% of the women with advanced malignancy, only 25% have evidence of complete pathological response at second-look laparotomy (Creasman and Eddy, 1989). Moreover, high relapse rates are encountered in women with histological evidence of complete remission (Creasman and Eddy, 1989). In contrast, the reported 5-year survival rates after diagnosis in women with stage I or II disease are much better, ranging from 50% (stage II) to 90% (stage I). Lead time bias should be borne in mind when interpreting such figures (see Chapter 1).

THE TEST

Serum CA-125 measurement.

What is the purpose of the test?

To identify at an early stage women with ovarian cancer and to differentiate between benign and malignant ovarian disease in women with a pelvic mass.

The nature of the test

The standard serum CA-125 assay (Centocor CA-125 immunoradiometric assay) was introduced in the early 1980s (Bast et al., 1983). The OC 125 monoclonal antibody was generated by the immunization of BALB/c mice with the OVCA 433 cell line derived from the ascitic fluid of a woman with a serous papillary cystadenocarcinoma of the ovary (Bast et al., 1981). It is postulated that the basement membrane of the normal ovary and the peritoneum prevent access of CA-125 to the circulation (Fleuren et al., 1987; Hilgers et al., 1988). Both benign and malignant growth disturbs these natural borders and may lead to an elevated serum CA-125 level. At present, various serum CA-125 assays are commercially available. These are not fully interchangeable (Pittaway, 1988; Yedema et al., 1992; van Kamp et al., 1993) and the user is to be cautioned. Recently, a heterologous double-determinant CA-125 II assay was developed using the M11 mcab as the capture antibody and OC 125 as the tracer antibody. This test has a higher signal to noise ratio, with test performance and cut-off levels similar to those of the original CA-125 assay. It can therefore be considered the new standard for CA-125 measurement (Kenemans et al., 1993).

Implications of testing

WHAT DOES AN ABNORMAL TEST RESULT MEAN?

Asymptomatic women: An elevated serum CA-125 level (greater than 35 U/ml) is found in 80% of women with ovarian cancer but in only 1–3% of healthy females (Bast et al., 1983; Yedema et al., 1994). Elevated levels have been observed from 10 months to more than 5 years before any clinical manifestation of disease (Bast et al., 1985; Zurawski et al., 1988). Only 41% of women with stage I disease have a serum CA-125 level greater than 35 U/ml (Yedema et al., 1994). The exact sensitivities are difficult to estimate since ovarian carcinoma is rare. For example, Zurawski et al. (1987) screened 915 women at risk but found no cases of ovarian cancer. However, Einhorn et al. (1992) identified 6 women with ovarian cancer in a study involving 5500 women; 3 women with ovarian carcinoma were missed (sensitivity 67%). Any calculation of sensitivity for CA-125 is compounded by incomplete data on the population screened, especially the duration of follow-up. Jacobs *et al.* (1993) detected 11 of the 19 women with ovarian carcinoma in their study of 22 000 women. Their sensitivity declined to 78% after 1 year and 58% after 2-year follow-up. Although the aim of screening with CA-125 is to detect women with ovarian cancer at an early – curable – stage, only 6 of the 18 women with ovarian cancer detected by screening had stage I disease at surgery (Jacobs *et al.*, 1988; 1993; Einhorn *et al.*, 1992). Hence, overall 11 of 29 women with ovarian cancer (38%) were missed at initial screening.

Malignancies other than ovarian cancer are often associated with an elevated serum CA-125 level. More than half of the women with non-ovarian pelvic malignancies have serum CA-125 levels exceeding 35 U/ml, particularly tumors metastatic to the ovaries and those originating from the endometrium and the colon (Yedema *et al.*, 1994). Pregnancy, menstruation and endometriosis are also well-known causes of elevated serum CA-125 levels (Mastropaolo *et al.*, 1986; Pittaway and Fayez, 1986, 1987; Seki *et al.*, 1986; Kenemans *et al.*, 1992). For example, an estimated 36% of women with endometriosis have CA-125 levels exceeding 35 U/ml (Yedema *et al.*, 1994). A wide variety of other nonmalignant disorders may cause an elevated serum CA-125 level, including pelvic inflammatory disease (Halila and Stenman, 1986; Duk *et al.*, 1989), pancreatitis, hepatitis, liver cirrhosis and congestive heart failure (Ruibal *et al.*, 1984; Bergmann *et al.*, 1987; Metzger *et al.*, 1987).

Women at increased risk: Bourne *et al.* (1994) assessed the value of serum CA-125 measurement as an adjunct to an ultrasound-based screening program for ovarian cancer in women with a history of familial ovarian cancer. Sixty per cent of the women were premenopausal. A vaginal ultrasound examination was performed at the first visit and the serum CA-125 level measured. Initially abnormal scans were repeated 3–8 weeks later. Of the 1502 women evaluated, 62 (4.1%) had an abnormal repeat ultrasound scan and were surgically evaluated. Ovarian cancer was found in 7 women, 6 of whom were premenopausal. One patient had advanced disease (stage III). Only 3 of the 7 patients had CA-125 levels above 35 U/ml. In fact, all women with ovarian cancer were detected using ultrasound alone. It was concluded that CA-125 measurements are not helpful for screening purposes in a high-risk population.

Women with a palpable pelvic mass: The serum CA-125 assay has been used to discriminate between benign and malignant pelvic mass. Eighty-five per cent of women with ovarian cancer have an elevated CA-125 level (> 35 U/ml) compared with 26% women with benign ovarian tumors (Yedema *et al.*, 1994). The sensitivity of CA-125 for the detection of ovarian cancer in women with a pelvic mass is not markedly altered, while the specificity remains close to 90%, if a higher cut-off value is used. If 65 U/ml is considered the upper limit of normal in premenopausal women with a pelvic mass, approximately 85% will be classified correctly (Yedema *et al.*, 1994) (Table 24.1). In postmenopausal women, the use of the lower cut-off level of 35 U/mL seems justified, with about 80% classified accurately (Table 24.1).

Jacobs *et al.* (1990) devised a malignancy index based on the product of several parameters including serum CA-125, the ultrasound score (0, 1 or 3) and the menopausal status (1 if premenopausal, 3 if postmenopausal). With a score above 250, they reported a 78% sensitivity at 1 year with a very high 99.8% specificity. The malignancy index is simple to apply, applicable to both premenopausal and postmenopausal women, and reproducible (Davies *et al.*, 1993). In post menopausal women, the effect of the combined use of CA-125 measurements and ultrasound on test accuracy is questionable (Schutter *et al.*, 1994; Maggino *et al.*, 1994). The additive value of color Doppler imaging and new tumor markers is limited and needs further evaluation (Yedema *et al.*, 1988; Einhorn *et al.*, 1989; Soper *et al.*, 1990; Bast *et al.*, 1991; Oram and Jeyarajah, 1994).

Table 24.1 Performance of the CA-125 test in discriminating a benign pelvic mass from ovarian cancer in premenopausal and postmenopausal women.

REFERENCE	n	SENS.	SPEC.	PPV	NPV	ACCURACY
PREMENOPAUSAL (cut-off level of 65 U/ml)						
Malkasian et al. (1988)	66	60	89	49	93	85
Gadducci et al. (1992)	213	50	87	24	96	84
POSTMENOPAUSAL (cut-off level of 35 U/ml)						
Finkler et al. (1988)	32	84	92	94	80	—
Malkasian et al. (1988)	92	81	91	94	74	85
Patsner and Mann (1988)	125	77	81	87	68	78
Schutter et al. (1994)	228	72	80	73	79	77
Maggino et al. (1994)	290	78	82	78	83	80

NPV, negative predictive value; PPV, positive predictive value; SENS., sensitivity; SPEC., specificity; n, number of women

Table 24.2 Reported specificities (%) in postmenopausal women, using the CA-125 assay as a primary screening test.

REFERENCE	CA-125			CA-125 > 30 U/ml plus US[a]
	> 30 U/ml	> 35 U/ml	> 65 U/ml	
Zurawski et al. (1987) (n = 915)	— —	93.3[b] 97.6[c]	98.8[b] 99.5[c]	— —
Jacobs et al. (1988) (n = 1010)	97.0	—	—	99.8
Einhorn et al. (1992) (n = 5500)	97.0	98.5	—	—
Jacobs et al. (1993) (n = 22 000)	98.5	—	—	99.9

[a] US refers to ultrasonography used as a secondary screening test; [b] Related to the subgroup of women less than 50 years old; [c] Related to the subgroup of women aged 50 years or more

WHAT DOES A NORMAL TEST RESULT MEAN?

Asymptomatic women: Menopausal status must be considered. The highest reported specificity in premenopausal women (98.8%) was achieved using a serum CA-125 threshold of 65 U/ml (Zurawski et al., 1987). If 16 per 100 000 screened women have ovarian cancer, for 100% sensitivity, the positive predictive value (PPV) of an elevated CA-125 level for ovarian malignancy would be 1.3% with a sensitivity of 100%. Given a specificity of 98.8%, of the 100 000 women screened 1200 would be falsely positive, implying that 75 laparotomies or laparoscopies would be performed per year to detect a single case of ovarian cancer. Using a 35 U/ml cut-off instead, specificity decreases below 95% and as a result the number of false positives would increase dramatically (Einhorn et al., 1992). In an attempt to circumvent the problem of low specificity, some investigators have combined serial CA-125 measurements for 'screen positive' with ultrasonography and a physical examination (Zurawski et al., 1990; Einhorn et al., 1992). The specificity of CA-125 for ovarian cancer screening could further be improved by the inclusion of the new tumor markers, such as CA-15.3 and TAG 72.3 assay (Jacobs et al., 1992), but at the cost of lower sensitivity, particularly in women with stage I disease (Yedema et al., 1988; Bast et al., 1991).

The specificity for CA-125 measurements tends to be better for postmenopausal women. In one study of 22 000 healthy postmenopausal volunteers, 299 women (1.4%) had raised levels (> 30 U/ml). Of these, 41 women had an abnormal ultrasound scan (0.2% of the total), and ovarian carcinoma was detected in 11 women. As specificity tends to improve, ultrasonography could be used as a secondary screening test in post-menopausal women. (Table 24.2). Given that 35 of 100 000 screened postmenopausal women have ovarian cancer, a sensitivity of 100%, and a specificity of 99.9%, the PPV is 26%. Hence, 100 of the 100 000 screened will be falsely positive, implying that four laparotomies or laparoscopies will be required to detect one case of ovarian cancer.

Women at increased risk: There are limited data on CA-125 and ultrasound screening in women with a history of familial ovarian cancer. Muto et al. (1993) screened women with both repeated serum CA-125 measurements and vaginal ultrasonography. If elevated, the CA-125 determinations were repeated after 3 months. A doubling over 3 months or a rise above 95 U/ml prompted further evaluation. Initially, 42 women (11%) had an elevated CA-125 (greater than 35 U/ml). Forty-one of these 42 women were premenopausal. Eventually 15 women had surgery; no malignancies were found. Bourne *et al.* (1994) detected 7 ovarian carcinoma by abnormal ultrasound, of which 3 cases showed elevated CA-125 levels. The authors concluded that screening using CA-125 and ultrasound was not helpful in detecting ovarian cancer in this high-risk, predominantly premenopausal population (Muto *et al.*, 1993).

What is the cost of testing?

The cost-effectiveness of screening has yet to be established in a large population. However, screening seems unlikely to be cost-effective considering the reported sensitivities and positive predictive values.

CONCLUSIONS AND RECOMMENDATIONS

In asymptomatic women the role of serum CA-125 measurement for screening purposes remains controversial. Skates and Singer (1991) developed a putative model using CA-125 in a screening setting in women aged 50–75 years. They concluded that survival was prolonged by 3.4 years per case detected if these women were screened annually. The survival advantage is primarily due to early detection of ovarian cancer, predominantly in the first year of screening. There are, however, concerns about the relatively high false positive rates, particularly in premenopausal women. For that reason, the CA-125 assay is not suitable as single screening test for ovarian cancer in asymptomatic premenopausal women. In postmenopausal women, the combination of serum CA-125 measurement as a primary screening test with ultrasonography as secondary test yields high specificities, approximately 99.9%. Preliminary data suggest that two-thirds of the ovarian cancers will be identified. Unfortunately, only one-third of the ovarian carcinomas identified are stage I. Even in women with a family history of ovarian cancer, the usefulness of CA-125 and ultrasound for the early detection of ovarian cancer remains unclear.

Measurement of CA-125 can be used in premenopausal women with a pelvic mass as a single test. About 85% of the pelvic masses in premenopausal women will be classified correctly if a cut-off of 65 U/ml is used. A serum CA-125 cut-off level of 35 U/ml is advocated in postmenopausal women, where 80% will be classified correctly. The malignancy index (Davies *et al.*, 1993) seems a relatively simple and reliable method to discriminate between benign and malignant pelvic masses in both premenopausal and postmenopausal women.

SUMMARY

1 WHAT IS THE PROBLEM THAT REQUIRES SCREENING?

OVARIAN CARCINOMA.

a What is the incidence/prevalence of the target condition?

Approximately 1 out of 80 female newborns will develop ovarian cancer during their lifetime. The median age is 53 years at detection. The incidence of ovarian cancer increases with age, from 15.7 per 100 000 women per year in the 40–44 year age group to an estimated 50 per 100 000 women per year in the higher age groups. Fewer than 25% of affected women have ovarian tumors confined to one ovary at diagnosis. Familial cases of ovarian cancer account for 3% to 5% of all women with the disease.

b What are the sequelae of the condition which are of interest in clinical medicine?

Ovarian cancer is the most common cause of death in women with genital tract malignancies. Since women with stage I or stage II disease usually do not have any clinical signs or symptoms, the majority of women with ovarian cancer are detected after their disease has progressed. Despite appropriate therapy, 5 year survival rates in women with stages III and IV disease range from 5% to 20%.

2 THE TEST

a What is the purpose of the test?

To identify at an early stage women with ovarian cancer and to differentiate between benign and malignant ovarian disease in women with a pelvic mass.

b The nature of the test

Standard serum CA-125 assay using a double-antibody radioimmunoassay.

c Implications of testing

1 What does an abnormal test result mean?

In postmenopausal women, about 2 out of 3 cases of ovarian carcinoma could be detected by annual serum CA-125 measurement. In premenopausal women, CA-125 is not a useful screening tool. Serum CA-125 screening in the postmenopausal age group will result in a relative low proportion (33%) of women with ovarian carcinoma being detected at an early, curable stage.

2 What does a normal test result mean?

A normal CA-125 measurement does not preclude the presence of an advanced ovarian carcinoma.

d What is the cost of testing?

Cost-effectiveness of screening has yet to be established in a large population. However, it seems unlikely to be cost-effective considering the reported low sensitivities and positive predictive values.

3 CONCLUSIONS AND RECOMMENDATIONS

Measurement CA-125 is not suitable as single screening test for ovarian cancer in asymptomatic premenopausal women because of a relatively high false positive rate. In postmenopausal women, the combination of serum CA-125 assay as the primary screening test with ultrasonography as a secondary test results in a high specificity. Preliminary data suggest that two-thirds of the ovarian cancers will be identified but only one-third of those identified are stage I. Even in women with a family history of ovarian cancer the usefulness of CA-125 and ultrasound screening for the early detection of ovarian cancer remains unclear.

Serum CA-125 assay can be used in premenopausal women with a pelvic mass as a single test. About 85% of the pelvic masses will be classified correctly if a cut-off of 65 U/ml is used. A serum CA-125 cut-off level of 35 U/ml is advocated in postmenopausal women where 80% will be classified correctly. The malignancy index seems a relative simple and reliable method to discriminate between benign and malignant pelvic masses in both premenopausal and post-menopausal women.

REFERENCES

Bast R, Feeney M, Lazarus H, Nadler L, Colvin R & Knapp R (1981) Reactivity of a monoclonal antibody with human ovarian carcinoma. *J Clin Invest* **68**: 1331–1337.

Bast R, Klug T, St John E *et al.* (1983) A radioimmunoassay using a monoclonal antibody to monitor the course of epithelial ovarian cancer. *N Engl J Med* **309**: 883–887.

Bast R, Siegal F, Runowicz C *et al.* (1985) Evaluation of serum CA-125 prior to diagnosis of an epithelial ovarian carcinoma. *Gynecol Oncol* **22**: 115–120.

Bast R, Knauf S, Epenetos A *et al.* (1991) Coordinate elevation of serum markers in ovarian cancer but not in benign disease. *Cancer* **68**: 1758–1763.

Bergmann J, Bidart J, George M, Beaugrand M, Levy V & Bohuon C (1987) Elevation of CA-125 in patients with benign and malignant ascites. *Cancer* **59**: 213–217.

Bourne T, Campbell S, Reynolds K *et al.* (1994) The potential role of serum CA-125 in an ultrasound-based screening program for familial ovarian cancer. *Gynecol Oncol* **52**:379–385.

Creasman W & Eddy G (1989) Prognostic factors in relation to second look laparotomy in ovarian cancer. *Baillières Clinical Obstetrics Gynaecology* **3**: 183–190.

Davies A, Jacobs I, Woolas R, Fish A & Oram D (1993) The adnexal mass: benign or malignant? Evaluation of a risk of malignancy index. *Br J Obstet Gynaecol* **100**: 927–931.

DiSaia P & Creasman W (1989) Advanced epithelial ovarian cancer. In DiSaia P & Creasman W (eds) *Clinical Gynecologic Oncology*, St Louis: CV Mosby. pp 325–416.

Duk J, Kauer F, Fleuren G & de Bruijn H (1989) Serum CA-125 levels in patients with a provisional diagnosis of pelvic inflammatory disease. *Acta Obstet Gynecol Scand* **68**: 637–641.

Einhorn N, Knapp R, Bast R & Zurawski V (1989) CA-125 assay used in conjunction with CA 15.3 and TAG-72 assays for discrimination between malignant and non-malignant diseases of the ovary. *Acta Oncol* **28**: 655–657.

Einhorn N, Sjövall K, Knapp R, Hall P, Scully R, Bast R & Zurawski V (1992) Prospective evaluation of serum CA-125 levels for early detection of ovarian cancer. *Obstet Gynecol* **80**: 14–18.

Finkler N, Benacerraf B, Lavin P, Wojciechowski C & Knapp R (1988) Comparison of serum CA-125, clinical impression and ultrasound in the preoperative evaluation of ovarian masses. *Obstet Gynecol* **72**: 659–664.

Fleuren G, Nap M, Aalders J, Trimbos B & de Bruijn H (1987) Explanation of the limited correlation between tumor CA-125 content and serum CA-125 antigen levels in patients with ovarian tumors. *Cancer* **60**: 2437–2442.

Friedlander M & Dembo A (1991) Prognostic factors in ovarian cancer. *Sem Oncol* **18**: 205–212.

Gadducci A, Ferdeghini M, Prontera C *et al.* (1992) The concomitant determination of different tumor markers in patients with epithelial ovarian cancer and benign ovarian masses: relevance for differential diagnosis. *Gynecol Oncol* **44**: 147–154.

Halila H, Stenman U & Seppala M (1986) Ovarian cancer antigen CA-125 levels in pelvic inflammatory disease and pregnancy. *Cancer* **57**: 1327–1329.

Henderson B, Ross R & Pike M (1991) Toward the prevention of cancer. *Science* **254**: 1131–1138.

Hilgers J, Zotter S & Kenemans P (1988) Polymorphic epithelial mucin and CA-125 bearing glycoprotein in basic and applied carcinoma research. *Cancer Rev* **11/12**: 3–10.

Houlston R, Bourne T, Davies A *et al.* (1992) Use of family history in a screening clinic for familial ovarian cancer. *Gynecol Oncol* **47**: 247–252.

Jacobs I, Stabile I, Bridges J, *et al.* (1988) Multimodal approach to screening for ovarian cancer. *Lancet* **ii**: 268–271.

Jacobs I, Oram D, Fairbanks J, Turner J, Frost C & Grudzinskas J (1990) A risk of malignancy index incorporating CA-125, ultrasound and menopausal status for the accurate preoperative diagnosis of ovarian cancer. *Br J Obstet Gynaecol* **97**: 922–929.

Jacobs I, Oram D & Bast R (1992) Strategies for improving the specificity of screening for ovarian cancer with tumor-associated antigens CA-125, CA 15.3 and TAG 72.3. *Obstet Gynecol* **80**: 396–399.

Jacobs I, Davies A, Bridges J, *et al.* (1993) Prevalence screening for ovarian cancer in postmenopausal women by CA-125 measurement and ultrasonography. *Br Med J* **306**: 1030–1034.

Kamp van G, Verstraeten A & Kenemans P (1993) Discordant serum CA-125 values in commercial immunoassays. *Eur J Obstet Gynecol Reprod Biol* **49:** 99–103.

Katsube Y, Berg J & Silverberg S (1982) Epidemiologic pathology of ovarian tumors. *Int J Gynecol Pathol* **1:** 3–16.

Kenemans P, Bon G, Kessler A, Verstraeten A & van Kamp G (1992) Technical and clinical evaluation of a new fully automated enzyme immunoassay for the detection of CA-125, a multicenter study. *Clin Chem* **38:** 1466–1471.

Kenemans P, van Kamp G, Oehr P & Verstraeten R (1993) Heterologous double-determinant immunoradiometric assay CA-125 II: reliable second-generation immunoassay for determining CA-125 in serum. *Clin Chem* **39:** 2509–2513.

Maggino T, Gadducci A, D'Addario V, *et al.* (1994) Prospective multicenter study on CA-125 in postmenopausal pelvic masses. *Gynecol Oncol* **54:** 117–123.

Malkasian G, Knapp R, Lavin P, *et al.* (1988) Preoperative evaluation of serum CA-125 levels in premenopausal and post-menopausal patients with pelvic masses: discrimination of benign from malignant disease. *Am J Obstet Gynecol* **159:** 341–346.

Mastropaolo W, Fernandez Z & Miller E (1986) Pronounced increases in the concentration of an ovarian tumor marker, CA-125, in serum of a healthy subject during menstruation. *Clin Chem* **32:** 2110–2111.

Metzger J, Haussinger K, Wilmanns W & Lamerz R (1987) Hohe CA-125-Serumspiegel bei benignem Aszites oder Pleuraerguss. *Geburtsh Frauenheilk* **47:** 463–465.

Muto M, Cramer D, Brown D, *et al.* (1993) Screening for ovarian cancer: The preliminary experience of a familial ovarian cancer centre. *Gynecol Oncol* **51:** 12–20.

Neijt J, ten Bokkel Huinink W, van der Burg M, *et al.* (1991) Long-term survival in ovarian cancer. *Eur J Cancer* **27:** 1367–1372.

Oram DH & Jeyarajah AR (1994) The role of ultrasound and tumour markers in the early detection of ovarian cancer. *Br J Obstet Gynaecol* **101:** 939–945.

Parkin D, Laara E & Muir C (1988) Estimates of the worldwide frequency of sixteen major cancers in 1980. *Int J Cancer* **41:** 184–197.

Patsner B & Mann W (1988) The value of preoperative serum CA-125 levels in patients with a pelvic mass. *Am J Obstet Gynecol* **159:** 873–876.

Petterson F, Kolstad P & Ludwig H (1988) *Annual Report on the Results of Treatment in Gynecological Cancer*, Vol. 20, Stockholm: International Federation of Gynecology and Obstetrics.

Pittaway D (1988) Correlation of an enzyme immunoassay with the radioimmunoassay for CA-125. *Am JObstet Gynecol* **158:** 62–64.

Pittaway D & Fayez J (1986) Serum CA-125 in the diagnosis and management of endometriosis. *Fertil Steril* **46:** 790–795.

Pittaway D & Fayez J (1987) Serum CA-125 antigen levels increase during menses. *Am J Obstet Gynecol* **156:** 75–76.

Ruibal A, Encabo G, Martinez-Miralles E *et al.* (1984) CA-125 seric levels in non-malignant pathologies. *Bull Cancer* **71:** 145–148.

Schiltkraut J & Thompson W (1988) Familial ovarian cancer: a population-based case-control study. *Am J Epidemiol* **128:** 456–466.

Schutter E, Kenemans P, Sohn C *et al.* (1994) Diagnostic value of pelvic examination, ultrasound and serum CA-125 in postmenopausal women with a pelvic mass: An international multicenter study. *Cancer* **74:** 1398–1406.

Seki K, Kikuchi Y, Uesatom T & Kato K (1986) Increased serum CA-125 levels during the first trimester of pregnancy. *Acta Obstet Gynecol Scand* **65:** 583–585.

Skates S & Singer D (1991) Quantifying the potential benefit of CA-125 screening for ovarian cancer. *J Clin Epidemiol* **44:** 365–380.

Soper J, Hunter V, Daly L, Tanner M, Creasman W, & Bast R (1990) Preoperative serum tumor-associated antigen levels in women with pelvic masses. *Obstet Gynecol* **75:** 249–254.

Yedema C, Massuger L, Hilgers J *et al.* (1988) Preoperative discrimination between benign and malignant ovarian tumors using a combination of CA-125 and CA 15.3 serum assays. *Int J Cancer* (suppl.) **3:** 61–67.

Yedema C, Thomas C, Segers M, Doesburg W & Kenemans P (1992) Comparison of five immunoassay procedures for the ovarian carcinoma-associated determinant CA-125 in serum. *Eur J Obstet Gynecol Reprod Biol* **47:** 245–251.

Yedema C, Von Mensdorff-Pouilly S, Kenemans P, Verheijen R, Bon G & Hilgers J (1994) Update on the serum tumour marker CA-125. In Bruhat M (ed.) *The Management of Adnexal Cysts*, pp 75–97. Oxford: Blackwell.

Zurawski V, Broderick S, Pickens P, Knapp R & Bast R (1987) Serum CA-125 levels in a group of non-hospitalized women: relevance for the early detection of ovarian cancer. *Obstet Gynecol* **69:** 606–611.

Zurawski V, Orjaseter H, Andersen A & Jellum E (1988) Elevated serum CA-125 levels prior to diagnosis of ovarian neoplasia: relevance for early detection of ovarian cancer. *Int J Cancer* **42:** 677–680.

Zurawski V, Sjovall K, Schoenfeld D, *et al.* (1990) Prospective evaluation of serum CA-125 levels in a normal population, phase I: the specificities of single and serial determinations in testing for ovarian cancer. *Gynecol Oncol* **36:** 299–305.

25

Mammography & Breast Self-Examination

Paul J. van der Maas & Harry J. de Koning

● ●

WHAT IS THE PROBLEM THAT REQUIRES SCREENING?

BREAST CANCER.

What is the incidence/prevalence of the target condition?

The highest incidence of breast cancer (60–90 per 100 000 women) is found in the USA, the Netherlands, the UK and several other European countries. In Asia (Japan, China) the incidence is typically 2–4 times lower (Table 25.1). Incidence differences between countries for premenopausal breast cancer are usually smaller than for postmenopausal breast cancer (Møller Jensen *et al.*, 1990; IARC and WHO, 1992; Netherlands Cancer Registry, 1992). In the Netherlands the prevalence of breast cancer is estimated to be approximately 7 times the incidence rate (Voogd *et al.*, 1993). The age-standardized breast cancer mortality rate is 40–50% of the incidence rate. Mortality rates for the different countries follow a pattern similar to that for incidence (Table 25.1) (Møller Jensen *et al.*, 1990; Vecchia *et al.*, 1992).

The incidence/mortality ratio varies between countries, depending on many factors

Table 25.1 World standardized incidence rates (per 100 000 women, 1983–1987).

BREAST CANCER	
USA (white)	89
The Netherlands (Eindhoven)	73
Canada	71
Italy	65
USA (black)	65
UK (Scotland)	63
Sweden	63
Australia (NSW)	60
Germany (Saarland)	56
Spain (Basque country)	47
Hong Kong	32
Japan (Osaka)	22
China (Shanghai)	21
India (Madras)	20

From: IARC and WHO (1992)

including differential survival and stage at diagnosis (Adami *et al.*, 1986). In the Netherlands the average relative survival is 70%, 55%, and 50% for 5 years, 10 and 20 years, respectively (Nab, 1995).

What are the sequelae of the condition which are of interest in clinical medicine?

Breast cancer is the most common form of cancer among women in many industrialized countries. It is typically diagnosed after the woman has felt a lump in her breast or has observed visible changes. These tumours generally have a diameter of at least 2 cm when diagnosed. They are treated either by surgery, radiotherapy, adjuvant systemic treatment, or any combination of these modalities. The typical length of survival after diagnosis without treatment is 3 years (Gullino, 1977). Both surgery that conserves the breast, and mastectomy with or without radiotherapy are intended to be curative. In addition, adjuvant systemic treatment improves survival, suggesting that treatment is effective against small or slow-growing micrometastases present at the time of primary diagnosis (Early Breast Cancer Trialists' Collaborative Group, 1992). The average survival after the diagnosis of distant metastases is 20 months (Koning *et al.*, 1992; Richards *et al.*, 1993).

THE TESTS

What is the purpose of the tests?

The purpose of mammography is to detect a malignant tumour before it has metastasized. In doing so, it is thought more likely that primary therapy will result in complete cure of the patient. In addition, both the size of the primary tumor at initial treatment and degree of angiogenesis are strongly related to the probability of metastasis (Horak *et al.*, 1992).

The nature of the tests

Mammography: Mammography consists of an X-ray examination of each breast, often from two different directions. The compression which occurs when the breasts are placed between two radiographic film plates can be painful for some women (Ellman *et al.*, 1989; Cockburn *et al.*, 1994). Screening mammography requires high-quality, specially calibrated equipment and experienced radiographers and radiologists who have been trained in screening mammography. The films are preferably read independently by two radiologists. Certain abnormalities on the mammogram may indicate early malignant lesions that are not yet clinically apparent.

Breast self-examination: The majority of breast masses in a population not screened by mammography are discovered by the patient. The breast self-examination is best performed the first few days after menstruation in premenopausal women and monthly in postmenopausal women. The examination begins with an inspection of the breasts in the mirror, looking for changes in shape and contour. It should then continue in the shower, where tactile sensation is increased. After showering the woman should lie on her side and, using the second through fourth fingers, systematically palpate the contralateral breast. Typical, the examination begins with the nipples and works away from them in a circular fashion. The process is repeated on the other side.

Implications of testing

WHAT DOES AN ABNORMAL TEST RESULT MEAN?

Many trials have demonstrated that the screening of women aged 50–69 years using mammography reduces breast cancer mortality (Shapiro *et al.*, 1982; Collette *et al.*, 1984; Verbeek *et al.*, 1984; Tabar *et al.*, 1985, 1992; Andersson *et al.*, 1988; UK Trial of Early Detection of Breast Cancer Group, 1988, 1993; Roberts *et al.*, 1990; Frisell *et al.*, 1991; Miller *et al.*, 1992; Nyström *et al.*, 1993). In premenopausal women, active glandular tissue makes the interpretation of the mammogram more difficult. At present, there is no firm proof that the screening of women under 50 years old reduces breast cancer mortality (Koning *et al.*, 1995). Though programs in which women are trained in periodical breast self-examination are associated with the somewhat earlier detection of breast cancer, the effect achieved is not sufficient to reduce mortality to a clinically significant degree (Gästrin *et al.*, 1994).

The sensitivity and specificity of mammography for the detection of breast cancer in women aged 50–69 years are approximately 85% and 95%, respectively. In younger women, the sensitivity is estimated to be 60–80% of the former value (Brekelmans *et al.*, 1992). The predictive value of an abnormal test result in a population with a high prevalence, such as the Netherlands, is at best about 50%. This means that half of the women with an abnormal test result have no malignancy proven. In order to limit the consequences of a false positive screening test result, a standardized sequential diagnostic work-up should be available to the woman without delay. As the suspect lesion will not be palpable in 40% of instances, this further diagnostic assessment should be done in centers with the required equipment and sufficient expertise. In some other countries, the predictive values are much lower (Ashby *et al.*, 1990; Chamberlain *et al.*, 1993). Because the lesion discovered by screening will be smaller on average, breast-conserving therapy is more often an option (Fisher *et al.*, 1989; Farrow *et al.*, 1992; Koning *et al.*, 1994).

The natural history of very small or very early breast cancer lesions is only partly known. The inevitable uncertainty about the prognostic improvement of major primary therapy should be weighed against its risks and drawbacks. Ductal carcinoma in situ (DCIS) constitutes 15–20% of all breast cancers detected in some series by mammography screening. In some cases this may result in overtreatment, although at present there is a growing understanding of prognostic factors in DCIS (Recht *et al.*, 1994).

About 30 of every 100 women aged 50–69 with screen-detected breast cancer will benefit in the sense that they will be cured instead of dying from their disease. The remaining 70 will not benefit from the earlier diagnosis: about 50 would have been cured anyway (i.e. the typical cure rate after primary therapy for symptomatic breast cancer is about 50%), another 15 will die of breast cancer despite the earlier diagnosis and about 5 will die from an unrelated problem before the breast cancer would have become clinically manifest without the screening. These 5 women represent an artificial increase in incidence of breast cancer owing to screening (Boer *et al.*, 1994). The total number of women who benefit from breast cancer screening is smaller than the number who die of their disease and must live extra years with the knowledge they have breast cancer. However, it is generally agreed that the benefit, about 15 life-years gained, outweighs the unfavorable effect (Haes *et al.*, 1991; Koning, 1993). This illustrates the subtle balance between the advantages and disadvantages of breast cancer screening. Table 25.2 gives an overview of favorable and unfavorable effects per 1 000 000 screens.

Table 25.2   Favorable and unfavorable effects when implementing nationwide breast cancer screening of women aged 50–69 every 2 years. Numbers are based on population screening 1990–2017 in the Netherlands (total of 15.8 million screens) and follow-up of effects until 2090.

UNFAVORABLE EFFECTS		FAVORABLE EFFECTS	
screens	1 million	life-years gained	16 500
screen false positives which have led to biopsy	2 100	breast cancer deaths prevented	1 080
increase in life-years after known diagnosis (earlier diagnosis without extra survival)	17 500	breast-conserving therapy instead of mastectomy	750
additional number of primary surgical treatments	590	decrease in biopsies outside program with benign result	3 200
additional number of primary radiation treatments	650	decrease in adjuvant hormonal treatment	525
		decrease in treatment of advanced disease	1 080

WHAT DOES A NORMAL TEST RESULT MEAN?

Though a sensitivity of about 85% can be reached after double reading of the films, about 15% of all breast cancers are still missed after screening with mammography. It is important to explain to women that if they feel or see an abnormality in their breasts after having a normal test result, they should not postpone a visit to the doctor or wait until the next round of screening.

What is the cost of testing?

The costs and cost-effectiveness of breast cancer screening have been examined in detail for several countries (Koning *et al.*, 1991; Brown and Fintor, 1993; Ineveld *et al.*, 1993; Beemsterboer *et al.*, 1994). The costs vary with the type of screening organization and the characteristics of the health care system. Table 25.3 illustrates some key figures about cost and cost-effectiveness for the centralized system in the Netherlands and for the decentralized system in Germany. The cost per screen per woman is approximately US $45 for the Netherlands and US $65 for Germany. The cost of further diagnostic evaluation will increase owing to the extra prevalence (see above) and the false positives. This increase may be partly offset by a decrease in preventive activity outside the screening program. The increased prevalence will also increase the frequency of primary therapy and follow-up (see also Table 25.2). However, major savings result from the prevented cases of advanced disease. Cost-effectiveness ratios show a wide variation among countries because they are not only sensitive to health care differences, but also to the effect of size which is directly related to the incidence and prevalence of the disease. Cost-effectiveness ratios are generally more favorable in countries with higher prevalence.

Table 25.3 Costs and cost-effectiveness of breast cancer screening of women aged 50–69 at 2-year intervals in the Netherlands and Germany during 27 years. Costs (rows 1–4) are expected differences between a situation with screening and one without screening (in millions of US$), 5% discount rate.

	NETHERLANDS SCREENING VS NO SCREENING	GERMANY SCREENING VS NO SCREENING
Costs:		
cost of screening	+300	+2 420
cost of assessment/treatment/follow-up	+60	+470
less cost of advanced disease	−130	−540
total cost	+230	+2 350
breast cancer deaths prevented	6 000	19 600
life-years gained	61 000	206 500
cost per life-year gained (CE ratio, US $)	3 800	11 400

From: de Koning et al. (1991), Beemsterboer et al. (1994).

CONCLUSIONS AND RECOMMENDATIONS

Systematic screening for breast cancer by mammography in women aged 50–69 years reduces the mortality from breast cancer and may be beneficial for even higher age groups. Until now, clinical trials have shown no clearcut benefit for women under 50 years old. Occasional clinical mammography for preventive purposes outside a systematic screening program is not recommended. The balance between the favorable and unfavorable effects of breast cancer screening is fragile. A favorable balance can only be reached in a systematic program with high-quality equipment, well-trained radiographers and radiologists and a system of continuous quality and effect control.

Whether breast cancer screening should be introduced in a country depends on at least three factors. First, the epidemiology of the disease: when incidence/prevalence is low the effectiveness and efficiency of the program will be less. Second, patient and physician behaviour: in areas where women with symptoms tend to postpone a visit to the doctor, or where doctors are reluctant to refer the patient to the specialist for further diagnostic evaluation and treatment, resulting in an unfavorable stage distribution in clinically diagnosed tumors, the gains of breast cancer screening will be larger than in areas where both women and doctors tend to be alert. Third, the screening organization and health care system: a centralized system with uniform procedures and quality control will generally be more effective and efficient than a decentralized system where screening mammography is performed in between a variety of diagnostic and therapeutic procedures. When mass screening is introduced, clinicians should be aware that the population of referred women differs fundamentally from the population that presents with symptoms. Such awareness is necessary in order to prevent overdiagnosis and overtreatment.

We would like to acknowledge the contribution made by GJ van Oortmarssen and R Boer to this work.

SUMMARY

1

WHAT IS THE PROBLEM THAT REQUIRES SCREENING?

BREAST CANCER.

a What is the incidence/prevalence of the target condition?

The highest incidence (60–90 per 100 000 women) is found in the USA, the Netherlands, the UK and several other European countries. In Asia, the incidence is typically 2–4 times lower. In the Netherlands, the prevalence of breast cancer is estimated to be about 7 times the incidence rate. This is likely to be a typical prevalence/incidence ratio in other, similar countries.

b What are the sequelae of the condition which are of interest in clinical medicine?

Breast cancer is the most common form of cancer among women in many industrialized countries. The typical length of survival after diagnosis without treatment is 3 years. Both surgery that conserves the breast and mastectomy with or without radiotherapy are intended to be curative. The average survival after diagnosis of distant metastases is 21 months.

2

THE TESTS

a What is the purpose of the tests?

To detect a malignant breast tumor before it has metastasized.

b The nature of the tests

Mammography consists of an X-ray of each breast, often viewed from two different directions. Screening mammography requires high-quality, specially calibrated equipment and experienced radiographers and radiologists who have been trained in screening mammography. Breast self-examination is performed monthly in a standing and supine position.

c Implications of testing

1 What does an abnormal test result mean?

The sensitivity and specificity of mammography for the detection of breast cancer in women aged 50–69 years are approximately 85% and 95%, respectively. In younger women, the sensitivity is estimated to be 60–80% of the former value. The positive predictive value of an abnormal test result in a population with a high prevalence is at best about 50%. About 30 of every 100 women aged 50–69 years with a screen-detected breast cancer will benefit in the sense that they will be cured instead of dying from their disease. The remaining 70 will not benefit from the earlier diagnosis; about 50 would have been cured anyway, another 15 will die of breast cancer despite the early diagnosis and about 5 will die from an unrelated problem before their breast cancer had become clinically apparent without the screening. Self-examination does not decrease the mortality from breast cancer.

2 What does a normal test result mean?

About 15% of all breast cancers are still missed by screening with mammography.

d What is the cost of testing?

The costs and cost-effectiveness of breast cancer screening with mammography varies with the type of screening organization and the characteristics of the health care system. The cost per screen per woman approximates US $45 for a centralized system and US $65 for a decentralized system.

3 CONCLUSIONS AND RECOMMENDATIONS

Systematic screening for breast cancer by mammography in women aged 50–69 years reduces the mortality from breast cancer and may be beneficial for even higher age groups. Until now, clinical trials have found no clear-cut benefit for women under age 50 years. Occasional clinical mammography for preventive purposes outside a systematic screening program is not recommended.

REFERENCES

Adami H-O, Malker B, Holmberg L, Persson I & Stone B (1986) The relation between survival and age at diagnosis in breast cancer. *N Engl J Med* **315:** 559–663.

Andersson I, Aspegren K, Janzon L *et al.* (1988) Mammographic screening and mortality from breast cancer: the Malmö mammographic screening trial. *Br Med J* **297:** 943–948.

Ashby J, Buxton M & Gravelle H (1990) Will a breast screening programme change the workload and referral practice of general practitioners? *J Epidemiol Comm Health* **44:** 36–38.

Beemsterboer PMM, Koning HJ de, Warmerdam PG *et al.* (1994) Prediction of the effects and costs of breast-cancer screening in Germany. *Int J Cancer* **58:** 623–628.

Boer R, Warmerdam P, Koning H de & Oortmarssen G van (1994) Extra incidence caused by mammographic screening (letter). *Lancet* **343:** 979.

Brekelmans CTM, Collette HJA, Collette C, Fracheboud J & Waard F de (1992). Breast cancer after a negative screen: follow-up of women participating in the DOM screening programme. *Eur J Cancer* **28A:** 893–895.

Brown ML & Fintor L (1993) Cost-effectiveness of breast cancer screening: preliminary results of a systematic review of the literature. *Breast Cancer Res Treat* **25:** 113–118.

Chamberlain J, Moss SM, Kirkpatrick AE, Michell M & Johns L (1993) National Health Service breast screening programme results for 1991–2. *Br Med J* **307:** 353–356.

Cockburn J, Staples M, Hurley SF & De Luise T (1994) Psychological consequences of screening mammography. *J Med Screen* **1:** 7–12.

Collette HJA, Rombach JJ, Day NE & Waard F de (1984) Evaluation of screening for breast cancer in a non-randomized study (the DOM project) by means of a case-control study. *Lancet* **i:** 1224–1226.

Early Breast Cancer Trialists' Collaborative Group (1992) Systemic treatment of early breast cancer by hormone, cytotoxic, or immune therapy. *Lancet* **339:** 1–15.

Ellman R, Angeli N, Christians A *et al.* (1989) Psychiatric morbidity associated with screening for breast cancer. *Br J Cancer* **60:** 781–784.

Farrow DC, Hunt WF & Samet JM (1992) Geographic variation in the treatment of localized breast cancer. *N Engl J Med* **326:** 1097–1101.

Fisher B, Redmond C, Poisson R *et al.* (1989) Eight-year results of a randomized clinical trial comparing total mastectomy and lumpectomy with or without irradiation in the treatment of breast cancer. *N Engl J Med* **320:** 822–828.

Frisell J, Eklund G, Hellström L *et al.* (1991) Randomized study of mammography screening – preliminary report on mortality in the Stockholm trial. *Breast Cancer Res Treat* **18:** 49–56.

Gästrin G, Miller AB, To T *et al.* (1994) Incidence and mortality from breast cancer in the Mama programme for breast screening in Finland, 1973–1986. *Cancer* **73:** 2168–2174.

Gullino PM (1977) Natural history of breast cancer. Progression from hyperplasia to neoplasia as predicted by angiogenesis. *Cancer* **39:** 2697–2703.

Haes JCJM de, Koning HJ de, Oortmarssen GJ van *et al.* (1991) The impact of a breast cancer screening programme on quality-adjusted life-years. *Int J Cancer* **49**: 538–544.

Horak ER, Leek R, Klenk N *et al.* (1992) Angiogenesis, assessed by platelet/endothelial cell adhesion molecule antibodies, as indicator of node metastases and survival in breast cancer. *Lancet* **340**: 1120–1124.

IARC (International Agency for Research on Cancer) & WHO (World Health Organization) (1992) Cancer incidence in five continents, Volume VI. Lyon: IARC Scientific Publications No. 120.

Ineveld BM van, Oortmarssen GJ van, Koning HJ de, Boer R & Maas PJ van der (1993). How cost-effective is breast cancer screening in different EC-countries? *Eur J Cancer* **29A**: 1663–1668.

Koning HJ de (1993) The effects and costs of breast cancer screening. Thesis, Erasmus University Rotterdam.

Koning HJ de, Ineveld BM van, Oortmarssen GJ van, *et al.* (1991) Breast cancer screening and cost-effectiveness; policy alternatives, quality of life considerations and the possible impact of uncertain factors. *Int J Cancer* **49**: 531–537.

Koning HJ de, Ineveld BM van, Haes JCJM de *et al.* (1992) Advanced breast cancer and its prevention by screening. *Br J Cancer* **65**: 950–955.

Koning HJ de, Dongen JA van & Maas PJ van der (1994) Changes in use of breast-conserving therapy in years 1978–2000. *Br J Cancer* **70**: 1165–1170.

Koning HJ de, Boer R, Warmerdam PG, Beemsterboer PMM & van der Maas PJ (1995) Quantitative interpretation of age-specific mortality reductions from the Swedish breast cancer screening trials. *J Natl Cancer Inst* **87**: 1217–1223.

Miller AB, Baines CJ, To T & Wall C (1992) Canadian National Breast Screening Study: 1. Breast cancer detection and death rates among women aged 40 to 49 years and 2. Breast cancer detection and death rates among women aged 50 to 59 years. *Can Med Assoc J* **147**: 1459–1471, 1477–1488.

Møller Jensen O, Estéve J, Møller H & Renard H (1990) Cancer in the European Community and its member states. *Eur J Cancer* **26**: 1167–1256.

Nab HW (1995) Trends in incidence and prognosis in female breast cancer since 1955. Thesis, Erasmus University, Rotterdam.

Netherlands Cancer Registry (1992) Incidence of cancer in The Netherlands 1989. Report, Utrecht.

Nyström L, Rutqvist LE, Wall S *et al.* (1993) Breast cancer screening with mammography: overview of Swedish randomised trials. *Lancet* **341**: 973–978.

Recht A, Dongen JA van, Fentiman IS, Holland R & Peterse JL (1994) Third meeting of the DCIS working party of the EORTC (Fondazione Cini, Isola S. Giorgio, Venezia, 28 February 1994). Conference Report. *Eur J Cancer* **30A**: 1895–1901.

Richards MA, Braysher S, Gregory WM & Rubens RD (1993) Advanced breast cancer: use of resources and cost implications. *Br J Cancer* **67**: 856–860.

Roberts MM, Alexander FE, Anderson TJ *et al.* (1990) Edinburgh trial of screening for breast cancer: mortality at seven years. *Lancet* **335**: 241–246.

Shapiro S, Venet W, Strax P, Venet L & Roeser R (1982) Ten- to fourteen-year effect of screening on breast cancer mortality. *J Natl Cancer Inst* **69**: 349–355.

Tabár L, Gad A, Holmberg LH *et al.* (1985) Reduction in mortality from breast cancer after mass screening with mammography. *Lancet* **i**: 829–832.

Tabár L, Fagerberg G, Day NE, Duffy SW & Kitchin RM (1992) Breast cancer treatment and natural history: new insights from results of screening. *Lancet* **339**: 412–414.

UK Trial of Early Detection of Breast Cancer Group (1988) First results on mortality reduction in the UK trial of early detection of breast cancer. *Lancet* **ii**: 411–416.

UK Trial of Early Detection of Breast Cancer Group (1993) Breast cancer mortality after ten years in the UK trial of the early detection of breast cancer. *Breast* **2**: 13–20.

Vecchia C La, Lucchini F, Negri E *et al.* (1992) Trends of cancer mortality in Europe, 1955–1989: III. Breast and genital sites. *Eur J Cancer* **28A**: 927–998.

Verbeek ALM, Hendriks JHCL, Holland R *et al.* (1984) Reduction of breast cancer mortality through mass screening with modern mammography. First results of the Nijmegen project, 1975–1981. *Lancet* **i**: 1222–1224.

Voogd AC, Coebergh JWW, Dongen JA van & Leeuwen FE van (1993) Borstkanker. In Ruwaard D & Kramers PGN (eds) *Volksgezondheid Toekomst Verkenning*, pp 280–287. Den Haag: Sdu Uitgeverij.

26

Screening Tests for Contraceptive Users

Jeffrey F. Peipert

Approximately 55% of the 39 million women at risk of unintended pregnancy in the USA use a reversible method of contraception. Thirty-five per cent rely on sterilization (vasectomy or tubal ligation), and the remaining 10% use no method of birth control (Forrest and Fordyce, 1993). Oral contraceptives (OCs) are the most popular form of reversible contraception among women, with nearly 40% of those at risk using them (Forrest and Fordyce, 1993). Other commonly used reversible methods of contraception include condoms and the diaphragm. The intrauterine device (IUD) is another highly effective method of contraception commonly used in Europe and throughout most of the world. While the number of IUD users worldwide increased from 60 million to 83 million between 1982 and 1988 (ACOG, 1992; Speroff and Darney, 1992), the number of users in the USA decreased from 2.2 million to 700 000 (Mosher and Pratt, 1990).

Before one can evaluate the appropriateness of screening tests for contraceptive users, a target condition must be first identified. This is not an easy task with over fifteen different types of contraception available and many potential target conditions. Furthermore, a screening test should target relatively common conditions. Given the age range of the population at risk, there are few conditions that would be considered both common and a contraindication to use of the contraceptive method. This chapter focuses on two methods of contraception commonly used in the USA and Europe – oral contraceptives and the intrauterine device.

Oral Contraceptives

WHAT IS THE PROBLEM THAT REQUIRES SCREENING?

THE INCREASED RISK OF THROMBOTIC AND LIPID DISORDERS IN WOMEN INGESTING ORAL CONTRACEPTIVES.

What is the incidence/prevalence of the target condition?

The prevalence of hypertension, thrombosis, diabetes, hyperlipidemia and hormone-sensitive malignancy in women using modern low-estradiol oral contraceptives (OCs) is similar to that of the noncontraceptive-using population.

What are the sequelae of the condition which are of interest in clinical medicine?

Possible sequelae of oral contraceptive use include arterial stroke, thrombosis and atherosclerosis.

THE TESTS

What is the purpose of the tests?

To identify conditions that might contraindicate hormonal contraception. Should screening practices for OC users differ from the routine screening practices applied to women of reproductive age and covered in other chapters of this book? Stated differently, what are the common complications of the OC that can effectively be screened for? Absolute contraindications to OC use include active (or history of) thrombosis or cerebral vascular disease, ischemic heart disease, markedly impaired liver function, known or suspected breast cancer, pregnancy, and undiagnosed abnormal vaginal bleeding (Hatcher *et al.*, 1994).

The nature of the tests

The 1994 edition of *Contraceptive Technology* (Hatcher *et al.*, 1994) states that 'weight, blood pressure, Pap smear, and pelvic examination should be done at the time of the initial examination' of potential oral contraceptive users. While family planning clinics often base their clinical protocols on such statements, there is little evidence to support the recommendations. In fact, there is little in the medical literature to permit an evaluation of which screening tests are prudent for either the prospective or current oral contraceptive user. Although some authors recommend blood testing prior to OC prescription (Serfaty, 1986; Baudet and Seguy, 1987), most English-language textbooks do not even mention routine blood screening (Speroff and Darney, 1992; Hatcher *et al.*, 1994). The US Food and Drug Administration only mentions the use of 'relevant laboratory tests' without any recommendation concerning systematic screening (Corfman, 1988).

Theoretically, there are two ways to address the issues of increased thrombotic and metabolic risks: a complete history and laboratory tests. Modern oral contraceptives have little impact on the lipid profile and carbohydrate metabolism. There are no screening tests for potential thrombosis. Thus, there are few if any tests that can detect a common condition that would contraindicate OC use, which would not be detected during the taking of a complete medical history including menstrual pattern, medical history, and smoking history. Most risk factors for cardiovascular disease are found among older women, in particular those who smoke. Thus, these conditions should be screened for using the same indications and guidelines that are applied to all women (ACOG, 1994).

What is the cost of testing?

Biochemical testing cannot be justified, since the likelihood of detecting a disorder not otherwise identified during either history taking or physical examination is small.

Intrauterine Device

THE DEVELOPMENT OF UPPER GENITAL TRACT INFECTION OR PELVIC INFLAMMATORY DISEASE (PID).

Screening tests prior to intrauterine device (IUD) insertion are controversial. Since the IUD has minimal systemic effect, routine blood screening is not justified.

What is the incidence/prevalence of the target condition?

The incidence of PID in IUD users is typically overestimated by medical practitioners. In the early 1980s, the annual incidence of PID in IUD users was estimated at 2% (Kessel, 1989). More recent studies have shown that the incidence is closely related to the time of IUD insertion. For example, the risk of PID has been observed to be five times higher during the first 20 days after insertion, compared with later periods (Farley et al., 1992). It is approximately 10 per 1000 woman years during the first 20 days after insertion dropping to less than 2 per 1000 woman years, where it remains steady for up to 8 years of follow-up. Thus, only 0.05% of women without a history of either PID, or a sexually transmitted disease within 6 months of insertion, develop genital upper tract disease within the first 20 days after the insertion of an IUD.

What are the sequelae of the condition which are of interest in clinical medicine?

The medical sequelae of PID include infertility, chronic pelvic pain, ectopic pregnancy, recurrent PID, and morbidity and mortality associated with tubo-ovarian abscesses. Active, recent, or recurrent pelvic infection are contraindications to the use of the IUD (Hatcher et al., 1994). The most important factor in patient selection for an IUD is the risk of sexually transmitted disease (STD) (Speroff and Darney, 1992). This factor requires the caregiver to take a careful sexual and reproductive history to determine that the woman is at low risk of contracting an STD.

What is the purpose of the tests?

Screening tests for prospective IUD users would seek to identify women at risk of the development of pelvic infection.

The nature of the tests

Since as many as 47% of women with evidence of mucopurulent cervicitis and 86% of women with cervicitis and positive chlamydial testing have evidence of upper genital tract infection on endometrical biopsy (Paavonen *et al.*, 1985), a case can be made for screening women for mucopurulent cervicitis and endocervical infection prior to IUD insertion. In addition, since bacterial vaginosis has been shown to increase the risk of postabortal infection (Larsson *et al.*, 1992), screening for bacterial vaginosis would be a cost-effective adjunct given the low cost of a saline wet preparation.

Microscopic examination of a saline wet mount of vaginal discharge would identify patients with either bacterial vaginosis or cervicitis. A wet mount or cervical Gram stain adds specificity to the diagnosis if clue cells or Gram-negative intracellular diplococci are identified.

Current rapid screening tests for chlamydia utilize an enzyme-linked immunosorbent assay (ELISA) and have sensitivities greater than 90% and specificities over 95% (Isada and Grossman, 1994).

Implications of testing

WHAT DOES AN ABNORMAL TEST RESULT MEAN?

Women with mucopurulent cervicitis are at increased risk for postinsertional PID. In populations with a high prevalence of chlamydia (such as 10%), 84% of positive ELISA tests results are associated with a positive chlamydia culture. In low-prevalence populations (2%), the positive predictive value drops considerably (to 50% or lower). Thus, a positive test will be erroneous in 1 out of 7 positive women from a high-prevalence population, and in 1 of 2 positive women from a low-prevalence population.

WHAT DOES A NORMAL TEST RESULT MEAN?

The risk of postinsertion PID in a woman with no evidence of genital tract disease in a monogamous relationship should be very low. Whether the prevalence of chlamydia is high or low, a negative ELISA is reassuring.

What is the cost of testing?

If we assume that universal screening of 700 000 IUD users in the USA for gonorrhea and chlamydia costs US $85 per women screened, the total cost of testing would be $59.5 million. Assuming an overall prevalence of endocervical infection of 4%, test sensitivity of 94% and specificity of 98%, a total of 26 320 cases of endocervical infection would be correctly identified (positive predictive value 66%). In addition, 658 560 cases would be correctly determined to be negative (negative predictive value 99.7%). However, 1680 cases of endocervical infection would be missed (false negatives) and at unknown risk for upper tract disease, and 13 440 cases would be falsely positive. Put another way, universal screening would correctly identify 26 000 cases of cervical infection and incorrectly inform over 13 000 women that they had a sexually transmitted disease, when in reality they did not. The benefits of screening must be carefully weighed against the psychological and emotional consequences of misclassification, which are potentially devastating – for example, to the monogamous woman in a stable relationship who is informed erroneously that she has a sexually transmitted disease. In a higher-risk group with a higher prevalence of disease, screening would appear to have greater potential.

Nonculture testing methods may be preferable and are certainly cheaper. Microscopic examination of a saline wet mount of vaginal discharge could identify women with either bacterial vaginosis, inflammatory vaginitis or cervicitis – women who are at high risk for upper genital tract infection following IUD insertion. A vaginal or cervical Gram stain, although slightly more time-consuming, increases the specificity of the diagnosis if clue cells or Gram-negative intracellular diplococci are identified. An endocervical swab test can also be performed to evaluate for mucopurulent cervicitis (Brunham *et al.*, 1988). If any of these tests were to be positive, IUD insertion could be delayed until treatment of cervicitis or vaginitis is completed or appropriate culture results are known. This approach would focus the use of other more expensive laboratory tests on high-risk women and should be a more cost-effective approach to screening IUD candidates.

OTHER CONTRACEPTIVE METHODS

Although this chapter has focused on only two reversible methods of contraception, similar arguments can be made for other contraceptive methods. Contraindications for depomedroxyprogesterone acetate (DMPA) and subdermal implants such as Norplant include unexplained vaginal bleeding and known or suspected pregnancy. As for all contraceptive methods, a thorough history is required and a pregnancy test should be performed if pregnancy is suspected. While active thrombophlebitis or pulmonary embolus are contraindications to Norplant, there are no accepted screening tests for these conditions. Contraindications to other methods of contraception can usually be determined by obtaining the medical and reproductive history. Screening tests should be employed as recommended for all women of reproductive age (ACOG, 1994), regardless of contraceptive choice.

CONCLUSIONS AND RECOMMENDATIONS

Laboratory tests for OC users should be ordered only when clinically indicated. The issue of screening tests for OC users came to the forefront because of the debate on whether OCs should be available without prescription (Trussel *et al.*, 1993). These authors point out that the broadest defense of the prescription status for OCs is that it ensures regular health examinations and screening. On the other hand, it has been convincingly argued that the availability of OCs without prescription would neither prevent nor discourage women from continuing to see physicians (Grimes, 1993). Rather, it would make physician visits related to oral contraception voluntary instead of mandatory.

The appropriateness of screening potential IUD candidates for genital tract infection seems clear, but the optimal approach is unknown. Women at high risk for sexually transmitted diseases should have a complete physical examination for vaginitis, cervicitis, and upper genital tract infection, incorporating the microscopic evaluation of vaginal flora and sexually transmitted disease testing when clinically indicated.

In summary, additional screening tests are rarely indicated for contraceptive users if their medical caregiver performs preventive health maintenance screening. There are little if any data to support additional screening tests for most contraceptive users. Routine cervical cytologic testing should be performed as is standard for all sexually active women in the reproductive age (see Chapter 21). Cholesterol and lipoprotein testing should be performed as is usual for women and as indicated by the risk status of the woman.

SUMMARY

1

WHAT IS THE PROBLEM THAT REQUIRES SCREENING?

CONDITIONS THAT MIGHT BE EXACERBATED BY CONTRACEPTIVE USE.

a What is the incidence/prevalence of the target condition?

The prevalence of hypertension, thrombosis, diabetes, hyperlipidemia, and hormone-sensitive malignancy is similar to that in the noncontraceptive-using population.

The incidence of pelvic inflammatory disease (PID) in intrauterine device (IUD) users is typically overestimated by medical practitioners. In the early 1980s, the annual incidence of PID in IUD users was estimated at 2%. It is approximately 10 per 1000 woman years during the first 20 days after insertion, dropping to less than 2 per 1000 woman years, where it remains steady for up to 8 years of follow-up.

b What are the sequelae of the condition which are of interest in clinical medicine?

Possible sequelae of oral contraceptive use include arterial stroke, thrombosis, and atherosclerosis. The medical sequelae of PID include infertility, chronic pelvic pain, ectopic pregnancy, recurrent PID, and morbidity and mortality associated with tubo-ovarian abscesses.

2

THE TESTS

a What is the purpose of the tests?

To identify conditions that might be exacerbated by hormonal manipulation. Screening tests for prospective IUD users seek to identify women at risk of the development of pelvic infection.

b The nature of the tests

See appropriate sections.

3

CONCLUSIONS AND RECOMMENDATIONS

Additional screening tests are rarely indicated for contraceptive users if their caregiver performs preventive health maintenance screening. There are little if any data to support additional screening tests for most contraceptive users. Women at high risk for sexually transmitted diseases should have a complete physical examination for vaginitis, cervicitis, and upper genital tract infection, incorporating the microscopic evaluation of vaginal flora to identify women in need of a more detailed (but costly) evaluation. Routine cervical cytologic testing should be performed as is standard for all sexually active women in the reproductive age. Cholesterol and lipoprotein testing should be performed as is usual for women and as indicated by the risk status of the patient.

REFERENCES

ACOG (1994) *Primary and Preventive Care. A Primer for Obstetricians and Gynecologists.* Washington, DC: American College of Obstetricians and Gynecologists.

ACOG (1992) *The Intrauterine Device.* ACOG Technical Bulletin 164, 1–4. Washington, DC: American College of Obstetricians and Gynecologists.

Baudet JH & Seguy B (1987) *Revision Accelerée en Gynecologie*, pp 58–60. Paris: Maloine.

Brunham RC, Paavonen J, Stevens C *et al.* (1988) Mucopurulent cervicitis – the ignored counterpart in women of urethritis in men. *N Engl J Med* 311: 1–6.

Corfman PA (1988) Labelling guidance text for combination oral contraceptives. *Contraception* 37 (5): 433–455.

Farley TMM, Rosenberg MJ, Rowe PJ, Chen J-H & Merik O (1992) Intrauterine devices and pelvic inflammatory disease: an international perspective. *Lancet* 339: 785–788.

Forrest JD & Fordyce RR (1993) Women's Contraceptive Attitudes and Use in 1992. *Fam Plann Perspect* 25: 178.

Grimes DA (1993) Over-the-counter oral contraceptives – an immodest proposal? (Editorial). *Am J Publ Health* 83: 1092–1093.

Hatcher RA, Trussell J, Stewart F, *et al.* (1994) *Contraceptive Technology*, 16th edn., 249 pp. New York: Irvington.

Isada NB & Grossman JH (1994) Rapid diagnostic tests: uses and limitations. In Pastorek JG (ed.) *Obstetric and Gynecologic Infectious Disease*, pp 736–737. New York: Raven Press.

Kessel E (1989) Pelvic inflammatory disease with intrauterine device use: a reassessment. *Fertil Steril;* 51: 1–11.

Larsson PG, Platz-Christensen JJ, Thejls H, Forsum U & Pahlson C (1992) Incidence of pelvic inflammatory disease after first-trimester legal abortion in women with bacterial vaginosis after treatment with metronidazole: a doubleblind, randomized study. *Am J Obstet Gynecol* 166: 100–3.

Mosher WD & Pratt WP (1990) Contraceptive use in the United States, 1973–1988. *Advance Data from Vital and Health Statistics 182.* Hyattsville, MD: National Center for Health Statistics.

Paavonen J, Kiviat N, Brunham RC, *et al.* (1985) Prevalence and manifestations of endometritis among women with cervicitis. *Am J Obstet Gynecol* 152: 280–286.

Serfaty D (1986) *La Contraception.* Paris: Doin.

Speroff L & Darney PA (1992). *A Clinical Guide for Contraception*, pp 157–182. Baltimore: Williams & Wilkins.

Trussel J, Stewart F, Potts M, Guest F, & Ellertson C (1993) Should oral contraceptives be available without prescription? *Am J Publ Health* 83: 1094–1099.

27

The Electrocardiogram

Rudolph W. Koster & Patrick M. M. Bossuyt

ASYMPTOMATIC DISTURBANCES OF CARDIAC RHYTHM OR
CONDUCTION, AND ISCHEMIC HEART DISEASE.

What is the incidence/prevalence of the target condition?

The prevalence of coronary heart disease (CHD) increases with age. The incidence of
all CHD in adults is 14.3 per 1000 per year for men and 7.2 per 1000 per year for
women (morbidity), and 3.1 per 1000 per year for men and 1.4 per 1000 per year
for women (mortality). This is true for all manifestations of CHD including angina
pectoris, myocardial infarction (MI) (Figure 27.1) and sudden death. However, the
gender ratio is not constant with advancing age (Lerner and Kannel, 1986). After
menopause, the male to female ratio of coronary heart disease declines from 7:1 to
3:1. It becomes equal by the 6th and 7th decades, and finally reverses slightly in the
8th and 9th decades. The proportions of silent (i.e. asymptomatic) MI are more or
less equal over the age groups: 35% in women, 28% in men (Figure 27.1) (Kannel
and Abbott, 1984). Atrial fibrillation may occur at any age, but its prevalence increases
with age from 2 per 1000 women aged 25–34 years to 30 per 1000 of women aged
55–64 years (Kannel *et al.*, 1982).

What are the sequelae of the condition which are of interest in clinical medicine?

Disturbances of rhythm: Most people are aware of occasional palpitations and
skipped beats which are not generally clinically significant. True arrhythmias rarely
go unnoticed. Paroxysmal tachycardias are generally sensed immediately, but occasionally a patient may be unaware of a paroxysmal or persistent tachycardia. Atrial
fibrillation is the single most important paroxysmal tachycardia. It can occur in the
presence or absence (lone atrial fibrillation) of organic heart disease. Atrial fibrillation
impairs the circulatory response to blood pressure changes during surgery, may cause
congestive heart failure and is often the source of arterial or pulmonary emboli. The
management of atrial fibrillation includes heart rate control, possibly by conversion to
sinus rhythm, and prevention of thrombosis development in the atria with subsequent
embolism.

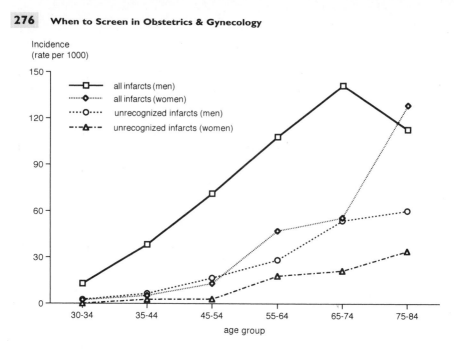

Figure 27.1 Ten-year incidence of myocardial infarction in the Framingham cohort. Unrecognized infarcts are those infarcts identified on the biannual electrocardiogram without previous clinical symptoms. In all age groups the proportion of unidentified infarcts is about one-third of all infarcts (data after Kannel and Abbott, 1984).

Premature atrial beats are usually benign and do not require medical intervention. Premature ventricular beats, especially when frequent, may be associated with ischemic myocardial disease and can trigger ventricular tachycardia. Ventricular tachycardia rarely goes unnoticed and is almost always associated with important heart disease. Other supraventricular tachycardias – such as the tachycardia associated with the Wolff–Parkinson–White syndrome and atrioventricular junction tachycardia – are not associated with organic heart disease, with rare exceptions.

Conduction disturbances: First-degree and second-degree atrioventricular nodal blocks are occasionally observed especially during sleep and are not necessarily associated with heart disease. A third-degree conduction block is usually associated with complaints of dizziness and fainting (Adams–Stokes attack) but may occasionally be found in asymptomatic individuals. The consequences of complete heart block depend on the location of the block, the ability of the heart to increase its rate with exercise, and the absence of disturbances in pump function. In general, complete heart block is considered an indication for implantation of a permanent pacemaker.

Ischemic heart disease: IHD is the most important reason for preoperative screening, as it is associated with much of the perioperative morbidity and mortality. The diagnosis of a silent MI can only be made by electrocardiogram (ECG), usually after the demonstration of pathological Q waves. In some patients chest pains have been absent, while in others the manifestations were mild or were perceived as another, self-limiting problem. Silent MI is associated with recurrent infarction, congestive heart failure and (sudden) death. The prognosis of a silent MI is similar to that of a symptomatic myocardial infarction.

THE TEST

What is the purpose of the test?

The preoperative identification of patients with potentially lethal cardiac pathology, including rhythm and conduction disturbances and ischemic heart disease, so that medical therapy may be initiated and nonemergency surgery avoided.

The nature of the test

The electrocardiogram (ECG) yields information on several, essentially independent functions of the heart. These include disturbances of rhythm, disturbances of impulse transmission through the conduction system, the presence of ischemic heart disease and congenital or acquired abnormalities of the heart chambers, and electrolyte disturbances. Disturbances of rhythm and conduction, and ischemic manifestations, can be present in apparently healthy people and thus detected for the first time at a preoperative screening. Throughout this chapter, it is assumed that a detailed history and physical examination have not revealed any important abnormal findings.

The ECG is a standardized, 12-lead recording of the electrical activity of the heart, lasting 12–60 seconds. It is simple and noninvasive. Since abnormalities of the heart such as ischemia, arrhythmias, and conduction disturbances are typically intermittent, the likelihood of one of these being recorded during this short interval is small. In general, myocardial ischemia cannot be identified by routine ECG in the absence of angina pectoris. Prolonged (24 hours) ECG recordings or recordings made during exercise improve the detection rate. On the other hand, if an abnormality is observed during this short period, it probably occurs frequently and is thus a more serious disorder.

Implications of testing

WHAT DOES AN ABNORMAL TEST RESULT MEAN?

The ECG diagnosis of acute myocardial infarction (AMI) of more than trivial size is relatively simple during the first weeks after occurrence, especially when serial ECGs are available. In the majority of patients, pathological Q waves remain visible. However, pathological Q waves may be absent in smaller infarcts making a diagnosis based solely on the ECG difficult. The timing of a MI cannot be determined with any certainty after the first 2–3 months, as the pathological Q waves become less obvious or even disappear, yielding a false negative rate of 33–62% (Smith and Hayes, 1965; Uusitupa et al, 1983). Other myocardial or neurological disorders may mimic an old MI leading to the unjustified diagnosis of an acute MI. Misinterpretation of a pathological Q wave is also possible. Though the frequency of false positive readings has not been studied in the context of screening, it is probably low.

Goldman et al. (1977) identified three preoperative cardiac risk factors for noncardiac surgery that could not be identified by either history or physical examination: (1) a MI less than 6 months prior to surgery; (2) a rhythm other than sinus rhythm or premature atrial beats on the preoperative ECG; and (3) more than 5 premature ventricular beats per minute at any time prior to surgery. The risk of surgery after a recent (under 6 months) symptomatic MI was reviewed in detail by Haagensen and Steen (1988). The

Table 27.1 The likelihood of silent myocardial infarction (MI) by age, together with the possible impact of ECG testing on mortality.

AGE GROUP (YEARS)	NUMBER OF SILENT MIs DETECTED (PER 100 000 ECGs)	NUMBER OF SILENT MIs OCCURRING IN THE LAST 6 MONTHS PRIOR TO ECG (PER 100 000 ECGs)	REDUCTION IN MORTALITY WHEN ALL PATIENTS WITH SILENT MI ARE RECOGNIZED AND THEIR OPERATION POSTPONED (PER 100 000 ECGs)
30–34	0	0	0
35–44	260	13	0.6
45–54	550	15	0.7
55–64	2330	90	4.5
65–74	4410	108	5.4
75–84	7660	173	8.6

risks of perioperative reinfarction ranged from 1.9% to 15.9%; subsequent mortality ranged from 28% to 72% (Haagensen and Steen, 1988). In general, the diagnosis of recent AMI is made by history and confirmed by a preoperative ECG.

It is unclear if the finding of a silent MI has the same prognosis during the perioperative period as a documented recent AMI. Nevertheless, many consider the finding of a silent MI on a routine preoperative ECG a contraindication to elective surgery for a 6-month period. It is assumed that postponement of surgery will reduce the excess risk of a perioperative cardiac complication to nil. Even if true, such a policy has a sizeable impact on the patient and society. As illustrated in Table 27.1, 260 of every 100 000 women aged 35–44 years screened preoperatively with an ECG would have their operation postponed for 6 months because of the diagnosis of a silent MI. Statistically, though, only 13 of the 260 (5%) would have actually suffered their MI in the preceding 6 months. As a result, the *maximum* reduction in perioperative mortality achieved by delaying surgery would be less than 1 for every 100 000 women screened (Table 27.1). In older age groups, these numbers are even less favorable in terms of number of women falsely labeled with MI in the preceding 6 months. For every 100 000 screened people of 60 years, 2330 would have their operation postponed for 6 months, yet only 90 patients (3.8%) would have had their MI in the preceding 6 months. The maximum reduction in mortality from this screening policy would be 4.5 per 100 000 women screened.

The most important arrhythmia is atrial fibrillation, which by itself is a concern if the ventricular rate is very high or very low. In addition, arrhythmias may reflect underlying heart disease (ischemia, congestive heart failure) which should be identified and treated, preferably before surgery.

First-degree or second-degree heart block needs no precautions prior to surgery. Neither is bundle branch block an independent risk factor for perioperative complications, even in the case of bifascicular bundle branch block (Pastore *et al.*, 1978). A temporary, transvenous pacemaker is indicated if a complete, third-degree heart block is diagnosed. However, it can be argued that definitive pacemaker implantation should be considered first in women who do not require emergency surgery. Complete heart block should be identifiable as a significant arrhythmia on physical examination.

WHAT DOES A NORMAL TEST RESULT MEAN?

The likelihood of perioperative cardiac complications in women with an uneventful medical history and normal ECG tracing is very small.

What is the cost of testing?

The direct costs of a routine ECG comprise the use of equipment, personnel and the fee for the cardiologist for assessment of the ECG tracing. In the Netherlands these costs total approximately 50 guilders (US $25). In many hospitals, the tracing is screened first by computer. The cost rises considerably should a consultation be needed in the case of abnormal findings on the ECG. The need for such a consultation largely depends on the age of the patient, as the likelihood of unexpected pathology, old or recent, increases with age.

The chance of finding a silent MI is given in Table 27.1. In the Netherlands the consultant fee is 83 guilders (US $40). Thus, in the range 45–54 years, routine preoperative ECG screening would cost $3.6 million dollars per life saved using these conservative Dutch financial estimates. In the USA, the typical ECG with interpretation approximates US $75. Thus, the total cost per life saved by routine preoperative ECG screening approximates $10.7 million if no additional consultant is used. It exceeds $800 000 even after age 75 years. Further assessment including exercise testing or nuclear scintigraphic studies would only increase the costs.

CONCLUSIONS AND RECOMMENDATIONS

Prior to surgery, rhythm and conduction disturbances can be detected by careful history and routine physical examination. The most important contributor to perioperative cardiac complications is a recent MI (within 6 months). The diagnosis of a silent MI is based on typical ECG changes. The timing of a silent MI cannot be determined from the ECG. Thus, it is impossible to differentiate a silent MI that occurred during the preceding 6 months from one that occurred more than 6 months previously. This inability has immense consequences. Based on the findings of Kannel and Abbott (1984), the calculated cost-benefit ratio for routine ECG screening in terms of deaths prevented is very high. The costs are even higher if one considers the negative medical effects and the costs to society of delaying surgery for 6 months.

It can be concluded that preoperative ECG screening is not warranted in gynecological surgery at any age, if history and physical examination do not give any evidence of the presence of heart disease.

SUMMARY

WHAT IS THE PROBLEM THAT REQUIRES SCREENING?

ASYMPTOMATIC DISTURBANCES OF CARDIAC RHYTHM OR CONDUCTION, AND ISCHEMIC HEART DISEASE.

a What is the incidence/prevalence of the target condition?

The incidence of coronary heart disease (CHD) is 14.3 per 1000 per year for men and 7.2 per 1000 per year for women (morbidity), and 3.1 per 1000 per year for men and 1.4 per 1000 per year for women (mortality). The incidence rises with age. This is true for all manifestations of CHD including angina pectoris, myocardial infarction (MI), and sudden death.

b What are the sequelae of the condition which are of interest in clinical medicine?

Atrial fibrillation impairs the circulatory response to blood pressure changes during surgery, may cause congestive heart failure and is often the source of arterial or pulmonary emboli. Ventricular tachycardia rarely goes unnoticed and is in almost all instances associated with important heart disease. Coronary heart disease is the most important reason for preoperative screening, as it is associated with much of the perioperative morbidity and mortality.

THE TEST

Electrocardiogram (ECG).

a What is the purpose of the test?

The preoperative identification of patients with potentially lethal cardiac pathology, including rhythm and conduction disturbances and ischemic heart disease, so that medical therapy may be initiated and nonemergency surgery avoided.

b The nature of the test

The ECG is a standardized, 12-lead recording of the electrical activity of the heart, lasting 12–60 seconds.

c Implications of testing

I   What does an abnormal test result mean?

Surgery should be delayed. There are three preoperative cardiac risk factors for noncardiac surgery not identifiable by either history or physical examination: (1) a MI within 6 months prior to surgery; (2) a rhythm other than sinus rhythm or premature atrial beats on the preoperative ECG; and (3) more than 5 premature ventricular beats/min at any time prior to surgery. The risk of surgery within 6 months of a symptomatic MI is perioperative reinfarction (1.9% to 15.9%) and death in the case of perioperative reinfarction (28% to 72%). The diagnosis of atrial fibrillation will lead to medical therapy. The discovery of complete heart block could end with the placement of a permanent pacemaker.

2   What does a normal test result mean?

The likelihood of perioperative cardiac complications in women with an uneventful medical history and normal ECG tracing is very small.

d **What is the cost of testing?**

The cost is $4–10 million dollars (US) per life saved in women aged 45–54 years. The cost exceeds $800 000 even after age 75 years.

3   CONCLUSIONS AND RECOMMENDATIONS

Preoperative ECG screening is not warranted in gynecological surgery at any age, if the history and physical examination do not give any evidence of the presence of heart disease.

REFERENCES

Goldman L, Caldera DL, Nussbaum SR *et al*. (1977) Multifactorial index of cardiac risk in noncardiac procedures. *N Engl J Med* **297:** 845–850.

Haagensen R & Steen PA (1988) Perioperative myocardial infarction. *Br J Anaesthesiol* **61:** 24–37.

Kannel WB & Abbott RD (1984) Incidence and prognosis of unrecognized myocardial infarction. An update of the Framingham study. *N Engl J Med* **311:** 1144–1147.

Kannel WB, Abbott RD, Savage DD & McNamara PM (1982) Epidemiologic features of chronic atrial fibrillation. The Framingham study. *N Engl J Med* **306:** 1018–1022.

Lerner DJ & Kannel WB (1986) Patterns of coronary heart disease morbidity and mortality in the sexes: 26-year follow-up of the Framingham population. *Am Heart J* **111:** 383–390.

Pastore JO, Yurchak PM, Janis KM, Murphy JD & Zir LM (1978) The risk of advanced heart block in surgical patients with right bundle branch block and left axis deviation. *Circulation* **57:** 677–680.

Smith S & Hayes WL (1965) The prognosis of complete left bundle branch block. *Am Heart J* **70:** 157–159.

Uusitupa M, Pyörälä K, Raunio H, Rissanen V & Lampainen E (1983) Sensitivity and specificity of Minnesota Code Q-QS abnormalities in the diagnosis of myocardial infarction verified at autopsy. *Am Heart J* **106:** 753–757.

28

Intravenous Pyelography

Joanne T. Piscitelli & David L. Simel

WHAT IS THE PROBLEM THAT REQUIRES SCREENING?

INJURIES TO THE URINARY TRACT DURING SURGERY FOR BENIGN GYNECOLOGIC DISEASE.

What is the incidence/prevalence of the target condition?

Ureteral injuries during hysterectomy occur in 0.1–2.5% of procedures (Solomons *et al.*, 1960; Freda and Tacchi, 1962; Schwartz *et al.*, 1964; Thompson and Benigno, 1971; Van Nagell and Roddick 1972; Amirikia and Evans, 1979; Sack, 1979; Naylor 1984; Larson *et al.*, 1987; Mann 1991). The injury rate is similar for both abdominal and vaginal procedures. Diseases that alter or obscure the normal anatomic relationships such as pelvic masses, pelvic adhesive disease, endometriosis or urinary tract anomalies may place the woman at greater risk of intraoperative ureteral injury. Knowledge of preexisting renal disease or urinary tract injury (for example, from previous surgery) may be useful to the surgeon.

What are the sequelae of the condition which are of interest in clinical medicine?

Unrecognized ureteral injury may result in pyelonephritis, sepsis, ileus, fistula formation and loss of renal function. Reoperation may be required with attendant morbidity. The condition for which the hysterectomy is being performed may have already caused urinary tract damage and imaging the urinary tract may prevent confusion. For example, untreated complete uterine prolapse results in 7.3% to 25% of ureteral obstruction progressing to renal failure (Rudin *et al.*, 1974; Moore *et al.*, 1978).

THE TEST

What is the purpose of the test?

The purpose of the preoperative intravenous pyelogram is to delineate the urinary tract anatomy and identify preexisting pathology.

The nature of the test

Intravenous pyelography sequences abdominal radiographs at timed intervals following intravenous injection of contrast agents. The radiographs outline the kidneys, renal calices, ureters and bladder. Ureteral dilatation, deviation (either laterally or more important medially), and congenital anomalies such as ureteral duplication or pelvic kidney are the primary abnormalities of interest to the gynecologic surgeon. Extrinsic compression of the bladder is a common finding in the presence of pelvic masses and generally is of little consequence. Most surgeons consider the intravenous pyelogram a suitable reference standard for identifying urinary tract abnormalities prior to surgery. Therefore, it is relevant for the surgeon to consider whether there are any features from the history or clinical examination that identify the patient as having an increased risk of a urinary tract abnormality.

Ultrasonography as a preoperative screening test of the urinary tract has been compared with intravenous pyelography (Aslaksen *et al.*, 1989). Each identified hydronephrosis equally, but with ultrasonography two out of five duplicated ureters were missed. Though it costs less and creates no contrast reactions, ultrasonography provides little information about the course of the pelvic ureter.

Implications of testing

WHAT DOES AN ABNORMAL TEST RESULT MEAN?

The rationale for preoperative intravenous pyelography has been that the recognition of anatomic abnormalities prior to surgery would reduce the risk of surgical injury. This has not been proven by any study to date. Retrospective studies (Sack, 1979; Piscitelli *et al.*, 1987) reveal similar ureteral injury rates in patients who underwent preoperative intravenous pyelography and in those who did not. Since intraoperative ureteral injuries occur infrequently, a randomized controlled trial to prove the effectiveness of the intravenous pyelogram in reducing ureteral injuries would require multiple study sites at prohibitive costs.

If one accepts the premise that 'forewarned is forearmed,' what is the likelihood of a preoperative pyelogram revealing an abnormality significant to the surgeon? In 455 patients undergoing major pelvic surgery, Roden *et al.* (1961) found 5.2% to have genitourinary anomalies, 7% hydronephrosis, and 3.1% ureteral deviation. Schwartz *et al.* (1964) found an 11.6% prevalence of ureteral dilatation or deviation, and 1.8% congenital anomalies. Both studies included some patients with gynecologic malignancies. Solomons *et al.* (1960) reported a 20% prevalence of hydronephrosis in patients undergoing hysterectomy for benign disease. In the largest study, Klissaristos *et al.* (1974) reported the findings of routine preoperative intravenous pyelograms for all types of gynecologic surgery and found a 5.2% prevalence of ureteral deviation, 7% of hydronephrosis, and 2% of congenital anomalies.

Several studies have investigated the relationships of a variety of clinical and physical examination findings with intravenous pyelography. Kretschmer and Kanter (1937) noted ureteral dilatation or displacement in 82% of patients with ovarian cysts, 71% with fibroids above the pelvic brim, 55% with fibroids below the pelvic brim, and 25% with uterine prolapse. Piscitelli *et al* (1987) found a 20% prevalence of ureteral dilatation and 10% prevalence of ureteral deviation in patients with a uterine size of 12 weeks' gestation or larger. In contrast, when the uterus was less than 12 weeks' size, no intravenous pyelograms showed dilatation and only 2.5% showed ureteral deviation. In 34 patients with adnexal mass, 21% had dilatation and 9% had deviations of the ureters (Piscitelli *et al.*, 1987). In patients with uterine prolapse, hydroureteronephrosis appeared in 7% to 66% (Rudin *et al.*, 1974; Jones and Evison, 1977; Piscitelli *et al.*, 1987). Phillips (1974) observed ureteral dilatation in 39% and deviation in 36% in 44 patients with tubo-ovarian abscesses. Six patients (14%) had medial deviation of the pelvic ureter. There are slightly over 100 reported cases of endometriosis involving the urinary tract (Moore *et al.*, 1979). In 16 patients with preoperative intravenous pyelograms and the diagnosis of endometriosis, Piscitelli *et al.* (1987) noted 18% with ureteral dilatation and 12% with ureteral duplication, a finding of particular interest to the surgeon. Previous abdominal surgery did not appear to increase the likelihood of an abnormal intravenous pyelogram.

WHAT DOES A NORMAL TEST RESULT MEAN?

A normal preoperative intravenous pyelogram reduces the likelihood of preexisting urinary tract disease and anatomic distortion. It does not obviate the need for direct intraoperative ureteral identification.

Do the history and physical examination findings predict urinary tract abnormalities? If intravenous pyelography serves as the pragmatic reference standard for identifying urinary tract abnormalities, the surgeon should be interested in screening tests that increase the likelihood of finding an abnormality. Taken in this context, the patient's history and physical examination findings do function as a screening test for urinary tract abnormalities. No retrospective study adequately allows precise estimation of the sensitivity and specificity of these features. However, reanalysis of the data to correct for verification bias does permit estimation of the sensitivity and specificity from data presented by Piscitelli *et al.* (1987). Virtually all retrospective studies of diagnostic tests are affected by verification bias, whereby patients with the abnormality of interest (e.g. uterine enlargement) are more likely to be referred for the reference test (e.g. intravenous pyelography) than those with normal examinations. These uncorrected biases generally function to overestimate sensitivity and underestimate specificity. Since the data of Piscitelli *et al.* (1987) were presented on consecutive patients and results were included for those with normal findings, we can mathematically correct for the verification bias as shown in Table 28.1. A likelihood ratio approaching 1 indicates that the test has no value. From these results, an adnexal mass or the presence of leiomyomas greater than 12 weeks' gestational size increases the likelihood of finding a urinary tract abnormality and are the only positive findings where the confidence interval around the estimate excludes 1.0. Smaller leiomyomas or normal uterine size decrease marginally the likeli-

Table 28.1 An adnexal mass or leiomyomas increase the likelihood of ureteral abnormalities

FINDING	SENSITIVITY (%)	SPECIFICITY (%)	LR(pos) (95% CI)	LR(neg) (95% CI)
adnexal mass	14	92	1.8 (1.1, 3.2)	0.9 (0.8, 1.0)
leiomyomas ⩾ 12 wks	35	78	1.6 (1.2, 2.2)	0.6 (0.7, 0.9)
endometriosis	6	96	1.3 (0.5, 2.9)	1.0 (0.9, 1.0)
uterine prolapse	5	95	0.9 (0.4, 2.0)	1.0 (0.9, 1.0)

CI, confidence interval; LR, likelihood ratio

hood of an abnormality by a factor of 0.6 and are the only negative finding where the confidence interval around the estimate excludes 1.0. The presence of endometriosis or uterine prolapse does not increase the underlying risk of a urinary tract abnormality. The absence of an adnexal mass, endometriosis, or uterine prolapse does not alter the chance of finding an abnormality beyond the baseline prevalence.

What is the cost of the testing?

The average total charge for an intravenous pyelogram is approximately US $200. The risk of death due to contrast reactions is approximately 1 per 40 000 contrast procedures (Ansell, 1970). Severe reactions requiring intensive therapy occur at a rate of 1 per 14 000 procedures (Mushlin and Thornbury, 1989). Nephrotoxicity occurs in about 0.6% of hospitalized patients without preexisting renal disease (Mushlin and Thornbury, 1989). Newer nonionic intravascular contrast agents reduce these risks markedly, but are 10–13 times more expensive.

Simel et al. (1988) used decision analysis techniques to evaluate the cost-effectiveness of preoperative screening intravenous pyelograms. Approximately $166 600 would be spent to avoid one ureteral injury, assuming a baseline ureteral injury rate of 0.5%, test efficacy of 25% (i.e. a preoperative intravenous pyelogram reduces the risk of injury by 25%), and a $200 cost. Approximately $3.33 million would be spent to prevent a single death. As the probability of injury increases, the marginal cost-effectiveness ratio is less dependent on the test efficacy and is more modest.

If abnormal ureteral anatomy increases the risk of injury and clinical findings are correlated with ureteral anatomy, selective use of preoperative intravenous pyelograms would be more cost-effective. The best clinical finding (an adnexal mass or leiomyoma greater than 12 weeks' gestational size) only increased the likelihood of an abnormality 1.8 and 1.6 times, respectively. Even if the probability of an injury is as high as 2.5% when the ureters are abnormal, the cost is still approximately US $31 700 to prevent a single injury (Simel et al., 1988).

CONCLUSIONS AND RECOMMENDATIONS

The intravenous pyelogram provides the opportunity for preoperative delineation of urinary tract anatomy and pathology. Ureteral abnormalities such as deviation, dilatation and duplication place the patient at increased risk for injury. However, it has never been proved that preoperative intravenous pyelography reduces the risk of such injury. Given the low probability of an intraoperative injury during a hysterectomy for benign disease, even if the intravenous pyelogram is effective, it clearly is expensive. Its use can only be justified in patients predicted on clinical grounds to have a high probability of abnormal findings. The only such category of patients identified from the literature are those with an adnexal mass or uterine leiomyoma of at least 12 weeks' gestational size. Unfortunately, the absence of any studied historical or physical examination finding does not rule out the presence of ureteral abnormalities, reminding the surgeon to use careful intraoperative techniques for visualizing the ureters.

SUMMARY

1

WHAT IS THE PROBLEM THAT REQUIRES SCREENING?

URINARY TRACT INJURY DURING BENIGN GYNECOLOGIC SURGERY.

a What is the incidence prevalence of the target condition?

Ureteral injuries occur during hysterectomy in 0.1–2.5% of procedures.

b What are the sequelae of the condition which are of interest in clinical medicine?

Unrecognized ureteral injury may result in pyelonephritis, sepsis, ileus, fistula formation, and loss of renal function. Reoperation may be required.

2

THE TEST

a What is the purpose of the test?

To delineate the urinary tract anatomy and identify preexisting pathology.

b The nature of the test

Intravenous pyelography (IVP) sequences abdominal radiographs at timed intervals after intra-. venous injection of contrast agents. Ultrasonography is less effective in identifying congenital duplication or an abnormal course of the ureter.

c Implications of testing

1 What does an abnormal test result mean?

The assumption is that awareness of anatomic abnormalities prior to surgery reduces the risk of inadvertent injury. This has not been proved by any study to date.

2 What does a normal test result mean?

A normal preoperative intravenous pyelogram reduces the likelihood of preexisting urinary tract disease and anatomic distortion. *It does not obviate the need for direct intraoperative ureteral identification.*

d What is the cost of testing?

Approximately US $ 166 600 would be spent to avoid one ureteral injury, assuming a baseline ureteral injury rate of 0.5%, test efficacy of 25% (i.e. a preoperative intravenous pyelogram reduces the risk of injury by 25%), and a $200 cost. Approximately $3.33 million would be spent to prevent a single death.

3   CONCLUSIONS AND RECOMMENDATIONS

Given the low risk of an intraoperative injury during a hysterectomy for benign disease, the intravenous pyelogram clearly is expensive even if it is effective. Its use can only be justified in patients predicted on clinical grounds to have a high probability of abnormal findings. The only such category of patients identified from the literature are those with an adnexal mass or uterine leiomyoma of at least 12 weeks' gestational size.

REFERENCES

Amirikia H & Evans TN (1979) Ten-year review of hysterectomies: trends, indications, and risks. *Am J Obstet Gynecol* **134**: 431–437.

Ansell G (1970) Adverse reactions to contrast agents. *Invest Radiol* **6**: 374–384.

Aslaksen A, Göthlin JH, Geitung JT & Anker C (1989) Ultrasonography versus urography as preoperative investigation prior to hysterectomy. *Acta Obstet Gynecol Scand* **68**: 443–445.

Freda V & Tacchi D (1962) Ureteral injury discovered after pelvic surgery. *Am J Obstet Gynecol* **83**: 406–409.

Jones JB & Evison G (1977) Excretion urography before and after surgical treatment of procidentia. *Br J Obstet Gynaecol* **84**: 304–308.

Klissaristos AA, Manouelides NS & Comninos AC (1974) Preoperative intravenous pyelography in gynecology. *Inter Surg* **59**: 31–32.

Kretschmer HL & Kanter AE (1937) Effect of certain gynecologic lesions on the upper urinary tract: a pyelographic study. *JAMA* **109**: 1097–1101.

Larson DM, Malone JM, Copeland LJ, Gershenson DM, Kline RC & Stringer CA (1987) Ureteral assessment after radical hysterectomy. *Obstet Gynecol* **69**: 612–616.

Mann WJ (1991) Intentional and unintentional ureteral surgical treatment in gynecologic procedures. *Surg Gynecol Obstet* **172**: 453–456.

Moore JG, Hibbard LT, Growdon WA & Schifrin BS (1979) Urinary tract endometriosis: enigmas in diagnosis and management. *Am J Obstet Gynecol* **134**: 162–170.

Moore S, Bailey RR, Maling TMJ & Little PJ (1978) Urinary tract obstruction and renal failure due to uterine prolapse. *NZ Med J* **87**: 429–431.

Mushlin AI & Thornbury JR (1989) Intravenous pyelography: the case against its routine use. *Ann Intern Med* **111**: 58–70.

Naylor AC (1984) Hysterectomy – analysis of 2901 personally performed procedures. *S Africa Med J* **65**: 242–245.

Phillips JC (1974) A spectrum of radiologic abnormalities due to tubo-ovarian abscess. *Radiology* **110**: 307–311.

Piscitelli JT, Simel DL & Addison WA (1987) Who should have intravenous pyelograms before hysterectomy for benign disease? *Obstet Gynecol* **69**: 541–545.

Roden JS, Haugen HM, Hall DG & Greenberg PA (1961) The value of intravenous pyelography prior to elective gynecologic operations. *Am J Obstet Gynecol* **82**: 568–571.

Rudin LJ, Megalli MR & Lattimer JK (1974) Obstructive uropathy associated with uterine prolapse. *Urology* **4**: 73–79.

Sack RA (1979) The value of intravenous urography prior to abdominal hysterectomy for gynecologic disease. *Am J Obstet Gynecol* **134**: 208–212.

Schwartz WR, Hofmeister FJ & Mattingly RF (1964) The value of intravenous urograms in pelvic surgery. *Obstet Gynecol* **23**: 584–588.

Simel DL, Matchar DB & Piscitelli JT (1988) Routine intravenous pyelograms before hysterectomy in cases of benign disease: possibly effective, definitely expensive. *Am J Obstet Gynecol* **159**: 1049–1053.

Solomons E, Levin EJ, Bauman J & Baron J (1960) A pyelographic study of ureteric injuries sustained during hysterectomy for benign conditions. *Surg Gynecol Obstet* **111**: 41–48.

Thompson JD & Benigno B (1971) Vaginal repair of ureteral injuries. *Am J Obstet Gynecol* **111**: 601–610.

Van Nagell JR & Roddick JW (1972) Vaginal hysterectomy, the ureter and excretory urography. *Obstet Gynecol* **39**: 784–786.

Index

Numbers in bold refer to main discussion; numbers in italic refer to illustrations or tables